SO-AFW-082

LANGUAGE DISORDERS IN OLDER STUDENTS:
PREADOLESCENTS AND ADOLESCENTS

Vicki Lord Larson, Ph.D. • Nancy McKinley, M.S.

Thinking Publications, Eau Claire, WI

© 1995 by Thinking Publications
A Division of McKinley Companies, Inc.

Thinking Publications grants limited rights to individual professionals to reproduce and distribute pages that indicate duplication is permissible. Pages can be used for student instruction only and must include Thinking Publications' copyright notice. All rights are reserved for pages without the permission-to-reprint notice. No part of these pages may be reproduced in any form, electronic or mechanical, including photocopy, recording, or any information storage and retrieval system without permission in writing from the publisher.

04   03   02   01   00   99   98   97   96   10   9   8   7   6   5   4   3   2

Larson, Vicki Lord.
     Language disorders in older students : preadolescents and adolescents / Vicki Lord Larson, Nancy McKinley.
          p. cm.
     Includes bibliographical references and index.
     ISBN 0-930599-29-2 (pbk.)
     1. Language disorders in adolescents. 2. Language disorders in children. I. McKinley, Nancy L. II. Title.
     [DNLM: 1. Language—in infancy & childhood. 2. Language Disorders—in adolescence. 3. Language Disorders—therapy. WL 340 L334L 1995]
RJ496.L35L37 1995
616.85'5'00835—dc20
DNLM/DLC
for Library of Congress
                                                                      94-34928
                                                                          CIP

Printed in the United States of America

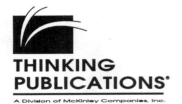

**THINKING
PUBLICATIONS®**
A Division of McKinley Companies, Inc.

424 Galloway Street
Eau Claire, WI 54703
(715) 832-2488
FAX (715) 832-9082

DEDICATION

To Our Sisters

Vivian Lord Joubert, who has carefully edited our writing for many years and who provides support and encouragement so that our books see completion.

Dottie Munsen, who has caringly taught children with language-learning and behavioral disabilities for many years and who provides support and encouragement for their development.

Sisters by Chance

Friends by Choice

TABLE OF CONTENTS

FIGURES AND TABLES

PREFACE

When we began revising our 1987 text, *Communication Assessment and Intervention Strategies for Adolescents*, we thought we were doing just that—revising. Now, several years later after hundreds of hours of reading, discussing, and writing, we offer you this substantially new text. *Language Disorders in Older Students: Preadolescents and Adolescents* is as different from our 1987 text as our 1987 text was from its original 1983 predecessor, *Adolescents' Communication: Development and Disorders*.

As our thinking and studying have evolved, so too have our viewpoints shifted on the topic of older students with language disorders. Those readers who have followed our work for the past twelve years hopefully will appreciate our evolution as we seek to stay current and responsive to meeting the needs of today's youth. Unfortunately, the tone of this book is not quite as optimistic as our past texts about the future of our at-risk youth given the world in which they are living. Meager progress is being made in creating better educational programs for them, not to mention the lack of progress in quelling the murder rate among youth, the suicide rate, the teenage pregnancy rate, and the high school dropout rate—to name just a few of the grim statistical categories still crying out for our attention and response.

And where do youth with language disorders fit in? They remain at risk for failure both at school and in their communities. Few speech-language pathologists are vocal in advocating for their rights, much less their needs. Attention remains focused on younger students, which is admirable to a point. Yes, professionals should be doing everything possible to intervene early and to ameliorate speech and language problems before children reach preadolescence and adolescence. However, early intervention never has and never will be the total solution for every child.

A certain group of students will need our ongoing help. A certain group will be able to compensate for their language disabilities for a long time, but then the demands become so great that they begin falling behind their peers. A certain group will experience environmental factors that suddenly surface when they are older students—possibly a car accident, an attempted homicide, or some other event that results in traumatic brain injury.

Whether the student has a long-standing language disorder or one that is suddenly acquired, the speech-language pathologist assigned to his or her school should assume responsibility for seeing that appropriate services get delivered. Quite the opposite occurs all too often. We hear grim tales from hospital-based clinicians who discharge adolescents back into communities with no speech-language services, or inadequate ones, available at the junior and senior high school levels. We read government reports that alert us to the fact that one-third of the students with speech-language identified as the primary disability area drop out of high school. We ask, "Where are the speech-language clinicians who would tolerate losing one in three of their students without crying out for major reform?"

"Well," you say, "one-third of the general education students drop out of high school. Why shouldn't we expect that one-third of our identified students would also drop out?" Because they should have an advocate in the speech-language pathologist getting programs adapted to meet their needs. Because these same clinicians should be teaching their students strategies for survival academically, socially, and vocationally. Because we have evidence from speech-language pathologists who have established appropriate, relevant programs for older students that the dropout rate can go to near zero percent.

That is why, in our evolution since our 1983 book, readers will find this text more emotional in spots, more passionate in some viewpoints, and more intense in pleading for involvement from our fellow colleagues. Too many youth are being lost. Too little change is occurring in too little time when it comes to creating, maintaining, and expanding speech-language programs for older youth. The time has come for a revolution in how speech-language pathologists serve preadolescents and adolescents who have language disorders.

Language Disorders in Older Students is "bookended" with two chapters that attempt to put speech-language services to preadolescents and adolescents into a broader context. Chapter 1 examines the youth-at-risk phenomenon and points out the overlap between language and at-risk behaviors. Chapter 8 summarizes the major transition points faced by youth and how they fit into a speech-language context.

A solid base of information about older students is supplied in Chapters 2, 3, and 4. Chapter 2 explains theories of adolescence along with their clinical/educational implications. Chapter 3 tackles the growing body of research documenting the cognitive and language development that continues into the preadolescent and adolescent years. Chapter 4 highlights the major language and communication deficits that are observable in older students who are labeled "language disordered."

Chapters 5 and 6 address the assessment process. Different procedures are needed for older students than for younger students, all the while being authentic, relevant, and dynamic. Sufficient detail is provided in these chapters, along with practical appendices of forms that can be copied, such that professionals can begin planning in-depth informal and formal assessment procedures.

Intervention with older students is the target topic in Chapter 7. Strategies are emphasized and, time and again, professionals are urged to put intervention in the context of helping students acquire the language needed for academic, social, and vocational settings.

In both the assessment and intervention chapters, we discuss the idea of direct services for the youth and indirect services for the people within the educational and environmental systems in which the student functions. Direct services alone are frequently insufficient. A holistic approach permits more accurate and thorough assessment findings and more supportive and effective intervention results.

More than ever, speech-language pathologists have the tools that they need to serve older students with language disorders. Chapters 6 and 7 provide extensive lists of commercially available tests and programs, many that are specifically designed with preadolescents and adolescents in mind. Excuses are running out as to why our profession can't or won't take the time to serve older students.

The fact that you are reading this book is a significant step in becoming the strong voice for youth that they so desperately need. The time for silence is gone. Your advocacy for strong speech-language programs is needed for a generation of students who have few adults even aware of their plight.

Our motivation in writing this book is to provide you with current information about how you might serve adolescents more effectively and efficiently. In short:

- Our older youth are at risk.

- As speech-language pathologists, each of us *can* make a difference.

- We show you *how* to make a difference in the context of your own communities.

Thank you for your vision for and your commitment to our country's youth.

A book would never see print if it were not for the "behind the scenes" assistants. Thank you to Linda Schreiber, our editor, who remained patient, supportive, and very helpful as we evolved from writing a revision to creating a substantially new text. We are indebted to our technical editor, Julie Poquette, who also shouldered the awesome task of subject indexing; for that, we are grateful. Graduate students Angie Sterling at the University of Wisconsin–Eau Claire and Deborah Yancy and Marion Peterson at the University of Wisconsin–Oshkosh helped us with hours of library work, including a review of the literature and countless reference checks. They all deserve to get great jobs upon graduation! Thank you to the faculty and staff at the University of Wisconsin–Oshkosh for supplying us with assessment and intervention materials to review.

We are grateful to our reviewers, Sue Schultz, Susan Backes, Carla Hess, Vivienne Ratner and her university students who were required to read several chapters, Christi Wujek Flores, and Bonnie Greenburg. Your feedback helped to shape this manuscript into a more cohesive text. We are also grateful to Robin Powell and Kellie Hiess, who endured many long hours at their word-processing stations entering batch after batch of changes and revisions.

Finally, we thank our husbands, Jim and Mike, who by now are used to being last in line to get our attention. We appreciate deeply their unconditional acceptance of our need to continue sounding the call on behalf of at-risk youth with our professional colleagues.

YOUTH AT RISK

GOALS:

To present definitions, symptoms, and problems of youth at risk

To define *adolescence*

To cite the prevalence of communication disorders in older students

To provide a rationale for speech-language services for older students

To challenge the need to label youth

Many adolescents with communication disorders remain undetected, unserved, and thus unable to realize their complete human potential. *Language Disorders in Older Students: Preadolescents and Adolescents* reviews the current information on preadolescent and adolescent development and communication disorders and presents alternative delivery models for serving our youth at risk. The terms *older students* and *youth* are used interchangeably and include preadolescents (9–11 years) and adolescents (12–20 years).

This book integrates theoretical knowledge and practical ideas for serving older students with communication disorders. Effective assessment and intervention strategies for preadolescents and adolescents are summarized. Infused throughout the book is

information on a multicultural perspective to assessment and intervention as well as how to apply computer technology to serving older students with language disorders. *Language Disorders in Older Students* is intended for educators providing services to youth at risk who have language disorders, but it could also be adopted as a text for university classes emphasizing services for older school-age students.

In Western society, the time span between the ages of approximately 9 and 11 years is called preadolescence, whereas the time span between the ages of 12 and 20 years is called adolescence. *Adolescence*, derived from the Latin word *adolescere*, means "to grow into maturity" (Turner and Helms, 1979). Adolescents are establishing their identities, making

1

career choices, learning how to think about their thinking, and realizing the potential of adult communication. The majority of adolescents are thriving, healthy beings who feel confident, happy, and self-satisfied (Offer, Ostrov, and Howard, 1981). However, a growing number of preadolescents and adolescents in the United States are youth at risk:

> While most young people are preparing to lead productive and responsible lives, it is estimated that one in four adolescents—about seven million youth—are seriously at risk of not making a successful transition from youth to adulthood. Another seven million may be at moderate risk. (Schubert and Gates, 1990, p. 1)

YOUTH AT RISK: WHO ARE THEY?

Hathaway, Sheldon, and McNamara (1989) stated that there is no set pattern when answering the question, "Who are these students at risk?" (p. 367). They go on to note that

> some are brilliant but bored; others have low ability and are undersupported or deterred by their home situation. Some are emotionally troubled, abused, on drugs, or prematurely pregnant; some are male and some are female; some are wealthy but most are poor. (p. 367)

There appears to be no one agreed-upon definition of *youth at risk*. As a result of the lack

of a common definition, statistics will vary as to how many youth are at risk and what it means to be at risk. The term *youth at risk* generally refers "to students who are at-risk of emerging from school unprepared for further education or the kind of work there is to do. Or they are ready only for lives of alienation and dependency" (MDC, 1988, p. 2). One point appears to be consistent within all the definitions—"the term is used to indicate individuals who are at risk of dropping out of the educational system" (Gross and Capuzzi, 1989, p. 5).

The reform of public education is one of the hottest national issues. Reducing the dropout rate has become the focal point of the push to help at-risk youth. Hamby (1989) notes that this goal is complicated by the fact that "there is no single national dropout rate" (p. 1); we have only estimates as opposed to direct measures. Reported dropout statistics—local, state, national—may be in error because different definitions and divergent databases may be used. Estimates of dropouts in urban schools may be as high as the 40 percent to 50 percent range. In an effort to establish a reliable national dropout rate, a general definition is needed. The definition proposed was "a student who (for any reason other than death) leaves school before graduation without transferring to another school/institution (Wittebols, 1986, p. 7)" (Hamby, 1989, p. 5). The federal definition parallels and expands slightly this definition:

> The federal government has defined a dropout as a student who leaves a school, for any reason except death, . . . who has been in membership during the

regular school term, and who withdraws . . . before graduating . . . or completing an equivalent program of studies . . . whether dropping out occurs before or after reaching compulsory school attendance age. (Barber and McClellan, 1987, p. 264)

Hahn (1987) noted that the dropout phenomenon is a multifaceted problem that "starts early, has many causes, and grows incrementally worse with each successive year" (p. 256).

A broader definition of *youth at risk* takes into account that the student may not only be at risk of dropping out of school or out of life but also there may be "a set of causal/behav-

ioral dynamics that place the individual in danger of a negative future event" (Gross and Capuzzi, 1989, p. 5). It is speculated that the way in which youth cope with the myriad of challenges that face them differentiates at-risk youth from their peers. Table 1.1 illustrates choice factors and delineates circumstances that may place youth at risk.

Given the choice factors and those related to circumstance, it becomes obvious that numerous factors contribute to youth being at risk. Clark (1988) noted that minority youth make up the preponderance of youth at risk, but they do not make up the entire population. Studies show that "the single common characteristic of at-risk youth is not race or economic disadvantage, but low scores on

TABLE 1.1	FACTORS CONTRIBUTING TO RISK
CHOICE FACTORS	**CIRCUMSTANCE FACTORS**
• The young person who chooses to drop out of school as a means of reducing both the stress and frustrations generated by the educational process.	• The young person who is forced to live in a disruptive, psychologically punitive family environment.
• The young person who chooses either alcohol or drugs or both as a remedy for the malaise he or she feels.	• The young person who is the victim of either or both physical and sexual abuse.
• The young person who chooses pregnancy as a means of escaping a negative home environment.	• The young person who, based upon family socioeconomic circumstances, is forced to leave school to support the family financially.
• The young person who chooses gang membership as a means of increasing his or her self-identity and need for acceptance.	• The young person who, based on family values, attitudes, and behaviors, develops dysfunctional coping strategies to deal with the challenges presented.
• The young person who chooses suicide as a means of escape from what is viewed as a hopeless situation.	• The young person who, based on academic ability, finds either no meaning or no success in the educative process.

From "Defining Youth at Risk," by D. Gross and D. Capuzzi, 1989, In *Youth at Risk: A Resource for Counselors, Teachers, and Parents*, p. 11. © 1989 by the American Association for Counseling and Development. Reprinted with permission.

tests of basic skills—reading, writing, and computing" (Clark, 1988, p. 3). The value of understanding these factors as well as the symptoms noted in the next section is to assist professionals in developing prevention rather than intervention plans.

YOUTH AT RISK: SYMPTOMS

When attempting to identify youth who are most likely to be at risk for dropping out of school, the 21 symptoms listed in Table 1.2, a number of which relate to language deficiencies, have been noted as indicators of who may drop out. (Caveat: One symptom does not appear to be more highly correlated than others with dropping out of school.)

Barber and McClellan (1987) developed a list of reasons why students drop out of school. This list provided in Table 1.3 presents reasons given by districts for students dropping out of school. The students' reasons for leaving school are listed from the most commonly cited to the least-often mentioned.

Knowing these symptoms may help us to identify youth who are most likely to become at risk for dropping out of school or society. According to Wells, Bechard, and Hamby (1989), "one of the most significant findings to emerge from research on dropouts is that early identification is vital to effective prevention and intervention" (p. 1). No one symptom or combination of symptoms may denote with certainty that a given youth is at risk. However, in some circumstances one symptom or combination of symptoms may result in a given youth being at risk. Each individual will react differently to a given set of circumstances. It is our responsibility as educators to monitor the individual exhibiting any one of these symptoms, so that we might assist our

TABLE 1.2	
WHO WILL DROP OUT? 21 SYMPTOMS	
Many absences	Verbal and language deficiencies
High truancy rate	Inability to tolerate structured activities
Frequent tardiness	Low family income
Poor grades	Poorly educated mother
Low math and reading scores	A fatherless home
Failure in one or more grades	A parent or sibling who dropped out
Limited extracurricular participation	Low self-esteem
Lack of identification with school	Numerous family relocations
Boredom with classes	Poor social adjustment
Failure to see relevance of education to life	An alcoholic parent
Rebellious attitudes	

From "Failure: Why Schools Must Help Children at Risk," by Sunburst Communications, 1988, *Solutions: News for Computer Educators*, 3(2), p. 1. © 1988 by Sunburst Communications. Reprinted with permission.

TABLE 1.3	
AMERICA'S DROPOUTS	
Student had attendance problems	School lacked desired program or course
Student lacked interest in school	Miscellaneous reasons
Student was bored with school	Student was pregnant
Student had academic problems or poor grades	Student had conflicts with employment
Student had problems with teachers	Student got married
Student had family problems or responsibilities	Student had enough education to work
Student had problems with assigned school	Illness in student's family
Student disliked a particular course	Student disliked discipline and rules
Student had problems with school administrators	Student had transportation problems
Student disliked everything	Student entered military service
Student had problems with counselors	Student moved and went to another school
Student had problems with other students	Student had achieved educational goals
Student had discipline problems and was suspended	Parents demanded that student leave school
Student felt too old for school	Don't know
Student had financial problems	Couldn't speak English
Student was ill	Student disliked some physical feature of school
	Student left because of gangs or racial problems

From "Looking at America's Dropouts: Who Are They?" by L. Barber and M. McClellan, 1987, *Phi Delta Kappan, 69,* p. 267. © 1987 by Phi Delta Kappa. Reprinted with permission.

youth in focusing their lives in more productive directions.

PROBLEMS FACING YOUTH AT RISK

A myriad of problems face youth at risk. According to Hamburg (1992), the common problems facing today's youth are substance abuse (experimentation with drugs, cigarettes, and alcohol); sexual activity, pregnancy, and disease (frequent sexual activity resulting in pregnancy and sexually transmitted diseases); nutrition, activity, and fitness (too much junk food, too little activity, and too much obesity); depression and suicide (many suffer depression and are driven to suicide by some combination of substance abuse, trouble with the law, intense anxiety in the face of social or academic challenges, feelings of personal worthlessness, impulsivity, guilt, and shame); delinquency and violence; and adolescent injury (from motor vehicle accidents, drowning, sport and recreational activities, etc.). These common problems are costly to the United States. For example, in the 1980s, alcohol and drug abuse cost about $150 billion per year in reduced productivity, treatment, crime, and related costs. Also, more than $19 billion was spent in 1987 in payments for income maintenance, health care, and nutrition to support families begun by adolescents.

According to statistics, the problems facing our youth are grim. Among industrialized nations, the United States leads the world in juvenile crime (given the present rate, 2 million juveniles will be arrested in the year 2000); substance abuse (the drug problem is 10 times greater than in Japan); and teen pregnancy (one in ten 15- to 19-year-olds becomes pregnant) (Schubert and Gates, 1990). Thirteen percent of high school students in the U.S. read below the sixth-grade level and one in four students drop out of school. "Eighty-five percent of teenagers appearing in juvenile court are functionally illiterate, as are 79 percent of welfare dependents, 85 percent of dropouts, 72 percent of the unemployed" (Schubert and Gates, 1990, p. 9).

Hechinger (1992), noting the crisis proportions that adolescent health in America has reached, claims:

Large numbers of ten- to fifteen-year-olds suffer from depression that may lead to suicide; they jeopardize their future by abusing illegal drugs and alcohol, and by smoking; they engage in premature, unprotected sexual activity; they are victims or perpetrators of violence; they lack proper nutrition and exercise. (p. 21)

Hechinger (1992) views these needs for health services as largely ignored. The leading cause of death among white youth is automobile accidents that are frequently related to drug or alcohol abuse (Schubert and Gates, 1990). The leading cause of death among black youth is homicide (Hechinger, 1992).

In an article written by U.S. Senator Dan Coats (1991), he stated that "suicide is now the second leading cause of death among adolescents, increasing 300 percent since 1950" (p. 1). Statistics on adolescent suicide vary: it may be more helpful to consider whether certain types of youth are more suicidal than others. The Los Angeles Suicide Prevention Center found that 50 percent of young victims (10 to 14 years of age) were diagnosed as learning disabled—specifically as hyperactive, perceptually impaired, and dyslexic. Some researchers suggest that being learning disabled is accompanied by feelings of low self-esteem; thus, these researchers suggested another reason for placing this population in a high-risk category (Peck, 1982).

Furthermore, the majority of case studies have shown that suicide victims feel they have no one with whom they can talk. This lack of a friend, of someone who will listen, can be a major concern for adolescents with learning or language disorders. Their communication problems often interfere with making and keeping friends (Donahue and Bryan, 1984) and with expressing their feelings; both are potential contributing factors in the total despair preceding suicide (Peck, 1982). Major attempts at preventing suicide rely on talking and listening as evidenced by the increasing number of hot lines available across the country. When oral language skills are impaired, and the adolescent is suicide-prone, there is cause for concern.

These are alarming statistics, but even more alarming is the fact that the "teen homicide rate has increased 232 percent since 1950. Homicide is now the leading cause of death among 15- to 19-year-old minority youth" (Coats, 1991, p. 1). The senator goes on to note that the average age for first-time drug use is 13 years old and that teen pregnancy has risen 621 percent since 1940.

AIDS (acquired immune deficiency syndrome), since it was publicly diagnosed in 1981, has presented a new and increasingly serious risk to adolescents. Because of no curative therapy, AIDS now ranks as the most serious epidemic of the past 50 years (Gray and House, 1989). It is projected that the number one killer of youth during the 1990s (exceeding the number of deaths resulting from automobile accidents in white adolescents and homicides in black adolescents) may be AIDS unless preventive measures are taken. Thus, it is important that school curricula incorporate discussions about what AIDS is, as well as prevention and treatment information. Likewise, common myths and misinformation about AIDS need to be dispelled.

Additional problems confronting youth are increasing numbers of students diagnosed with attention deficit disorders (ADD), car and other accidents resulting in traumatic brain injury (TBI), and fetal alcohol syndrome (FAS). These problems are mentioned here because ADD may not be diagnosed until preadolescence or adolescence, TBI may not occur until adolescence, and FAS is present from birth but the symptoms persist into preadolescence and adolescence.

Attention Deficit Disorders (ADD)

ADD is a cluster of syndromes that includes a short attention span, difficulty concentrating, poor impulse control, distractibility, moods that quickly change, and sometimes hyperactivity and a learning disability. Frequently, students with ADD have oral and written language disorders; are poorly organized; and scramble information, which leads to reaching wrong conclusions.

According to Weaver (1993), "The American Psychiatric Association's forthcoming Diagnostic and Statistical Manual-IV will list the defining characteristics under two relatively separate behavior dimensions: inattention-disorganization, and impulsivity-hyperactivity" (p. 80). She goes on to state that ADD is not simply a neurological condition but a social construct (i.e., a dysfunctional relationship between an individual with a biological predisposition and an environment that has certain expectations, demands, and reactions).

Traumatic Brain Injuries (TBI)

TBI occurs with an increased incidence in preadolescents and adolescents, particularly in the latter as a result of car accidents resulting in closed head injury (CHI). According to Blosser and DePompei (1989), the CHI student is not a "peer" of other handicapped students. Characteristics of CHI students that make them different from other students with language disorders are listed in Table 1.4.

When working with students who have a CHI, it is important to keep in mind how they are similar to and different from other older students with language disorders. According

TABLE 1.4

CHARACTERISTICS OF CHI STUDENTS

- A sense of being normal that persists from the premorbid period

- Discrepancies in ability levels

- A previous history of successful experiences in academic and social settings

- Inconsistent patterns of performance

- Variability and fluctuation in the recovery process, resulting in unpredictable and unexpected spurts of recovery

- More extreme problems with generalizing, integrating, or structuring information

- Poor judgment and loss of emotional control, which cause the student to appear to be emotionally disturbed at times

- Cognitive deficits that, although present in other handicaps, are more uneven in extent of damage and rate of recovery

- Combinations of handicapping conditions that do not fall into usual categories of disabilities

- Inappropriate behaviors that may be more exaggerated than the behaviors of students with other handicaps (e.g., greater impulsivity or distractibility)

- A learning style that requires the use of a variety of compensatory and adaptive strategies

- Some intact high-level skills (making it difficult to understand why the student will have problems in performing lower-level tasks)

From "The Head-Injured Student Returns to School: Recognizing and Treating Deficits," by J. Blosser and R. DePompei, 1989, *Topics in Language Disorders*, 9(2), p. 69. © 1989 by Aspen Publishers. Reprinted with permission.

to Gruen and Gruen (1994), numerous cognitive-linguistic disorders are common to individuals with TBI: "These impairments include deficits in concentration, sustained attention, memory, nonverbal problem solving, part/whole analysis and synthesis, conceptual organization and abstraction" (p. 3).

The student with a CHI may suffer from psychological difficulties as well as physical impairment and cognitive-communication problems. Psychological difficulties may include depression, anger, and behavior inappropriate to the situation. The National Institutes of Health (1984) has cited three types of personality change in CHI individuals. One common personality change is apathy—a reduced interest in life's activities and challenges. This can be devastating for a student, since such apathy may lead to teachers and family members ignoring these individuals because they are not behavior problems in the classroom or home. Such ignoring only reinforces the adolescent's or young adult's apathy. Another personality change common among CHI individuals is to become overly optimistic (i.e., believing that things are better than they are or underestimating their disabilities). A third common personality change is loss of social restraint and judgment. Some CHI clients become tactless, talkative, and hurtful, and they may have outbursts of rage in response to trivial frustrations.

Fetal Alcohol Syndrome (FAS)

Abel (1990) noted that confirmed heavy and frequent drinking by a mother during pregnancy can be responsible for the pattern of abnormalities known as FAS. FAS includes such features as unusual facial formation; prematurity; low birth weight; postnatal growth retardation; malformation, especially of the heart, limbs, and palate; delayed intellectual development; and delayed language development (Ratner and Harris, 1994). Infants who are exposed to alcohol in utero may exhibit some but not all the characteristics associated with FAS. They are known as children with fetal alcohol effects (FAE). Sparks (1993) estimates that FAE occurs at two or three times the frequency of FAS. Ratner and Harris (1994) describe characteristic behaviors of children with FAS and FAE:

- lack of social skills;
- hyperactive, distractible, inattentive, and impulsive;
- delayed motor development;
- uninhibited behavior;
- lack of attachment or indiscriminate attachment;
- difficulty making transitions to new activities;

- poor judgment, poor recognition of cause-effect relationships;
- inappropriate language use in context;
- conceptual confusion; and
- temper tantrums and defiance of authority.

Ratner and Harris (1994) also present characteristics of FAS and FAE in adolescents. These include sexual difficulties, depression (due to social isolation), restlessness, and the tendency to be truant or drop out of school.

In discussing academic behaviors of FAS and FAE students, Ratner and Harris (1994) state that academic difficulties occur in such areas as listening and reading comprehension; abstract thinking; memory (visual and spatial); basic problem solving; and time, space, and causal concepts. The types of communication difficulties noted are poor pragmatic language skills; difficulty comprehending social language rules and expectations; and ineffective communication because it lacks substance, cohesion, meaning, and relevance. FAS and FAE impacts adolescents in that they seem to plateau in daily and academic functions. Later, their behaviors such as attention deficits, poor judgment, and impulsiveness make successful employment difficult (Ratner and Harris, 1994). It is not uncommon for children with FAS or FAE to become alcoholic themselves, and the cycle repeats itself.

Attention to these problems among adolescents must begin with knowing that this age group is not homogeneous. There are many subgroups which, although they face common problems, have different degrees of risk dependent upon their social, ethnic, or racial backgrounds. "For example, black male adolescents are five to six times as likely to die as a result of homicide as white males, and black girls are two to three times as likely to become homicide victims as white girls" (Hechinger, 1992, p. 29). Thus, the degree of risk to adolescents will depend on their ethnicity and how society responds.

COSTS AND RESPONSES

The costs of juvenile problems are astronomical. The average cost of one youth in a public juvenile facility for one year is $27,000 (Schubert and Gates, 1990). The cost of dropouts per year in lost earnings and foregone taxes is $260 billion. In 1983, alcohol and drug abuse cost America more than $175 billion in reduced productivity, crime, and related costs. Greater than the economic costs are the costs in human terms—ruined lives for our young people, a lower quality of life in our communities, and the threatened loss of America's continued prosperity and standard of living (Schubert and Gates, 1990).

It has long been noted and recently documented that to prevent youth from being at risk, both family and community members must share the responsibility (Search Institute, 1991). "The family provides rules, discipline, encouragement, and caring. The community makes available such things as educational experiences, community rules and expectations, friends, recreational experiences, and spiritual nurture" (Search Institute, 1991, p. 1). These are external assets that collectively form a scaffold around our youth while they are developing their own set of internal supports (Search Institute, 1991). The internal support

or backbone needed to make healthy choices is depicted in Figure 1.1. The backbone is composed of 14 vertebrae that are divided into three categories:

1. *Educational commitment*—The student cares about school performance, is motivated to achieve, takes schoolwork/ homework seriously, and aspires to go on to some form of postsecondary school.

2. *Positive values*—The student values sexual restraint, helping others, solving world hunger, and caring about others' feelings.

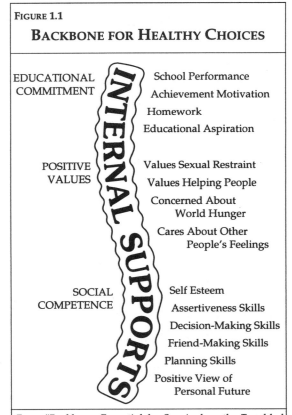

FIGURE 1.1
BACKBONE FOR HEALTHY CHOICES

EDUCATIONAL COMMITMENT

INTERNAL SUPPORTS

School Performance
Achievement Motivation
Homework
Educational Aspiration

POSITIVE VALUES

Values Sexual Restraint
Values Helping People
Concerned About World Hunger
Cares About Other People's Feelings

SOCIAL COMPETENCE

Self Esteem
Assertiveness Skills
Decision-Making Skills
Friend-Making Skills
Planning Skills
Positive View of Personal Future

From "Backbone: Essential for Survival on the Troubled Journey," by the Search Institute, 1991, *Source*, 7(1), p. 1. © 1991 by the Search Institute. Reprinted with permission.

3. *Social competence*—The student exhibits self-esteem, displays assertiveness skills, applies good decision-making skills, uses good friend-making skills, possesses planning skills, and has a positive view of a personal future.

The more external and internal assets a youth has, the fewer at-risk behaviors he or she will possess. However, it should be noted that "there are no quick fixes or simple solutions for the problems that place learners at risk" (Wood, 1988, p. 7). The developmental period most descriptive of youth at risk is adolescence. This developmental period is further explored in the next section.

DEFINITIONS OF ADOLESCENCE

An extensive review of the literature reveals numerous definitions of *adolescence*. It has been defined as a transitional period between childhood and adulthood (Lewin, 1939; Turner and Helms, 1979); as a rite of passage into adulthood (Kett, 1977); as a time of identity crisis and psychosocial moratorium (Erikson, 1968); as a coming of age (Freeman, 1983; Mead, 1950); and as the age of commitment and a move toward interdependence (Konopka, 1973). However, at the root of these definitions is the heated debate on whether adolescence is a natural developmental stage or purely sociologically determined, and thus a product of Western society (Konopka, 1971). Elder (1975) emphasized that adolescence

must be discussed from a socio-historical perspective, that is, relative to the current decade or to a specific moment in time.

How do these definitions agree with those applied by professionals who work with adolescents? Adolescents are often stereotyped by professionals as rebellious, irrational beings to be tolerated and endured. They are looked upon as a homogeneous age group, discontinuous from the remainder of the life cycle (Lipsitz, 1980).

ADOLESCENCE AS A DEVELOPMENTAL PERIOD

We need to view adolescence, as do Konopka (1971) and Lipsitz (1980), as just one of the developmental periods within the overall life cycle. Adolescents must be perceived first as unique individuals and second as people going through a period of development called *adolescence*. Adolescence involves biological, sociocultural, and psychological aspects, and each interacts with the others. No single aspect is sufficient to explain adolescence, but all are necessary; collectively, they may describe adolescence.

Biologically, adolescence spans the years between the onset of puberty and the completion of bone growth (Lipsitz, 1980). Puberty, according to Tanner (1974), includes the following factors: (1) adolescent growth spurt, which can occur in the individual with variations in onset, intensity, magnitude, and duration, resulting in an increase in the skeleton, muscles, and viscera; (2) changes in body composition such as bone, fat, and muscles;

(3) sex-specific growth rate, varying between the sexes, and leading to differences in body dimensions; and (4) development of the adult reproductive system and secondary sex characteristics.

Socioculturally, adolescence is influenced by cultural values, attitudes, and beliefs, as well as by socioeconomic class and by Western society's laws on compulsory education, child labor, and juvenile proceedings (Bakan, 1971). Most societies use functional criteria (e.g., the ability to support oneself) or status criteria (e.g., voting rights) to mark the end of adolescence. These sociocultural dimensions influence society's tolerance range for what is the time length for "typical adolescence." Researchers note that the more sophisticated a society's technology, the more prolonged is the period of adolescence (Eisenberg, 1965).

Psychologically, adolescents attain the ability to think at an abstract level (Inhelder and Piaget, 1958) and to establish a personal identity (Erikson, 1968). Thus, this is a time of accelerated cognitive growth (Alley and Deshler, 1979; Epstein, 1978) and of personality formation (Ferguson, 1970). Both of these domains will continue to evolve in later stages of adulthood, but at a lesser rate.

The critical aspect of a definition of adolescence is that it emphasizes an interrelationship among biological, sociocultural, and psychological dimensions. For example, as people mature physically and thus sexually, they learn, through their culture and social class, a specific sex role, which in turn is made a part of their personality—or it is rejected and may result in some personal confusion.

In summary, any cohesive definition of adolescence must accommodate the fact that adolescence as a developmental period is constantly changing, contingent upon the sociocultural environment and upon the function of time. Adolescence, therefore, must be perceived as a concept in transition.

MYTHS ABOUT ADOLESCENTS

The failure to perceive adolescence as a concept in transition can lead to myths that may impair perception and consequently lead to erroneous assumptions about this period of development. The following myths may be evident:

1. The "continuous growth" myth implies that development is uniform and synchronized during adolescence (Lipsitz, 1979). Frequently, however, a mismatch occurs in development. Physical growth may spurt without a corresponding psychological change. Rather than being uniform, growth tends to be characterized by spurts, troughs, and plateaus. Adolescent growth and development should be considered neither continuous nor stagelike, since both patterns are possible (Muuss, 1975).

2. The "generation gap" myth states that vast differences exist between youth and adults (Mitchell, 1979). But generational differences are often dissimilarities in outlook for achieving the same goal, and they have to do with specific preferences rather than general beliefs. In other words, parents may struggle with the adolescent over dress code, curfew, and

peer group choice, but these conflicts are fundamentally the same as when that child was a toddler and conflict arose over bedtime and bath time—they concern the struggle for independence. The change is that all participants are a decade or so older. Adult-adolescent conflict is no more unusual than adult-adult conflict or conflict arising between adolescents. In fact, the rift between early and late adolescents is often much stronger than between adolescents and adults (Mitchell, 1979).

3. The "life skills incompetence" myth promotes the image of adolescents who are incompetent in performing important tasks (Mitchell, 1979). However, competence may be difficult to determine because adolescents have been excluded from any important work where competence might be demonstrated. Laws prohibit most jobs before age 16; even after that age, business and labor usually refuse to hire adolescents for anything except menial jobs. Projections for the year 2000 are that jobs will require a workforce whose median level of education is 13.5 years (MDC, 1988), thus continuing to put our youth at a disadvantage for employment. Few adolescents, particularly those in early adolescence, are trained in a specific skill area that would make them marketable to business and labor.

Mitchell (1979) argues that many constructive uses of youth talent in the community are currently being ignored. Exemplary community work projects exist such as Habitat for Humanity, a nationwide project that uses volunteer adolescents and others to build houses for low-income families. Such programs recognize and capitalize upon the competence and talents of adolescents.

4. The "turmoil" myth suggests that adolescents are in constant psychological turmoil. Mitchell (1979) believes that this myth may stem from the negative way that many social scientists describe the adolescent experience. A quick check of article and book titles containing information about adolescents carries through the turmoil theme: *The Turbulent Teens* (Gardner, 1982), "The Age of Insolence: Those Terrible Teens" (Coles, 1983), *The Transition of Youth to Adulthood: A Bridge Too Long* (National Commission on Youth, 1980); "America's Youth: A Crisis of Character" (Coats, 1991). Not all adolescents experience turmoil; yet adults may expect it. Mental health professionals were asked to complete the Offer Self-Image Questionnaire (Offer, Ostrov, and Howard, 1977) the way they thought normal adolescents would complete it. On 7 out of 10 scales, professionals described the normal adolescent as significantly more disturbed than normal adolescents viewed themselves (Offer et al., 1981). Much of the turmoil appears to be created in the minds of adults, although some adolescents do experience turmoil.

Adults might consider assuming some responsibility for whatever problems these youth are encountering. For example, by age 14, the average adolescent has witnessed 11,000 murders on television (National Commission on Youth, 1980). The "throw away population," those adolescents disposed of by parents who can no longer cope, is on the increase (Wellborn, 1981). Today's adolescents, growing up in a crowded world, are in strong competition with the baby boom generation of adults who are demanding jobs, goods, and services at record levels. Although the majority of adolescents are not in turmoil, those who are should not go unnoticed by adults.

The professional's belief in any one of these common myths can lead to erroneous assumptions about adolescents. Professionals must examine their beliefs about and attitudes toward adolescence and then determine whether objective evidence substantiates or contradicts their beliefs and attitudes. This examination of beliefs will ensure a more objective approach to working with adolescents.

5. Finally, we believe that a fifth myth specific to the field of speech-language pathology needs to be dispelled. The "there's nothing more to do" myth, widely held by speech-language pathologists, says that little can be done past the fourth grade for the student with an oral language disorder. Many developmental charts for language end at 10 years; thus professionals may question what more can be accomplished if the child has not already been "cured" by that age. This myth is fueled by current diagnostic batteries. Many times formal

tests seem to indicate that the student's language deficit has been cured, when in fact it has not. While clinical intuition might suspect continuation of certain language deficits into the middle school grades and beyond, many formal tests are not sensitive to the functional aspects of communication that affect the older student (Damico, 1991, 1993). Current assessment instruments overemphasize superficial aspects of language and artificially fragment language into separate parts (Damico, 1991, 1993), therefore yielding an inaccurate or partial picture of the adolescent.

The "discrete point" testing approach, which evaluates isolated finite aspects of language, contributes to the disparity between formal test observations and what students do in actual conversation. Older students may perform within norms on standardized tests, but they may display deficits in discourse that severely impede them academically, socially, or vocationally. "As a function of this testing procedure, these older children [are] classified according to a different set of guidelines and [are] labeled as having learning disorders rather than language disorders. They [are], in effect, taken out of our professional domain" (Damico, 1991, p. 126).

It is not that speech-language pathologists *cannot* do anything more for older students, but that frequently they *have not* done anything more. In the past, other professionals have served older students with language disorders, or these youth have been unserved. Yet the prevalence of adolescents with communication disorders is sufficiently documented to warrant speech-language pathologists' attention as service providers to this population. Students past the age of 9 should no longer go unserved or underserved.

PREVALENCE OF COMMUNICATION DISORDERS

Statistics on the number of older students with impairments of speech, language, or hearing are scattered because specific data on this age group have not often been gathered. The one exception has been data gathered in juvenile detention centers. In these centers, a disproportionately large number of adolescents with communication disorders has been evident. Taylor (1969) found that 84 percent of the incarcerated youth she studied had communication disorders. Although these data are more than two decades old, they remain the most comprehensive available. Since prison populations are on the increase, current data are direly needed on the prevalence of communication disorders in incarcerated youth.

Gillespie and Cooper (1973) reported the prevalence of speech problems in junior and senior high schools to be 5.5 percent. A report from the American Speech-Language-Hearing Association (ASHA) (Fein, 1983) documented that 1.94 percent of individuals 5 to 14 years of age and 0.67 percent of individuals 15 to 24 years of age were speech-language impaired.

These data excluded cleft palate cases, deaf people who cannot speak, and any institutionalized individuals. Based on available data, researchers cannot derive a specific prevalence figure for the entire adolescent population.

In late 1983, we attempted a national survey of state consultants for speech-language programs to determine the prevalence of communication disorders among adolescents. The return rate of the questionnaires was 26 percent. The majority of the surveys returned indicated that consultants had no means to retrieve statistics specifically for adolescents with communication disorders in their states. Thus, we could not compute a national prevalence figure. However, one reporting state, Florida, computed prevalence figures and reported that 1.4 percent of students aged 13 to 21 years were receiving services. Florida implemented Project Adolang (Task Force on Secondary Programs for the Speech-Language Impaired, 1983) to identify adolescent language problems and their implications for education.

An update to the aforementioned 1983 national survey was conducted in 1992. Only 8 of 50 states (16 percent) responded, and the majority of those reported that their states still had no way to retrieve statistics specifically for the 12- to 20-year-old age group. The several who were able to derive numbers showed a considerable difference between those receiving speech-language services in the 6- to 11-year-old range versus the 12- to 20-year-old range (e.g., 5.3 percent for the 6- to 11-year-old group versus 0.8 percent for the 12- to 20-year-old group of students receiving speech-language services; of these, 2.9 percent of the 6- to 12-year-old group had speech-language identified as their only disability, compared to 0.4 percent of the 12- to 20-year-old group). Another state could report only the unduplicated count (i.e., students who have speech-language as their primary disability) and cited that 4.1 percent of their 6- to 11-year-olds received speech-language services compared to 0.8 percent of their 12- to 20-year-olds.

One state "translated" the age ranges to grades 1–6 versus grades 7–12 and reported that 4.7 percent of the younger group received speech-language services compared to 1.5 percent of the older age group. Particularly striking is the observation that only a fraction of students between 12 and 20 years of age receive speech-language services compared to those between the ages of 6 and 11 years; percentages ranged from 0.07 to 0.25 among the reporting states. The implication is that relatively few students continue to receive speech-language services beyond age 12. An unanswered question is whether the overwhelming decline in secondary students receiving speech-language services is due primarily to "curing" communication disorders by age 12 or to other factors.

To obtain additional data on prevalence, we surveyed 200 speech-language pathologists randomly selected from an original pool of 600 people who had attended one of our 1983–85 workshops (Larson and McKinley, 1985a). The original pool of 600 people was selected because they had demonstrated an interest in serving adolescents. Of the 200 sampled, 55 percent returned their questionnaires. The average prevalence of secondary school students being served by these speech-language pathologists was 2 percent. The range of adolescents being served was from .04 percent to 10 percent of the secondary-level population. Sixty-one percent of these secondary-level students were receiving dual services (e.g., services from both a speech-language pathologist and a learning disabilities specialist), and 39 percent were receiving speech-language services exclusively.

After reviewing the literature on prevalence of communication disorders among older students and then attempting to collect data specific to that population, we have concluded that perhaps as many youths as the 5 percent figure often quoted by the American Speech-Language-Hearing Association are in need of services. Even using the conservative unduplicated count statistic from the 15th Annual Report to Congress (U.S. Department of Education, 1993) that 2.34 percent of school-age children are communicatively handicapped, speech-language pathologists can expect that a high school of 1,000 students would have at least 23 students with significant oral communication deficits (i.e., language deficits, hearing impairment, articulation disorders, voice problems, and stuttering). By far the largest proportion of students will be those with language disorders (Shewan, 1989). This conservative estimate does not include those students who are classified in other categories (e.g., learning disabilities, behavioral disorders) who have concomitant speech-language disorders in need of services.

Unfortunately, wide discrepancies among school districts exist in the provision of services for these preadolescents and adolescents with communication disorders. One program with which we have consulted has a full-time speech-language pathologist at a junior high school with a school census of 1,200 students. Another school that we know in the same geographical area has a school census of 1,800 and only 3 hours of services a week.

RATIONALE FOR SPEECH-LANGUAGE SERVICES

Decision makers often ask, "If students with communication disorders couldn't be 'cured' during elementary years, why should additional services be provided by speech-language pathologists during adolescence? Why isn't the language work they receive in English and other classes enough?" Speech-language pathologists committed to older students should be offering these counterarguments:

1. Many students with language disorders need continued assistance from speech-language pathologists to learn the higher-level concepts and vocabulary demanded at each grade. Many of these students require special services to remain in the mainstream through the elementary grades; their need does not stop upon entrance into junior- and senior-high levels. In fact, these very transitions may heighten students' needs as they move from one educational level to the next or from one educational setting to another.

2. "Turning over" language instruction to other professionals usually ensures that students will be taught communication for academics, but not for social and vocational areas. The speech-language pathologist is the only professional who is concerned primarily with communication, using content (academic, social, vocational) to achieve speaking, listening, reading, writing, and thinking goals.

Other professionals are concerned primarily with academic content, using communication as a vehicle to achieve their curriculum goals. Moreover, these educators are expected to teach this content in restricted time frames to large groups of students with varied needs.

3. Students generally make the transition from the concrete into the formal period of cognitive development at the adolescent level (Piaget and Inhelder, 1969). The formal level of thinking permits students to consider the realm of possibilities; they are no longer tied to the present. Learning abstract concepts that require formal operational thought is now possible.

4. Strong speech-language programs in combination with other special programs (e.g., those for learning disabilities and vocational education) have proven effective in reducing dropout rates. For instance, one rural Wisconsin high school went from 45 students dropping out in a five-year period to 14 students dropping out in the next five years following implementation of the prototype speech-language program

(McKinley and Larson, 1989), which will be explained in Chapter 7. These promising statistics have held in subsequent years. Only four students dropped out in the next four years. Another urban Illinois district's "Communication Development Program" at the senior-high level has had only two dropouts in the 14-year history of the program (C. Wujek, personal communication, 1991). Every potential dropout who is retained will earn an additional $200,000 over his or her lifetime (Rukeyser, 1988). Conversely, by the year 2000, dropouts may not be able to gain employment. More specifically, Gillespie (1990) cited statistics from the National Alliance of Business indicating that currently one job in three can be done by a dropout, whereas in the year 2000 one job in ten will be able to be done by a dropout. He goes on to state that America cannot move into the 21st century with a competitive edge in the marketplace if our workforce is educationally unprepared.

5. Speech-language pathologists need to document precisely the growth in language development that occurs over time with adolescents who are receiving language intervention. This documentation of language growth would be convincing evidence that intervention does make a difference for these students and that significant progress can be made in oral and written communication skills.

6. Taxpayers will ultimately pay for these students at some point (if not in high school, then during their later years) in the form of adult literacy programs, welfare, basic job training, and many other attempts to reverse the pattern of failure. Business is spending billions of dollars in remedial education every year (Naisbitt, 1988; Rukeyser, 1988). According to John Naisbitt's *Trend Letter* (1988), U.S. companies spend $21 billion a year on remedial education and fundamental job skills; some of these monies are used to teach basic language skills.

Despite the passage more than a decade ago of the original PL 94-142 legislation, the Education for All Handicapped Children Act, many junior and senior high schools provide little or no direct speech-language services. In addition to the legal issues that could arise, failure to provide adequate services contributes to the problem of at-risk children (Simon, 1990, 1991). Although speech-language clinicians are busy serving younger children, this is no excuse for failure to provide adequate services for junior and senior high school students. Additional staff, if needed, is a small price to pay for reduced dropout rates, improved functioning of students, and prevention of legal suits.

When involved with serving older students, speech-language pathologists should function as part of a team. Under PL 94-142 and its revisions under the Individuals with Disabilities Education Act (IDEA), both the assessment and intervention processes are required to utilize a multidisciplinary approach. The team members need to consist of regular educator(s), parent(s), and the youth at risk and may also include any one or more of the following: administrators, special educators, speech-language pathologists, audiologists, occupational therapists, physical therapists, social workers, school psychologists, counselors, etc. Youth at risk will benefit from a multidisciplinary approach wherein each team member brings his or her expertise to help solve problems that place youth at risk (Wood, 1988). As a professional, if you choose to work with youth at risk, you will find many challenges, numerous frustrations, and numbers increasing daily.

ARE LABELS NEEDED?

The major focus of this book is to provide a framework for working with youth at risk (preadolescents and adolescents) who have some type of language disorder that interferes with achieving academic progress, reaching vocational potential, or enhancing personal-social interactions. Since labels like *language disordered* or *learning disabled* provide no information about the nature of the communication disorder, we use labels sparingly.

Labels set up negative expectations for performance. Affixing a label that indicates a diagnostic category may be the most powerful determining force in the individual's personality and social interactions, virtually guaranteeing the formulation of a prognosis that will continue to justify the diagnosis and the continued application of the label (Feuerstein, 1979). As such, labels are a disservice.

Although only specific aspects of the person's behavior lead to a label, in practice the whole person is labeled, and he or she is treated accordingly. Unfortunately, "the process of labeling is a formal procedure, [but] the removal of labels is not" (Goldstein, Arkell, Ashcroft, Hurley, and Lilly, 1975, p. 36). Mercer (1975) found, in the community she studied, that public schools were the predominant label users among 241 agencies serving people with retardation. This is probably because state and federal laws mandate the use of these labels for reimbursement purposes.

A whole series of behavioral expectations, beliefs, and images operate under the rubric of the label. "Normal" people develop an explicit set of negative expectations, beliefs, and images about "disabled" people, especially those with physical, mental, or emotional disorders. Often "disabled" people develop similar beliefs about themselves that restrict their potential to overcome or to accept their limitations. When this set of beliefs is operating, the "disabled" view themselves as "handicapped." These labels, and others, undermine one of the essential premises of categorizing youth: that students are benefited. Findings suggest that adverse categorization stigmatizes students and reduces both their self-image and their worth in the eyes of others (Kirp, 1974). Categorizing also tends to separate students along racial and social class lines, and this segregation may cause educational injury to minority students (Rivers, Henderson, Jones, Ladner, and Williams, 1975).

While the labels *language disordered* and *speech impaired* may not carry the emotional impact of the labels *mentally retarded* and *emotionally disturbed*, we have chosen to use labels cautiously and to talk about students with language disorders rather than about "the language disordered adolescent." Emphasis is placed first upon the normality of the individual, and second upon the communication disorder. Although labeling may be necessary in certain agencies to procure funding or to ensure services under PL 94-142 and IDEA, it serves little utility in education past that point.

SUMMARY

This chapter attempted to define youth at risk and to discuss the symptoms and problems facing these youth and society. The developmental period most commonly associated with youth at risk is adolescence. In Western society, *adolescence* is a concept in transition.

Several common myths of adolescence were discussed and, we hope, dispelled. A rationale was presented as to why professionals need to provide speech-language services to older students who have language disorders, using a team approach to assessing, intervening, and solving problems facing youth at risk.

Finally, professionals were urged to apply categorical labels cautiously to students with language disorders. Labels may actually be a disservice to youth, in that they may lower professionals' expectations and create negative self-images.

DISCUSSION QUESTIONS

1. In what additional myths of adolescence do you believe? Are there any cited in this chapter with which you disagree?

2. What do you perceive to be a functional definition of *youth at risk?* How will this definition help you to identify, assess, and intervene with this population?

3. What advantages and disadvantages do you see in labeling students by categories?

SUGGESTED READINGS

Hechinger, F. (1992). *Fateful choices: Healthy youth for the 21st century.* New York: Hill and Wang.

MDC. (1988). *America's shame, America's hope: Twelve million youth at risk.* Chapel Hill, NC: Author.

THEORIES OF ADOLESCENCE

GOALS:

To describe theories of adolescence

To present a theory of adolescence as it relates to older students with language disorders

Knowles (1973) isolated the most salient features of a theory when he stated, "A theory is a comprehensive, coherent, and internally consistent system of ideas about a set of phenomena" (p. 6). A theory should unify, relate, and explain diverse phenomena that were previously viewed as separate, unrelated, and unaccountable (Eisner, 1965). Theories provide an explanation of phenomena and guidelines for action (Knowles, 1973). In communication sciences and disorders, theories should provide the framework upon which procedures are based. In summary, a theory provides a basis for action, a rationale for practice, and a roadmap for exploring unfamiliar terrain.

THEORIES OF ADOLESCENCE

A number of theorists and theoretical positions have contributed to professionals' knowledge of adolescence. In turn, how these theorists impact upon the speech-language pathologist's work with adolescents who have language disorders will be discussed later in this chapter. Muuss (1975) considered various theories of adolescence and isolated the following theoretical viewpoints: biological, anthropological, sociological, and psychological. The major theoretical positions and their theorists or major contributors are presented in Table 2.1.

Table 2.1			
	THEORIES OF ADOLESCENCE		
BIOLOGICAL	**ANTHROPOLOGICAL**	**SOCIOLOGICAL**	**PSYCHOLOGICAL**

Hall (1904)	Mead (1950)
	Benedict (1954)
	Freeman (1983)
		Davis (1944)
		Havighurst (1953)
			Central European Theories
			    Kroh (1944)
			    Kretschmer (1951)
			    Zeller (1952)
			    Spranger (1955)
			    Remplein (1956)
			Psychoanalytic Theory
			    Rank (1945)
			    Freud, A. (1948)
			    Freud, S. (1953)
			Field Theory
			    Lewin (1939)
			Social Learning Theory
			    Miller and Dollard (1941)
			    Bandura and Walters (1963)
			Stage Theories
			    General Development
			        Gesell, Ilg, and Ames (1956)
			        Mitchell (1979)
			    Identity Development
			        Erickson (1968)
			        Marcia (1980)
			    Cognitive
			        Inhelder and Piaget (1958)
			        Elkind (1974, 1978)
			        Feuerstein (1979, 1980)
			        Selman (1980)
			    Moral
			        Kohlberg (1975)

Each of these theoretical positions has influenced how adolescents are viewed in the latter part of the 20th century.

BIOLOGICAL THEORY

In 1904, Hall perceived adolescence as a period of *sturm und drang* (storm and stress), a myth that remains to the present day. Hall's (1904) recapitulation theory (i.e., ontogeny recapitulates phylogeny) presented adolescence as a genetically predetermined time that corresponds to a turbulent transitional stage in the human race. Today, many people con-tinue to view adolescence as "turbulent" and "transitional," due mainly to the major physiological changes that teenagers experience.

Educational/Clinical Implications

According to Hall's biological theory, environmental influences are limited by a biological clock. Miller (1989) states that the main message of the biological theory for educators is "that they should be sensitive to when all children as individuals, directed by their own innate growth potential, have reached a state of readiness for acquiring new behaviors . . . or concepts . . . via training" (p. 18).

ANTHROPOLOGICAL THEORIES

Anthropologists (Benedict, 1954; Mead, 1950) have argued that adolescence is culturally determined. Stress and turmoil, if experienced during adolescence, are the result of one's culture, not of biological changes in the body. Mead (1950), for example, argued that cultures, such as the Samoan, perceived the overall cycle from birth to death as gradual and continuous, because the adolescent girls she studied did not experience stress and turmoil. Benedict (1954), supporting Mead's position, maintained that growth was a gradual, continuous process from infantile dependence to adult independence, unless altered by the culture. The implication in Benedict's and in Mead's work is that Western society, unlike the Samoan culture, has created a phenomenon called "adolescence" and has decreed that this time is filled with stress and turmoil. It should be noted that Mead's work has recently received severe criticism from Freeman (1983), who believes that Mead's cultural determinism ideology biased her observations.

Educational/Clinical Implications

An anthropological perspective emphasizes the need to take a more multicultural perspective on adolescent development. According to this theory, educators need to account for and accommodate differences in each adolescent's culture as educational/clinical assessment and intervention strategies are developed.

SOCIOLOGICAL THEORIES

In contrast with the biologists and anthropologists, sociologists have not concerned themselves with whether adolescence is biologically or culturally determined. Instead, the primary contribution of sociologists (Davis, 1944; Havighurst, 1953) has been their description of social development during adolescence. Davis (1944) emphasized the emergence of "internalizing socialized anxiety" during adolescence. He postulated that adolescents control their behavior because of their anticipation and fear of punishment. Havighurst (1953) emphasized developmental tasks of adolescents, such as achieving a masculine or feminine social role, achieving emotional independence from parents and other adults, desiring and achieving socially responsible behavior, and so forth. Both Davis and Havighurst emphasized how social class differences affect expectations of social development, an ongoing topic of interest in the late 20th century.

Educational/Clinical Implications

Based on the sociological theories of adolescent development, educators would account for contrasts in adolescents' behaviors by social class differences. Educators should investigate how social class differences warrant different educational and clinical approaches.

PSYCHOLOGICAL THEORIES

Like the sociologists, psychologists (see Table 2.1) have not debated whether adolescence is primarily determined by biological or cultural factors; instead, psychologists have attempted to document theories of psychological development, both personality and cognitive, during adolescence. Psychological theories of adolescent development have been grouped according to Central European theories, psychoanalytic theory, field theory, social learning theory, and developmental stage theory. Each of these theoretical groups will be discussed, except for Central European theories (Kretschmer, 1951; Kroh, 1944; Remplein, 1956; Spranger, 1955; Zeller, 1952), which have had minimal influence upon American psychologists and educators.

Sigmund Freud (1953) catalyzed American inquiry into psychoanalytic theory by documenting universal psychosexual stages that he believed are genetically, not environmentally, determined. Freud believed that character formation during adolescence results from a struggle between two forces: the id (i.e., the biological-instinctual force) and the superego (i.e., the socially oriented force). Anna Freud (1948) placed greater emphasis on adolescent development and the role of puberty in character formation than did her father. Rank (1945), unlike Sigmund and Anna Freud, placed more emphasis on positive human dimensions of creativity and productivity, the conscious ego, and the present than on human repression and neurosis, the unconscious ego, and the past.

An alternate explanation of psychological development during adolescence has been offered by field theory (Lewin, 1939). In this theory, adolescence is viewed as a period of transition during which the individual changes group membership. The adolescent belongs partly to the child group and partly to the adult group, without belonging completely to either. It should be noted that this viewpoint of adolescence has been expressed frequently by speech-language pathologists attending our workshops. Lewin believes that various cultures differ regarding their requirements for changing from the child to the adult group. Muuss (1975), who offered an interpretation of Lewin, noted that the greater the differentiation between the adult group and the child group in a given culture or social class, the more difficult the transition.

A third alternative to explain psychological development during adolescence has been offered by social learning theorists (Bandura and Walters, 1963; Miller and Dollard, 1941). These theorists attempted to integrate psychoanalytic and behavioristic theory by stressing a reliance upon environmental events (e.g., imitation of parents, teachers, peers) rather than biological factors to explain development. They seem to agree with the anthropologists in that they view adolescence as part of the continuous development from childhood to adulthood, not as a separate stage of development.

Finally, stage theories attempted to explain psychological development during adolescence (Elkind, 1974, 1978; Erikson, 1968; Feuerstein, 1979, 1980; Gesell, Ilg, and Ames, 1956; Inhelder and Piaget, 1958; Kohlberg, 1975; Mitchell, 1979). Some theories concentrated attention on general development (Gesell et al., 1956; Mitchell, 1979), while others focused on specific aspects of development, notably identity development (Erikson, 1968), moral development (Kohlberg, 1975), and cognitive development (Elkind, 1974, 1978; Feuerstein, 1979, 1980; Inhelder and Piaget, 1958). From these stage theories in particular, information on adolescents has been extrapolated by speech-language pathologists.

For this reason, these theories will be discussed in greater depth than preceding theories.

General Development Stage Theories

According to Muuss (1975), Gesell's theory of adolescence (Gesell et al., 1956) drew heavily from his general theory of recapitulation. Gesell's theory incorporated the concept that developmental trends and behavioral traits are biologically determined. The environment can only stimulate, modify, and support growth; it cannot sequence it. Gesell was mainly interested in studying overt behaviors as they are manifested in gradual stages or cycles of development. He studied both mental and physical growth from a normative, descriptive, and chronological age perspective.

Gesell explained that his sequential patterns of development oscillate along a spiral course toward maturity: The child begins to master a skill, then reverts to earlier forms of behavior, and then may plateau before totally mastering the new skill and moving forward.

Gesell considered adolescence to be a transitional period from childhood to adulthood. The adolescent period begins at approximately 11 years and ends in the early 20s, although he believes that girls go through this period more rapidly than boys and that the most important changes occur in the first five years of adolescence. Gesell et al. (1956) described the specific aspects of adolescence through a series of maturity profiles at each age level.

Gesell, unlike Hall (1904), did not see adolescence as a time of "storm and stress," but as a process of enrichment with some inconsistencies. Although Gesell stated that the chronological ages used are only approximates, his tables of averages are frequently criticized. His critics believe that these tables do not take into account the diversity and variability in human behavior and development. Also, the subjects used to derive the behavioral characteristics at each age level were from one geographical area and from a high-average to a superior intellectual population.

Mitchell (1979), who is not a theorist per se, advocated that adolescence covers too many years and too much growth to be considered one developmental period. Instead, Mitchell subdivided adolescence into three stages: the early or child-adolescence stage, the middle or adolescence stage, and the late or adult-adolescence stage. He emphasized that the differences between early and late adolescence are profound and that professionals should treat these differences with more respect. Mitchell used chronological age clusters for each stage, but emphasized the overlap between the upper limits of one age group and the lower limits of the next. He did this to indicate that general age clusters are more important than rigid chronological years. The major characteristics in each of the three stages of adolescence are as follows:

Stage I—
Early or Child Adolescence

Chronological ages for Stage I are 12, 13, and 14 years for boys and 11, 12, and 13 years for girls. This stage is dominated more than the other stages by body growth spurts in height and weight and in primary and secondary sex characteristics. As a result of rapid body growth, the psychological response of the adolescent is one of concern about how the body looks and feels. These individuals are childlike and limited in their emotional range. Of the three stages, this is the time the adolescent is the most egocentric. Socially, the peer group exerts influence, but the home and family still remain the most important social and emotional factors in the adolescent's life. Moral outlook is at the conventional level (Kohlberg, 1975). (The conventional level is explained in the section entitled "Moral Stage Theory" on page 30.) The future carries less importance during this stage than it does during the next two stages.

Stage II—
Middle Adolescence or Adolescence

This stage most closely resembles the typical image of adolescents. Mitchell maintains that the individual in this stage is neither a child nor an adult. Chronological ages for both boys and girls in this stage include 13, 14, and 15 years. Physical growth continues, but not at as rapid a pace as during early adolescence. Mental growth increases dramatically: It is now more abstract, theoretical, and idealistic. Because of the mental growth factor, the person shows more awareness of the outside world, engages in introspection, and experiences an increase in self-doubt. Along with introspection, idealism is tested. The person is more interested in the opposite sex, and dating is more common than during early adolescence. The individual's social life is primarily with peers. This is the time in which Erikson's (1968) psychosocial moratorium, part of his "identity development stage theory" (explained in the next section), is most likely to take place.

Stage III—
Late or Adult Adolescence

The ages for both boys and girls in this stage are 16, 17, and 18 years. Physically and mentally, these individuals are adults and have achieved most of their adult growth. However, in terms of their social roles, they remain primarily adolescents. In Western society, Stage III is more a social phenomenon than a biological fact. During this stage, sexual intimacy increases and the person is more capable of dealing with interpersonal complexities. In addition, the individual becomes increasingly concerned about the future.

Identity Development Stage Theory

Erikson (1968) studied with Sigmund and Anna Freud and was influenced by their psychoanalytic training. However, his theory of identity development went beyond their theories by encompassing socialization. The main concept in Erikson's theory was the acquisition of an ego-identity, and the most important characteristic of adolescence was identity crisis. Erikson (1968) maintained that the adolescent must search out an identity by asking, "Who am I?" Identity, then, is not given by society, nor is it a maturational phenomenon.

Identity can be found only through interaction with, and feedback from, other people. Under this theory, peer group conformity is a means of testing roles. Erikson also noted that pubescence is a time of rapid body changes; hence the identity crisis is partly the result of psychophysiological factors. Erickson believed that personal identity is achieved during adolescence through acceptance of the past, integration of the present, and orientation toward the future in terms of a decision about a career.

Another phenomenon occurring during adolescence is that of a psychosocial moratorium, or an "as if" period when the adolescent can try on different roles as if not fully committed and accountable. Experimentation with various roles in life can occur without penalty. The moratorium is an essential prerequisite for identity achievement, Erickson maintains.

An individual influenced by Erikson's (1968) work on identity development was James Marcia. According to Miller (1989), Marcia (1980) expanded two of Erikson's notions: crisis and commitment. Marcia defined crisis as those times during adolescence when the individual is actively involved in choosing among alternative occupations and beliefs. Commitment is the degree of personal investment the individual expresses in an occupation or belief. The presence or absence of crisis or commitment results in one of the four potential "identity statuses" (Miller, 1989):

1. *Identity diffused*—These types of adolescents have not experienced an identity crisis or commitment. They are easily influenced by others and they change from one belief or behavior to another in rapid succession. Often their self-esteem fluctuates rapidly from low to high, depending on how others react to them.

2. *Foreclosure*—These are adolescents who have made commitments without experiencing an identity crisis. The person has a set of consistent beliefs and goals.

These beliefs, attitudes, and knowledge of occupations usually come from others and have been accepted without question. They usually are people who over-identify with and conform to their peer group or parents.

3. *Moratorium*—These adolescents are usually in a severe state of identity crisis but cannot yet make a commitment. They may make several tentative commitments and thus explore occupational alternatives.

4. *Identity achieved*—These are adolescents who have experienced an identity crisis and resolved it by making personal commitments. This level of identity development results in a synthesis of one's past, present, and future. It "involves self-acceptance, ego strength, and the ability to achieve heterosexual intimacy" (Miller, 1989, p. 24).

These four identity statuses appear to form a developmental sequence; however, the only actual sequence is that *moratorium* must be experienced before *identity achieved*. The first three identity statuses are normal phases of adolescence and only become a problem if they extend into adulthood. It should be noted that some people do not develop through all four phases. Also, some people may experience all four phases in some aspects of their lives but not in other areas.

Cognitive Stage Theories

Piaget's theory of cognitive development (Piaget, 1970) has two interrelated aspects: a description of the four periods of development (sensorimotor, preoperational, concrete operational, and formal operational) and an explanation of concepts such as *assimilation, accommodation,* and *equilibrium,* which are as applicable to the formal operational period as to the sensorimotor period.

The formal operational period is the most relevant to adolescence. According to Inhelder and Piaget (1958), this period has two stages: IIIA (approximately ages 11 or 12 to 14 or 15 years) and IIIB (approximately ages 14 or 15 years and upward). Stage IIIA appears to be a preparatory stage in which the adolescent can handle some formal operations, but in a cumbersome way, and with systematic, rigorous proof. However, in Stage IIIB the adolescent is capable of performing formal operational tasks in a spontaneous, systematic, rigorous way. Some of the characteristics of adolescents in the formal period are that they can reason on the basis of verbal propositions, leave the world of reality behind and enter the world of ideas, and think about their thinking.

The formal operational period is characterized by propositional and combinatorial operations: (1) combining by conjunction (i.e., both A and B make a difference); (2) combining by disjunction (i.e., it has to be this or that); (3) combining by implications (i.e., when this happens, then that happens); and (4) combining by incompatibility (i.e., when this happens, then that does not) (Inhelder and Piaget, 1958).

A second set of formal groupings, in the propositional logic of the adolescent, is the INCR group. Each of the four letters stands for one of the logical transformations that can be performed on a propositional operation (Inhelder and Piaget, 1958): I=identity trans-

formation, in which the original proposition retains its identity; N=negation transformation, in which everything in a given proposition is changed into the opposite of the original proposition; R=reciprocal transformation, in which one factor in a proposition compensates for another (e.g., the student sees the relationships among rods of various lengths and weights and how much they will bend); and C=correlative transformation, in which conjunction is changed to disjunction, and vice versa, but leaves everything else unchanged.

David Elkind (1974, 1978) has written extensively on children and adolescents and has done much to popularize Inhelder and Piaget's (1958) theory in the United States. He has described two developmental phenomena that emerge at adolescence as a result of higher levels of thinking. One is the imaginary audience. Adolescents, with their newly acquired skill of thinking about what others are thinking of them, act as though they are constantly on stage performing for everyone. The imaginary audience phenomenon is a new form of egocentrism through which adolescents must pass.

The second phenomenon is the personal fable, which maintains adolescents think that they are not like other people. Others might die in a car accident, but they could not; nothing bad could happen to them. Elkind's ideas supplement, rather that supplant, Inhelder and Piaget's theory of cognitive development.

Feuerstein (1980), who worked with Piaget, has made a significant contribution to adolescents with learning problems. His theory of cognitive modifiability holds that the human organism, even one judged to be severely impaired, is capable of change at any age. This is true even if adolescents had inadequate development earlier in life or were exposed to conditions typically considered as barriers to change. Some of these barriers are exogenic (e.g., poverty, lack of stimulation at early ages), and others are endogenic (e.g., genetic defects, sensory impairments).

Cognitive modifiability results from direct exposure to stimuli and mediated learning experiences. However, while direct exposure to stimuli may explain some learning, it does not explain the diversity of learning that occurs within different individuals given the same situation. People who have the same biological parents and similar environmental stimuli turn out to be very different individuals. According to Feuerstein, differences in mediated learning experiences are the primary way to explain this phenomenon.

In a mediated learning experience, an adult selects and organizes stimuli for the youth. An experience becomes mediated when there is an intention on the part of the adult to focus on an experience and to transmit the meaning of the object or event. An attempt to generalize the learning should occur. The adult needs to think continually, "How can I make the adolescent acquire alone what I now need to facilitate?" The cognitive structure of the individual is affected through this process of mediation, and as learning sets are acquired, the capacity to become modified through direct exposure to stimuli increases in efficiency.

According to Feuerstein (1980), the more and the earlier that children are subjected to mediated learning experiences, the greater will be their capacity to be affected by and to learn from direct exposure to stimuli. Normal adolescents have had consistent mediated learning experiences, according to Feuerstein, and have benefited from direct exposure to stimuli. In essence, they have learned how to continue learning on their own. Feuerstein's theory maintained that when barriers obstruct learning, they can be overcome or bypassed, thus making it possible to restore a normal pattern of cognitive growth during adolescence.

Like Piaget and Elkind, Selman (1980) views the development of social cognition as movement through an invariant sequence of stages of perspective taking (Miller, 1989). The sequence of stages is as follows:

- Differentiate the self from others while confusing the psychological and physical aspects of the social world (Level 0).

- Differentiate the social perspectives of the self and others (Level 1).

- Coordinate the two viewpoints (self and others) by reflecting on one's own thoughts and feelings from another's perspective (Level 2).

In summary, "the child knows that people are aware of each other's perspectives and are evaluating these perspectives" (Miller, 1989, p. 36). During preadolescence (roughly 10 to 12 years), the child realizes "that reciprocal perspectives can form an infinite chain" (Miller, 1989, p. 36). Preadolescents can remove themselves from an interaction and view it objectively while simultaneously coordinating the perspectives of each individual. During adolescence, the individual comes to realize various levels of mutuality between people, for example, a superficial level, common interest level, or in-depth feeling level. It should be noted that "the development of formal operations is necessary (but not sufficient) for this most advanced level of interpersonal understanding, and some adults never reach it" (Miller, 1989, p. 36).

In summary, Selman's (1980) theoretical model is a social cognitive one, which maintains:

> People develop an underlying cognitive structure or set of cognitive skills that allow them (1) to infer what other people are thinking, feeling, intending, and seeing and what they are like as a person . . . and (2) to understand social relationships or social institutions. (Miller, 1989, p. 39)

Piaget, Elkind, and Selman all focus on the development of the cognitive structures underlying the understanding of the self within a context of human relationships.

Moral Stage Theory

Kohlberg's (1975) theory of moral development was greatly influenced by Piaget's (1970) cognitive development approach. Kohlberg advanced three levels of moral development: the preconventional or premoral level, the conventional or moral level, and the postconventional or autonomous level. Each level is divided into two stages. The conventional level is where most adolescents and many adults function. At this level, the person conforms to authority and obeys laws and social rules.

Kohlberg's (1975) theory of moral development incorporated the following principles:

Moral stages form an invariant sequence of development, and moral development can terminate at any stage. Kohlberg maintained that the advancement through the stages of moral reasoning depends upon the interplay of three factors: cognitive developmental level, ability to empathize, and cognitive disequilibrium. He also maintained that these stages are universal and cut across cultures and socioeconomic levels.

Kohlberg's theory has been criticized by several of his colleagues. Siegal (1980) questioned the invariant sequence of the early stages and the methodology that posed moral dilemmas outside the subjects' personal experiences. Gilligan (1982) criticized Kohlberg's theory for failing to consider differences in stages of moral development between boys and girls during early adolescence. In Gilligan's research, young girls have not adhered to the stages postulated by Kohlberg.

Educational/Clinical Implications

The psychological theories are extremely diverse and therefore will be discussed as to their educational/clinical implications in the following categories: psychoanalytic theory, field theory, social learning theory, and stage theory. A psychoanalytical theory takes the position that

> educators can help by not making rules or expectations more frustrating than necessary and by discouraging heavy reliance on defense mechanisms. Educators also can look beyond a problem behavior to the underlying psychological conflict and encourage teenagers

to talk about and try to understand their feelings. (Miller, 1989, pp. 20–21)

According to field theory, educators should be concerned about environmental factors, such as high school class size and number of school clubs available, that affect students' behavior. Social learning theory maintains that educators need to recognize that behaviors are learned by watching others or having one's behavior reinforced by others. Thus, educators are important role models who can influence and shape adolescents' behavior.

According to stage theory, educators need to be aware of the developmental level of the adolescent and not skip over stages but realize one stage serves as the foundation for the next level of development. Curriculum and other school activities are designed and implemented in a developmental hierarchy.

One of the major thrusts of cognitive stage theorists is that educators should look at events and situations from the adolescent's point of view. Educators need to assess whether the adolescent is cognitively ready to learn a new concept. Materials must be at appropriate levels. Adolescents need to be actively involved in the learning process, manipulating materials and ideas. As adolescents develop more advanced thinking skills, they are ready to develop a more advanced moral philosophy (Miller, 1989). Educators need to be aware of the interaction between thinking skills and moral development and choices. The adolescent is creating a value system from which to operate on a daily basis.

SUMMARY OF THEORIES OF ADOLESCENCE

This section summarizes the viewpoints of major contributors to the theoretical positions on adolescent development. With this summary, professionals should better understand how these theoretical positions have influenced, historically and currently, the concept of normal adolescence.

Muuss (1975) compared and contrasted the various theoretical positions. He noted disagreements in definitions, characteristics, and general patterns of adolescent development among the different theories. However, once the older and more extreme theoretical positions are eliminated, agreement does exist.

All theorists agree on the existence of endocrinological changes during early adolescence and on behavioral changes due to an increase in sexual interests, awarenesses, and tensions. They disagree on the amount of importance placed on the endocrine changes, and on the extent to which the behavioral changes are caused by physiological or sociological events.

Most theorists discuss physiological changes that result in the individual's need to adjust to a new body image, and they view adolescence as a transitional period. The exceptions are those social learning theorists who view human development as a continuous process. A few theorists agree that adolescence is a multistage period of development, but they disagree as to the number, characteristics, and psychological meaning of each of the stages. Lipsitz (1980) stated that all theories of adolescence emphasize physical growth, sexual maturation, increased autonomy, and cognitive sophistication. The various theoretical positions collectively postulate that adolescence is a time of rapid physiological and psychological changes influenced by sociocultural determinants.

COPING WITH DIFFERENT THEORIES

When confronted with varying theoretical perspectives, a professional might select one of the following options.

Ignore all theories—This option has been advocated by some professionals who believe theories are too impractical, abstract, and obtuse to be of any clinical value. Perhaps this attitude is responsible for the lack of a theoretical framework in many tests and educational materials. For example, when critiquing standardized tests and commercial intervention programs used with adolescents, we discovered how frequently professionals either do not state, or do not have, a theoretical model on which they base their test or program. However, stating the theory or theories upon which a test or program is developed is essential for providing a rationale as to why it is being used. Knowles (1973) states the following:

> There is a cliche in the applied social sciences, often attributed to Kurt Lewin, that nothing is as practical as a good theory to enable you to make choices confidently and consistently, and to explain or defend why you are making the choices you make. (p. 93)

Select one theory—Another option is to conclude that one theory is the most appropriate, regardless of any conflicting evidence. Picking one theory may be initially advantageous in that it might minimize confusion. The disadvantage is that this option reflects a rigid position and may be erroneous, thus resulting in negative consequences. The state of the art is such that concepts, assumptions, and hypotheses about adolescents are constantly changing; therefore, a single theoretical position may result in a narrow perspective of the problem and the assessment and intervention procedures.

Select one theory for research and another for clinical application—This option is selected by professionals who view research and clinical application as opposing or mutually exclusive entities. Individuals are seen not as whole people, but as fragments to be either investigated or treated. Selecting one theory for research and another for clinical application creates false dichotomies within a discipline. This results in researchers and clinicians failing to communicate and work cooperatively for the benefit of the person with a communication disorder.

Select precepts from a variety of theories and develop a more comprehensive, synthesized perspective—Currently, no one theory exists to account for the wide array of adolescent behaviors that require the speech-language pathologist's assessment and intervention. For example, cognitive functions of adolescents may be accounted for by one theory, while syntactic and semantic features may be accounted for by other theories.

Although selecting precepts from a variety of theories may prove to be time consuming, this alternative may ultimately prove to be the most effective. The selection of precepts, when thought through carefully, avoids a superficial eclecticism. If professionals select this option of incorporating features from a variety of prevailing theories into a unified whole, they must do so in a systematic fashion to guarantee compatibility and consistency among the various theoretical constructs. For example, according to Lipsitz (1980), one of the problems of categorizing adolescence into a biological, anthropological, or sociological camp is that there is little dialogue among these disciplines. Each theoretical position is insufficient by itself, but each may be necessary when developing a comprehensive theoretical perspective of adolescence.

In conclusion, nothing is as practical as a good theory to provide a rationale as to why professionals are doing what they are doing. If professionals do not spend the necessary time building a theoretical perspective into research and clinical services, the result will be a confusing, invalid, and unreliable database.

OUR THEORETICAL POSITION

We chose the last option above (i.e., to "select precepts from a variety of theories and develop a more comprehensive, synthesized perspective") when developing the theoretical base for this text. No one theoretical position adequately explains what we believe about adolescents.

Our theory of adolescence holds that both biological and environmental factors influence adolescent development, although environmental factors may be stronger. This viewpoint

has been influenced by Feuerstein (1980), who has documented bringing some individuals to near normal levels of functioning, despite negatively loaded genetics, by bombarding them with mediated learning experiences.

Adolescence involves unique and genetically predetermined bodily changes (e.g., puberty) to which the American culture has had different responses across racial and socioeconomic stratas. For example, in some lower and middle socioeconomic strata, adolescence marks the time when children are expected to contribute significantly to family finances by getting a job or working in the family business; in some middle and higher socioeconomic strata, adolescents are not expected to work, but rather are sent away to private high schools to better prepare themselves for future careers. These responses constantly change as new generations of adults seek to improve their communication with adolescents.

We view the life cycle as a series of developmental phases of which adolescence is one period. To us, adolescence is no more "transitional" than are the periods from infancy to toddlerhood to childhood. It can be said that any period of time in human development is transitional (Sheehy, 1981). Furthermore, we concur with Muuss (1975), who has argued that adolescence manifests both continuous and stagelike patterns. Adolescence is continuous (i.e., part of a continuum from infancy to adulthood), but there are stages within the adolescent period (i.e., early, middle, and late).

We also question whether adolescence is filled with more stresses than other developmental periods. We believe that adolescence is a major developmental period within the life cycle, filled with its own unique challenges and stressful moments.

We concur with Mitchell (1979) that adolescence is an extended time period encompassing several stages. We believe that speech-language pathologists should be guided in their assessment and intervention decisions by a student's stage of adolescence (i.e., Stage I—early; Stage II—middle; Stage III—late). We also extrapolate from the psychological theories of Inhelder and Piaget (1958) and Feuerstein (1980) when making decisions about cognitive functioning of adolescents. This cognitive functioning in turn influences intervention procedures. Adolescents at lower cognitive levels will probably need more concrete, hands-on activities; adolescents at higher levels may participate in communication activities requiring abstract reasoning.

Finally, we have observed that the physical development of adolescents influences their psychosocial development and, in turn, these two domains impact upon communication development. It would be artificial to assume that only biological or only environmental factors affect the adolescent's overall development. Rather, a combination of developmental factors, both biological and environmental, occur simultaneously. These developmental milestones are highlighted in the next chapter.

SUMMARY

This chapter presented information on theories of adolescence. The four major theoretical positions concerning adolescence (biological, anthropological, sociological, and psychological) have each contributed to how adolescents are viewed today. A rationale was presented for why knowledge of theories is important, as well as the theoretical framework to which we, the authors, subscribe.

DISCUSSION QUESTIONS

1. How does your own comprehensive theory of adolescence interact with your theory(s) of cognition, language, and communication development?

2. What relevance do the various theoretical educational/clinical implications have upon the older student's communication behaviors?

SUGGESTED READINGS

Muuss, R. (1975). *Theories of adolescence.* New York: Random House.

Miller, P. (1989). Theories of adolescent development. In J. Worell and F. Danner (Eds.), *The adolescent as decision-maker: Applications to development and education* (pp. 13–49). San Diego, CA: Academic Press.

DEVELOPMENTAL MILESTONES IN OLDER STUDENTS

3

GOALS:

To summarize information on normal physical and psychological development

To compare early and later language development

To describe normal language development during preadolescence and adolescence

PHYSICAL DEVELOPMENT

Adolescence is a time when children experience drastic physical changes (Hamburg, 1992). Early adolescence involves a more rapid period of growth than any other period in life, including infancy and early childhood (Lipsitz, 1979). These rapid bodily changes have a profound effect on how adolescents perceive themselves and communicate with others.

Professionals working with adolescents need to be cognizant of how preoccupied adolescents can be with their own bodily changes. For example, the adolescent who is late in making bodily changes (described later in this section) may feel very uncomfortable being grouped with peers who have already begun those changes. Adolescents, desiring peer conformity, do not easily tolerate noticeable developmental differences. The adolescent with an obvious physical disability, delayed development, or accelerated development is often at a disadvantage when it comes to peer acceptance and peer popularity. While the differences in physical development during adolescence may not seem important to adults, those differences may be of singular importance to some adolescents.

Failure by professionals to recognize the impact of physical development can undermine attempts to communicate with adolescents. Professionals need to empathize with the growing pains of adolescence.

During adolescence, pronounced bodily changes take place because of the presence of testosterone in males and estrogen in females. This time of rapid biological growth, which gives way to the first indications of sexual maturity, is known as puberty (Turner and Helms, 1979). Puberty now begins earlier than it used to, probably because of better nutrition and fewer serious infections (Hamburg, 1992). For example, in the United States, the onset of menstruation now occurs, on average, at 12½ years, whereas 150 years ago it occurred at 16 years of age (Hamburg, 1992). Reproductively mature youth now spend years in childlike roles, thus extending the transition period we call "adolescence." Therefore, today's adolescents undergo their transition from childhood to adulthood under circumstances unique in the long history of our species (Hamburg, 1992).

Certainly the age range for the onset of puberty varies. One only needs to observe an eighth or ninth grade class to realize the physical variability among the students. According to Papalia and Olds (1975), "the normal age range for puberty is ten to sixteen years for girls, with an average age of twelve, and twelve to eighteen years for boys, with an average age of fourteen" (p. 554). While individual variability is normal, the sequence of pubertal events is similar. The trend is toward adolescents being slightly taller and heavier than their parents and females experiencing menarche 10 months earlier than their mothers. This trend is probably influenced by a higher standard of living today than a century ago (Papalia and Olds, 1975).

In particular, the adolescent growth spurt is characterized by a sharp increase in height—in girls, usually between 11 and 13 years, and in boys, between 13 and 15 years (Papalia and Olds, 1975). Weight follows a similar curve, but this data may not be as informative, because weight reflects a combination of developmental events such as skeletal growth, increased muscle and fat tissue, and size of various organs (Conger, 1973). Almost all skeletal and muscular dimensions are growing, but not to an equal degree, with greater changes in males than in females (Tanner, 1974).

Differences in body composition between the sexes (sexual dimorphism) are evident prior to adolescence, even during fetal development. However, some of the most notable differences arise during adolescence: the male's greater height and shoulder width, and the female's wider hips (Tanner, 1974). Adolescent males show a decrease in adipose mass as a percentage of body weight, whereas females do not lose any fat, but show a slower accumulation (Adams, 1980).

The adolescent body also undergoes changes in primary and secondary sex characteristics. Primary sex characteristics involve those physiological features related to the sex organs (Turner and Helms, 1979); secondary sex characteristics serve to distinguish mature males from mature females. Hair growth is one of the obvious secondary sex characteristics of adolescence. Papalia and Olds (1975) state that one of the meanings of the Latin word *pubescere* is "to grow hairy." Other secondary sex characteristics are breast development and increased width and depth of the pelvis in females, and voice changes in males. Voice changes in both males and females are characterized by a lowering of fundamental frequency.

Epstein (1974, 1978) studied brain growth stages and concluded that the first four stages of brain growth (i.e., 3 to 10 months, 2 to 4 years, 6 to 8 years, and 10 to 12 years) coincide with mental growth (i.e., Piaget's four periods of cognitive development). Epstein hypothesized a fifth stage of brain growth (i.e., 14 to 16-plus years) that has no identifiable counterpart in Piaget's periods of cognitive development. Arlin (1975) investigated this notion and reported that such a cognitive period does exist, having its onset in the 14- to 16-year-old period.

Epstein (1974, 1978) suggested that brain growth data may reveal why some children fail to learn in certain intervention programs such as Head Start: the 4- to 6-year age period is one of minimal brain and cognitive growth. Therefore, for biological reasons, the results of intervention do not indicate improved intellectual functioning for children in those programs. Epstein and Toepfer (1978) also speculated that the adjustment problems and the social and educational difficulties of junior high students may be tied to a brain-related growth plateau. These difficulties have been commonly blamed on sexual maturation.

In summary, a discussion of adolescent physical development is incomplete without acknowledging its interaction with psychological development. Adolescents appear to be self-conscious about their bodily changes whether they mature early or late. Generally, those who mature early are found to be more adept in overall social adjustments than those who mature late (Turner and Helms, 1979). Boys

appear to be more affected by the timing of maturation than girls (Papalia and Olds, 1975).

PSYCHOLOGICAL DEVELOPMENT

DEVELOPMENTAL TASKS

Preadolescents and adolescents face a specific set of developmental tasks as they approach maturity. According to Miller (1989), some of these tasks begin during childhood and continue into adolescence, whereas others are primarily a concern of adolescence. Each developmental task involves some degree of problem solving and personal decision making. The developmental tasks are these (Miller, 1989):

1. Develop a sense of self-identity that is a unique combination of values, attitudes, beliefs, and behaviors.

2. Adapt to a physically changing body, as well as make psychological adjustments, including gender identity.

3. Develop a more abstract thought process about the physical world as well as the social world of people, events, and social structures.

4. Acquire interpersonal skills that will allow the adolescent to build strong relationships with people of the same and opposite sex.

5. Establish a new relationship with one's family members that is the result of

needing autonomy and having less emotional dependence while still needing psychological and financial support.

6. Formulate a personal value system that guides decision making and interpersonal interactions.

7. Set goals for future achievement in terms of education, career, marriage, etc.

Obviously, these tasks are interrelated and not mutually exclusive. Progress in one task results in progress in another. For example, cognitive development will assist in moral development and thus the building of a value system that will be applied to various aspects of one's life.

STAGES

Mitchell (1979) noted that adolescents should be viewed in terms of early, middle, and late stages of adolescence. We concur with this point of view. Table 3.1 presents the characteristics of stages and tasks of normal adolescence from the perspective of early, middle, and late stages of adolescent development and the approximate age of emergence.

Four developmental tasks are also presented in Table 3.1. They are stated more succinctly than those just presented from Miller (1989) and include (1) acceptance of the physical changes of puberty, (2) attainment of independence, (3) emergence of a stable identity, and (4) development of cognitive patterns (Adams, Montemayor, and Gullotta, 1989).

SELF-CONCEPT AND SELF-ESTEEM

Self-concept refers to the attributes that the individual believes characterize himself or herself; *self-esteem* refers to the evaluative notions one holds about oneself (i.e., "Who am I?" versus "How do I feel about myself?") (Suls, 1989).

Rosenberg (1986) noted that self-concept in older students shifts from an emphasis on the social exterior to psychological elements. When Montemeyer and Eisen (1977) asked youth in grades 4, 6, 8, 10, and 12 to answer "Who am I?" in 20 words or less, the younger subjects identified themselves in these categories: possessions, physical self-body image, and territoriality (where they lived). In contrast, older subjects (grades 10 and 12) described themselves in terms of internal beliefs and standards and stable personality traits. These changes in self-concept are gradual rather than abrupt (Suls, 1989).

Self-esteem can be treated as a global concept (i.e., the overall evaluation of oneself either in positive or negative terms) and/or as a domain-specific concept (i.e., one's perceived worth academically, socially, athletically, etc.). Children show relative stability in global self-esteem between ages 8 and 11, lowered scores between 12 and 14, and a rise again from ages 15 to 18 (Harter and Connell, 1984; Rosenberg, 1979). Self-esteem continues to rise during the five years post-high school (ages 18 to 23) as well (O'Malley and Bachman, 1983).

In discussing the dip in self-esteem during early adolescence, Suls (1989) concluded that the transition from elementary to junior high

TABLE 3.1			
CHARACTERISTICS OF STAGES AND TASKS OF NORMAL ADOLESCENCE			
	STAGE OF ADOLESCENCE		
TASK	**EARLY (10–14)**	**MIDDLE (14–16)**	**LATE (16–20)**
Acceptance of the Physical Changes of Puberty	• Physical changes occur rapidly but with wide person-to-person variability. • Self-consciousness, insecurity, and worry about being different from peers.	• Pubertal changes almost complete for girls; boys still undergoing physical changes. • Girls more confident; boys more awkward.	• Adult appearance, comfortable with physical changes. • Physical strength continues to increase, especially for males.
Attainment of Independence	• Changes of puberty distinguish early adolescents from children, but do not provide independence. • Ambivalence (childhood dependency unattractive, but unprepared for the independence of adulthood) leads to vacillation between parents and peers for support.	• Ability to work, drive, date; appear more mature; dependency lessens and peer bonds increase. • Conflict with authority, limit testing, experimental and risk-taking behaviors at a maximum.	• Independence a realistic social expectation. • Continuing education, becoming employed, getting married—all possibilities that often lead to ambivalence about independence.
Emergence of a Stable Identity	• Am I OK? Am I normal? • How do I fit into my peer group? • Paradoxical loss of identity in becoming a member of a peer group.	• Who am I? • How am I different from other people? • What makes me special or unique?	• Who am I in relation to other people? • What is my role with respect to education, work, sexuality, community, religion, and family?
Development of Cognitive Patterns	• Concrete operational thought: present more real than future, concrete more real than abstract. • Egocentrism. • Personal fable. • Imaginary audience.	• Emerging formal operations: abstractions, hypotheses, and thinking about future personal interests and emerging identity.	• Formal operations: thinking about the future, things as they should be, options, consequences can be considered.

school is a time of uncertainty, particularly for girls, as they "sort out" their position in a new school. As an aside, Simmons, Blyth, Van Cleave, and Bush (1979), when studying children in a K–8 school, found no decrease in self-esteem when the shift from sixth to seventh grade did not involve a change in schools. This finding has major implications for how schools are structured for preadolescents and adolescents and for how transitions are orchestrated. (Chapter 8 will address these transitions further.)

LANGUAGE DEVELOPMENT

And we . . . like we found this really like awesome CD and we . . . um . . . we decided to play it and um. . . . Jeremy's mom come in and she was SO mad, like she was yelling and screaming at us. And all we did was play her CD!

Is this normal language, or is it disordered? For the particular adolescent quoted, the language was determined to be normal. Knowledge of language development is crucial to making this determination.

Professionals skilled in language assessment and intervention with adolescents are often called upon to sort out what's "normal" and what's not. At first glance, normal adolescent language may appear disordered from an adult perspective. Astute professionals observe large numbers of adolescents in a variety of situations to develop awareness and knowledge of what's "normal" in the

fluctuating language world of youth. They also amass information on later language development. In the past decade, a considerable amount of research has documented semantic, syntactic, and pragmatic aspects of normal and disordered language.

The linguistic development that occurs during preadolescence and adolescence is much more subtle than the rapid language acquisition during early childhood (Nippold, 1988a). From ages 9 to 19, language development unfolds in a slow and protracted manner, and changes become obvious only when nonadjacent age groups are compared and sophisticated linguistic phenomena are studied (Nippold, 1988a). Increasing individualism in language development (as a result of variability in course work, extracurricular activities, and social contacts) also makes it difficult for researchers to establish guidelines for "normal" linguistic performance in preadolescents and adolescents (Kamhi and Lee, 1988; Nippold, 1988a).

Major contrasts between early language learning and later language development include these (Nippold, 1988a):

- The major language goal for young children is to acquire spoken language. The major language goal for school-age students is to acquire written communication skills.

- The primary source of language stimulation for young children is spoken communication. For preadolescents and adolescents, both spoken and written communication forms are significant sources of language stimulation.

- Young children learn language in nondirected, informal settings. Older children and adolescents learn a great amount of language through formal instruction.

- Language development in younger children does not require metalinguistic competency. Metalinguistic competency is required for language development in older children and adolescents, especially as they learn to read and write (Grunwell, 1986).

- Young children are literal in their interpretations of language. Older children demonstrate increasing ability to appreciate figurative meanings.

- Young children's language and reasoning are concrete. Preadolescents and adolescents are learning language and acquiring reasoning processes that are abstract.

- Young children do not always take the perspective of others when communicating. Preadolescents and adolescents are more aware of listeners' and readers' needs and adjust their spoken and written messages accordingly.

The remainder of this chapter provides empirical data on normal language during adolescence. Definitions of various language components are provided. Cognition is also discussed because of its integral link with language. This information should provide professionals with considerable knowledge about adolescent communication development.

COGNITION

Cognition is the mental organization of experience. Cognition subsumes thinking, which is the application of cognition for a purpose, such as reasoning, judging, analyzing, recalling, inferring, imagining, problem solving, and so forth. Labels such as *propositional thinking, reflective thinking,* and *abstract thinking* have emerged in the literature.

Metacognition involves knowing what one knows, and what needs to be known, to achieve a goal (Wallach and Miller, 1988); it refers to a collection of means by which individuals assess the successes and failures of their problem-solving strategies (Flavell, 1976, 1977).

We recommend the use of the term *thinking,* rather than *cognition,* with preadolescents and adolescents because *thinking* is a term with which they are familiar. *Think about your thinking* might also be used instead of *metacognition.*

The relationship of language and cognition is open to debate. Rice (1983) provided a summary of the range of hypotheses about the relationship between cognition and language to which professionals might ascribe:

1. *Strong cognition hypothesis*—Cognition precedes and accounts for language acquisition.

2. *Local homologies hypothesis*—Simultaneous emergence of parallel cognitive and linguistic knowledge.

3. *Interaction hypothesis*—Language and cognition mutually influence each other's development.

4. *Cognition-anchored-in-language hypothesis*—Concepts are unstable until anchored with linguistic forms.

5. *Weak cognition hypothesis*—Cognition does not account for all language development.

6. *Mental-processes-not-rooted-in-meanings hypothesis*—Language disorders are associated with perceptual processing and/or memory problems.

Theorists supporting these different hypotheses have cited varying levels of linguistic competence and varying kinds of linguistic phenomena. The hypotheses that emphasize the strength of cognition focus on the earlier stages of language acquisition. Those hypotheses that emphasize linguistic influence tend to be based on later stages. In essence, the cognition and language relationship may vary as a function of age, type of cognitive task, and linguistic ability (Rice, 1983; Schlesinger, 1977). Of the six primary possibilities, our stance centers around the interaction hypothesis.

Preadolescents and adolescents experience significant cognitive and metacognitive changes. To describe these changes, developmental theorists have taken two general approaches—the Piagetian approach and the information processing approach (Kamhi and Lee, 1988). Both approaches describe cognitive development marked by quantitative and qualitative changes.

Piagetian Approach

An abundance of research studies, journal articles, and book chapters have debated the existence of Piaget's formal operational thought during adolescence, as well as who engages in such thinking, when, and under what experimental conditions (Berzonsky, 1978; Broughton, 1977; Elkind, 1975; Ellsworth and Sindt, 1991; Hains and Miller, 1980; Kamhi and Lee, 1988; Lawson and Wollman, 1976; Leadbeater and Dionne, 1981; Martorano, 1977; Neimark, 1979; Overton and Meehan, 1982). Formal operational thought includes the ability to reason systematically and logically about abstract ideas, which may have no basis in reality. Several studies found that adolescents apply formal operational thought in some contexts but not in others (Bart, 1971; Martorano, 1977). For example, formal operational thought may be applied in English literature but not in chemistry. Some researchers found that the transition from concrete to formal operational thought may never be complete across all content areas and that as many as half of the adults in the United States either do not engage in formal operational thought, or do so only in their field of expertise (Labinowicz, 1980; Lawson and Wollman, 1976).

On traditional Piagetian tasks requiring application of formal operational thought, Elkind (1975) found that adolescent boys consistently outperform girls. However, he found that adolescent girls are more likely to apply their formal operational thinking to interpersonal matters, perhaps for social role reasons. Adolescents of average intellectual ability probably attain formal operations but do not apply them equally to all aspects of reality (Elkind, 1975). Martorano (1977), in her research, found that mean scores on formal operational tasks completed by girls increased consistently during grades 6 through 12.

Formal operational thinking begins to emerge between 12 and 15 years, although not even the oldest age group tested showed formal operational performance across all tasks. Other researchers found no sex differences when formal operational tasks were attempted (Jackson, 1965; Killian, 1979; Kishta, 1979). Overton and Meehan (1982) found that *learned helplessness*, the perception of a lack of control over response outcomes, combined with feminine sex roles, resulted in inconsistent formal operational deficits. However, with most problems presented during their research, no sex differences were found. Hains and Miller (1980) found steady cognitive growth for normal adolescents but a lack of such growth in delinquent youth.

Thus, while research on attaining formal operational thought would indicate that most adolescents achieve hypothetic-deductive reasoning in some situations, in a few individuals and in some settings, abstract thinking does not occur. Empirical research would indicate that to expect formal operational thought to occur consistently within the adolescent population, across a variety of contexts, is unrealistic, even though teachers of secondary curricula in American schools supposedly expect formal operational thought across all content areas.

Ellsworth and Sindt (1991) addressed this mismatch between school curricula, which appear to demand formal operational thought, and cognitive levels of preadolescents and adolescents, which seem to indicate that the majority of students fail to perform the abstract thinking tasks required in the curricula. Table 3.2 summarizes the cognitive levels found by Epstein (1979) in each grade level. Ellsworth and Sindt (1991) reason that students still graduate from high school, despite their lack of abstract reasoning, because teachers sense that the majority of their students do not have the reasoning abilities to succeed in

TABLE 3.2	COGNITIVE LEVELS				
AGE (YEARS)	PREOPERATIONAL	CONCRETE ONSET	CONCRETE MATURE	FORMAL ONSET	FORMAL MATURE
5	85	15			
6	60	35	5		
7	35	55	10		
8	25	55	20		
9	15	55	30		
10	12	52	35	1	
11	6	49	40	5	
12	5	32	51	12	
13	2	34	44	14	6
14	1	32	43	15	9
15	1	14	53	19	13
16	1	15	54	17	13
17	3	19	47	19	12
18	1	15	50	15	19

From *What Every Teacher Should Know About How Students Think: A Survival Guide for Adults* (p. 28), by P. Ellsworth and V. Sindt, 1991, Eau Claire, WI: Thinking Publications. © 1991 by Thinking Publications. Reprinted with permission.

the established curriculum and accommodate these students by providing lower-level tasks (e.g., testing memory for facts rather than application of ideas).

Higher-level language behaviors have had an uncertain relationship with formal operational thought. Piaget's view that the level of cognitive development is not dependent on concurrent language development has been supported by empirical research (Davelaar, 1977; Jones, 1972). Performance on formal operational reasoning tasks, for example, has not been found to be related significantly to subordinate clause use or to tentative statement use such as "it looks like" (Davelaar, 1977). However, Rosenthal (1979) found a relationship between formal operational thought and use of dimensional language. Concrete operational thinkers describe events by using comparatives and superlatives, while formal operational thinkers cite the most general statement possible (e.g., "The most important thing is the length of the string"). Kamhi and Lee (1988) summarized the debate by stating, "It is generally agreed that language plays a more important role in thinking as children get older" (p. 155).

Information Processing Approach

Developmental theorists who embrace information processing theories are concerned with how information is taken into the organism, interpreted, represented, transformed, and acted upon (Gross, 1985). Three of the more fully developed approaches are neo-Piagetian theory (Case, 1984, 1985), skill theory (Fischer, 1980; Fischer and Corrigan, 1981; Fischer and Pipp, 1984), and triarchic theory (Sternberg, 1985).

Neo-Piagetian theory postulates that an executive system governs the way humans process and use information (Case, 1984, 1985; Pascual-Leone, 1980). As children grow, they assemble executive control structures (i.e., a mental plan) for solving various problems. Similar to Piagetian theory, neo-Piagetian theory specifies age-related restrictions on processing capacity (e.g., Case's [1985] stages are 0 to 18 months, 18 months to 5 years, 5 years to 11 years, and 11 years to 18 years). Four substages of cognitive development during the preadolescent and adolescent years have been proposed by Case (1985): ages 9–11, 11–13, 13–15, and 15–18. According to neo-Piagetian theory, preadolescents use increasingly complex dimensional operations, and adolescents use increasingly complex and abstract operations.

Skill theory postulates 10 developmental levels that occur in three tiers (sensorimotor, representational, and abstract) (Fischer, 1980; Fischer and Corrigan, 1981; Fischer, Hand, and Russell, 1984; Fischer and Pipp, 1984). Preadolescents (i.e., around the age of 10 or 11) demonstrate Level 7 single abstractions, which is the most primitive form of abstractions. Not until approximately 14 or 15 years of age, according to Fischer et al. (1984), can adolescents coordinate two or more abstractions in a single skill (i.e., Level 8 abstract mapping). Level 9 abstract systems emerge at about age 18 or 19, which means the adolescent now understands the complexities of relations between abstractions. Integrating abstract systems to form Level 10 general principles occurs around age 25; individuals at this level are now capable of fully mature organization of identity, morality, political ideology, etc. What sets skill theory apart from Piagetian and neo-Piagetian stage theories is its emphasis on the different paths children and adolescents follow in acquiring skills. Stage theories assume that when a particular stage is reached, most of the skills exist at that level. Skill theories assume behavior may vary widely across levels below the optimal level, which sets the upper limit on skills. According to skill theory, environmental differences also contribute to the varied paths adolescents follow in acquiring skills. Different experiences among adolescents lead to unevenness in development (e.g., there is more diversity in high school courses than during elementary years, so a student taking a literature course might show advanced performance in critical reading skills and average performance in chemistry).

Triarchic theory (Sternberg, 1985) does not specify developmental stages or levels. Rather, it describes mechanisms that underlie developmental changes, as well as the three kinds of components involved in intelligent thinking: metacomponents, performance components, and knowledge-acquisition components. Metacomponents (i.e., higher-order executive processes) are used in planning, monitoring, and decision making and are crucial mechanisms in cognitive development.

Seven metacomponents are identified by Sternberg (1985):

- recognition of the problem to be solved;
- selection of the components that execute the task;
- selection of the mental representations on which the components or strategy can operate;

- selection of a strategy for combining lower-order components into a working algorithm for problem solving;
- deciding how to allocate attentional resources;
- monitoring what one has done, what one is doing, and what one still needs to do in problem solving; and
- sensitivity to external feedback.

According to Sternberg (1985), a crucial aspect of adolescent thought is the ability to monitor and evaluate the effectiveness of problem-solving strategies. Improved monitoring of the function of the metacomponents also underlies cognitive development during adolescence.

Cognition Summarized

In general, the cognitive developmental changes that occur from childhood to adolescence can be summarized as follows:

1. a growing ability to think about one's own thinking (metacognition);

2. the ability to consider events removed in time or space, real or imagined;

3. the ability to consider all possible alternatives to a problem or situation; and

4. the ability to formulate hypotheses and test them.

The development of metacognitive and metalinguistic abilities is marked by increases in children's ability to engage in deliberate, controlled mental activities (Hakes, 1980). Metalinguistic abilities show their greatest development during middle childhood (i.e., 4 to 8 years of age) (Hakes, 1980). However, development continues through adolescence.

Use of "meta" abilities is optional (i.e., we choose whether or not to use our metacognitive and metalinguistic abilities). When we need them, we invoke them (James, 1990). Metalinguistic awareness depends on linguistic knowledge.

CONCEPT DEVELOPMENT

The adolescent's conceptual ability is more flexible than that of the child's, as conceptual orientation in the former can shift back and forth between abstract-categorical and perceptual (Crager and Spriggs, 1969; Elkind, Barocas, and Johnsen, 1969; Kagan, Rosman, Day, Albert, and Phillips, 1964; Olver and Hornsby, 1966). Olver and Hornsby (1966) concluded that adolescents' thinking becomes increasingly freed from perception. However, there remains the flexibility to classify perceptual characteristics at an analytic level (e.g., both a ruler and a watch have numbers) (Elkind et al., 1969; Kagan et al., 1964). Adolescents have a greater ability than children to classify by homogeneous functions (e.g., a lighter and a match go together because they can start fires) and abstract functions (e.g., a camera and a pencil go together because they can make a record of events) (Crager and Spriggs, 1969).

It appears that the adolescent has an increasing ability to use words as a means of conceptualizing. Vygotsky (1962) suggested that the ability of the adolescent to use language as a vehicle for the acquisition of new concepts is the major intellectual advance-

ment during this period. He also observed that while the young child thinks by remembering, an adolescent remembers by thinking. Acquisition of concepts becomes increasingly important for the adolescent as the secondary-school curriculum focuses almost exclusively on the acquisition of conceptual knowledge in the content areas (Wiig and Semel, 1980).

Wiig and Secord (1992) note that older children and adolescents translate their word knowledge into world knowledge. This is in contrast to early concept development (i.e., up to age 7), when the child's world knowledge translates into word knowledge (Crais, 1990).

From ages 9 to 19, new words and concepts are added to the lexicon, old words take on new and subtle meanings, and it becomes easier to organize the lexicon's content (Nippold, 1988b). For example, double-function terms such as *cold* and *bright* are understood by 6-year-olds when physical meanings are intended, but their psychological meanings may not be understood until preadolescence (Asch and Nerlove, 1960). Nippold (1988b) reports, "On graduating from high school, the average adolescent has learned the meaning of at least 80,000 different words" (p. 29).

COMPREHENSION AND PRODUCTION OF LINGUISTIC FEATURES

Comprehension of linguistic features includes the understanding of morphological, syntactic, and semantic components of language. The term *listening* will be used in this discussion because of its predominance in textbooks used by adolescents and in professional literature involving adolescents. The literature also distinguishes between comprehension of a message and monitoring comprehension of a message. The latter task "is a metacognitive skill that allows listeners to notice and respond when they encounter messages that are difficult to comprehend" (Dollaghan, 1987, p. 46).

Listening is difficult to define because of the complexity of the behavior. As many definitions of listening exist as persons who have written about the topic (Barker, 1971; Nichols and Lewis, 1954; Weaver, 1972; Wolff, Marsnik, Tacey, and Nichols, 1983). Listening must be considered an integral part of the total communication process: The function of the listener is to derive meaning from the speaker's intent.

Listening is the basic language skill that is used the highest percentage of the time. Markgraf (1966) determined that high school students were expected to spend 46 percent of their classroom time listening. Rankin (1926) was one of the first to study how adults spend their verbal communication time. The study revealed that adults spent 42 percent of their time listening, 32 percent speaking, 15 percent reading, and 11 percent writing. In 1975, Werner conducted an update of the Rankin study. She found that 55 percent of verbal communication time was spent listening, 23 percent speaking, 13 percent reading, and 9 percent writing. Clearly, the need for listening spans a lifetime.

The production of linguistic features includes the appropriate expression of mor-

phological, syntactic, and semantic components during speaking. The term *speaking* is being used in this book because preadolescents and adolescents understand the term, since it is part of their curriculum.

Normal Development: Comprehension of Linguistic Features

Until the 1980s, child language researchers focused most of their efforts on charting and analyzing linguistic developments that occur between birth and age 6. Since then, interest in aspects of later language development have begun to escalate, and researchers have posed questions concerning differences between early and later development (Nippold, Schwarz, and Undlin, 1992).

Subtle changes occur in the adolescent's ability to understand oral communication. Professionals should not expect preadolescents and adolescents to comprehend everything that is spoken to them, since certain linguistic features may not be entirely understood even by adults. For example, it has been found in both children and adults that sentences with relative clauses in the middle are more difficult to comprehend than sentences with such clauses at the end (Sheldon, 1977). Also, sentences that violate the minimal distance principle are persistently treated as if they adhered to it (Chomsky, 1969; Reed, 1977; Sanders, 1971). (A sentence that adheres to the minimal distance principle contains a subject and a verb in reasonably close proximity, thus allowing accurate comprehension.) Also, comprehension of the ask/tell distinction is late developing and is never fully resolved by some individuals (Kramer, Koff, and Luria, 1972). Using ninth graders as subjects in a pilot study, Thomas and Walmsley (1976) found that the students made errors in sentences with *ask* and *tell*, *promise*, *persuade*, and *threaten*. The investigators reported that errors may have been caused by the students' linguistic deficiencies or by their current level of metalinguistic development.

The development of figurative language comprehension is particularly important to adolescents (Reed, 1994). They frequently encounter figurative language in textbooks and classroom discourse (Nippold, 1991, 1993) and in the slang and jargon of their peers. The ability to comprehend and use slang and jargon has been linked to peer acceptance and the ability to establish friendships during adolescence (Donahue and Bryan, 1984; Nippold, 1985, 1993).

Researchers have investigated the development of the comprehension of metaphors in normal students between the ages of 4 and 15 years. (Galda, 1981). Results indicate that metaphoric understanding increases with age. Once students are in the concrete operational period, their metaphoric understanding and linguistic abilities increase, resulting in their ability to comprehend and explain abstract metaphors.

Similarly, comprehension of idioms is acquired gradually during adolescence and remains incomplete even at the age of 19 (Nippold, 1988c). Preadolescents tend to understand novel idioms at a literal level, although even 8-year-olds interpret sentences figuratively if familiar idioms and/or idiomatically biasing contexts are used (Ackerman, 1982). The

degree of success in idiom comprehension depends on numerous factors, including the frequency of exposure to specific idioms, the manner in which understanding is to be indicated, and the degree of supporting contextual information (Abkarian, Jones, and West, 1992; Nippold and Martin, 1989).

Some researchers claim youth have little or no comprehension of proverbs before adolescence (Douglas and Peel, 1979; Lutzer, 1988). However, a study by Nippold, Martin, and Erskine (1988) found proverb comprehension among preadolescents to be markedly better than have other studies. Their task did not demand explanation of proverbs, nor were proverbs presented out of context. Thus, when task demands are simplified, it appears preadolescents comprehend proverbs reasonably well, a finding consistent with the development of metaphors and idioms. In general, 9-year-olds have a basic understanding of the various figurative language types, but major improvements occur throughout adolescence (Nippold, 1988c).

Normal Development: Production of Linguistic Features

One of the most extensive studies to date that explored language production was that of Loban (1976). He completed a 13-year longitudinal study on 211 normal subjects from kindergarten through grade 12. He selected a group high in language ability as reported by teachers, a group low in language ability, and a random group of subjects representative of the total group. The characteristics that teachers used to describe those in the high group included the use of a varied vocabulary, the adjustment of speaking pace to listeners' needs, and the ability to remain in control of ideas expressed. Subjects in the high language ability group spoke freely, fluently, and effectively, and listened attentively. The characteristics that teachers used to describe those in the low group included unawareness of listeners' needs and meagerness of vocabulary. Their language rambled without apparent purpose and projected a hesitant, faltering style.

Each year, Loban (1976) completed an oral interview with all subjects, and from grade 3 on, he collected one or more written compositions. The purpose of Loban's research was to determine if differences existed between pupils who ranked high in language proficiency compared with those who ranked low. He also wanted to know if growth in language followed a predictable year-by-year sequence.

Using communication units as his basic measurement, Loban (1976) charted the average number of words per unit during oral language. (See Table 3.3.) A *communication unit* was defined as an independent clause with its modifiers. Loban found that those students with a high average number of words per communication unit were the same

TABLE 3.3

AVERAGE NUMBER OF WORDS PER COMMUNICATION UNIT—ORAL LANGUAGE

Grade	AVERAGE NUMBER OF WORDS PER COMMUNICATION UNIT (MEAN)			RELATIVE GROWTH* (IN PERCENT)			YEAR-TO-YEAR VELOCITY** (IN PERCENT)		
	High Group	Random Group	Low Group	High Group	Random Group	Low Group	High Group	Random Group	Low Group
1	7.91	6.88	5.91	67.61	58.80	50.51	—	—	—
2	8.10	7.56	6.65	69.23	64.62	56.84	+1.62	+5.82	+6.33
3	8.38	7.62	7.08	71.62	65.13	60.51	+2.39	+0.51	+3.67
4	9.28	9.00	7.55	79.32	76.92	64.53	+7.70	+11.79	+4.02
5	9.59	8.82	7.90	81.97	75.38	67.52	+2.65	-1.54	+2.99
6	10.32	9.82	8.57	88.21	83.93	73.25	+6.24	+8.55	+5.73
7	11.14	9.75	9.01	95.21	83.33	77.01	+7.00	-0.60	+3.76
8	11.59	10.71	9.52	99.06	91.54	81.37	+3.85	+8.21	+4.36
9	11.73	10.96	9.26	100.26	93.68	79.15	+1.20	+2.14	+2.22
10	12.34	10.68	9.41	105.47	91.28	80.43	+5.21	-2.40	+1.28
11	13.00	11.17	10.18	111.11	95.47	87.01	+5.64	+4.19	+6.58
12	12.84	11.70	10.65	109.74	100.00	91.03	-1.37	+4.53	+4.02

* Relative Growth uses the scores of the Random Group at grade 12 to equal 100 percent.
** Year-to-Year Velocity is the percentage change in any given group from one year to the following year.

From *Language Development: Kindergarten Through Grade Twelve* (p. 27), by W. Loban, 1976, Urbana, IL: National Council of Teachers of English. © 1976 by the National Council of Teachers of English. Reprinted with permission.

students who were rated high on a checklist of language skills by teachers.

Loban's (1976) investigation of a random group of subjects (i.e., a mixture of students rated high or low on language skills by teachers) revealed that a year of language growth was typically followed by a plateau, then by another year of growth. See Table 3.3 for a comparison of the relative growth of the three groups during grades 1 through 12.

In addition to examining the average number of words per communication unit, Loban analyzed the percentage of total words that were in mazes. When a maze is removed from a communication unit, "the remaining material constitutes a straightforward, acceptable communication unit" (Loban, 1976, p. 102). All groups ended grade 12 with virtually identical percentages of verbal mazes used in grade 1, with erratic fluctuations evidenced during the middle years of school. These percentages are summarized in Table 3.4.

The average number of words per maze was also relatively stable throughout all 12 grades. (See Table 3.5.) The high language ability group consistently showed the smallest degree of maze behavior as a percentage of total words, and the lowest average number

---

TABLE 3.4

MAZE WORDS AS A PERCENTAGE OF TOTAL WORDS—ORAL LANGUAGE

Grade	High Group	Random Group	Low Group
1	7.61	7.46	9.04
2	6.21	8.03	8.31
3	4.71	6.39	7.98
4	6.39	8.38	11.06
5	6.41	7.53	9.04
6	6.98	8.29	10.33
7	5.82	7.76	11.08
8	6.08	8.12	9.30
9	5.31	7.29	10.18
10	7.45	7.40	7.51
11	7.32	7.04	9.01
12	7.25	7.04	9.19

From *Language Development: Kindergarten Through Grade Twelve* (p. 29), by W. Loban, 1976, Urbana, IL: National Council of Teachers of English. © 1976 by the National Council of Teachers of English. Reprinted with permission.

TABLE 3.5

AVERAGE NUMBER OF WORDS PER MAZE—ORAL LANGUAGE

Grade	High Group	Random Group	Low Group
1	1.94	2.09	1.81
2	1.89	1.89	1.90
3	1.88	1.85	1.98
4	1.97	2.06	1.99
5	1.93	2.09	2.07
6	2.15	2.21	2.16
7	1.90	2.06	2.17
8	1.96	2.01	2.11
9	1.78	1.98	2.18
10	1.85	1.92	1.92
11	1.94	1.97	1.97
12	1.77	1.99	2.24

From *Language Development: Kindergarten Through Grade Twelve* (p. 31), by W. Loban, 1976, Urbana, IL: National Council of Teachers of English. © 1976 by the National Council of Teachers of English. Reprinted with permission.

of words per maze. Although students in the low language ability group used a lower average number of words, they simultaneously used a larger amount of verbal maze behavior.

In comparing the average number of communication units in oral language with those in written language, Loban (1976) found that his subjects tended to speak and write in units that had similar average lengths. He found that those students who were superior in oral language skills in kindergarten and first grade, before they learned to read and write, were the same students who excelled in reading and writing by the time they were in sixth grade. The inclusion of longer and more complex adjectival clauses was a primary mark of increasing language development, both oral and written. The growth of adjectival clauses was centered mainly in junior high school, grades 7 through 9.

In most oral language measurements taken by Loban (1976), the high language ability subjects were approximately four to five years advanced in comparison with low language ability subjects. There was a strong correlation between high socioeconomic status and entry into the high language ability group. A similar correlation existed between the low language ability group and low socioeconomic status. While subjects from minority ethnic groups (i.e., Oriental, Mexican, Black Americans) comprised a disproportionately high percentage of the low group and a low percentage of the high group, social inequity, not ethnic background, affected language proficiency. As Loban stated, "Minority students who came from securely affluent home backgrounds did not show up in the low proficiency group. The

problem is poverty, not ethnic affiliation" (Loban, 1976, p. 23).

Language production during preadolescence and adolescence has also been discussed extensively by Nippold (1988d). Syntactic growth during adolescence is subtle (Scott, 1988). Between the ages of 8 and 12, the frequency of phrases *like and, everything, and stuff,* and *or something* increases threefold. Connectives are gradually mastered, with these being more difficult than others: *although, which, yet* (intrasentential), and *thus* and *however* (intersentential).

Production of figurative language also shows gradual improvement throughout preadolescence and adolescence. Nippold (1988c) notes, "It has been suggested that growth in figurative language production follows a U-shaped curve, i.e., novel, imaginative expressions are frequently produced by preschoolers, decrease during the elementary years, but increase during adolescence" (p. 180). The ability to explain sentential ambiguity also improves steadily during the preadolescent and adolescent years (Nippold, 1988e).

DISCOURSE

According to Austin (1962), discourse is composed not of words or sentences but of speech acts. Austin maintained that speech acts can be analyzed in three parts: (1) locutions, or propositions; (2) illocutions, or the speaker's intentions; and (3) perlocutions, or the listener's interpretations. "The ways in which normally developing children link consecutive utterances within discourse to maintain coherency and to clarify messages"

(Craig, 1983, p. 106) is referred to as *pragmatics*. This definition of pragmatics considers the integrated nature of structural and conversational rules. Hymes, writing in 1971 before the popularity of the term *pragmatics*, discussed the importance of sentence acceptability, or "who can say what, in what way, where, and when, by what means and to whom?" (p. 15). His insight into "sentence acceptability" in the 1970s paved the way to pragmatics in the 1980s and to social communication skills in the 1990s. As Gallagher (1991) so astutely noted, "Social cognition, social skills, and the attainment of age-appropriate friendship skills provide the foundation on which peer relationships are built. Central to each of these is language skill" (p. 13).

There are two types of discourse: narrations and conversations. Several primary differences exist between the two (Roth and Spekman, 1986):

1. Narrations have more extended or elaborated units of text than conversations.

2. Narrations are expected to have story markers (e.g., an introduction and closing) and an orderly presentation of events leading to a logical resolution.

3. Narrations carry the expectation that the speaker will engage in an oral monologue and that the listener's role can be more passive. More responsibility is placed on the speaker to be organized, coherent, and interesting.

Narratives can be further broken down into personal narratives and expository language (i.e., instructional discourse). Both types will be discussed in a later section of this chapter.

Numerous studies have investigated the discourse of older students. Data are presented in the following sections on conversations and narrations.

Conversations

Definition

The term *conversation* frequently "is used loosely and non-technically to refer to any interactional stretch of talk involving at least two participants, and taking place in a non-formalized setting" (Edmondson, 1981, p. 6).

Normal Development

Grice (1975) proposed four fundamental rules of conversations that summarize expectations held by speakers and listeners. These rules are intact by late adolescence and frequently emerge by the middle grades:

A. Quantity: Informativeness

"1. Make your contribution as informative as is required (for the current purposes of the exchange).

2. Do not make your contribution more informative than is required" (p. 45).

B. Quality: Sincerity

"1. Do not say what you believe to be false.

2. Do not say that for which you lack adequate evidence" (p. 46).

C. Relationship: Topic Management

"1. Be relevant" (p. 46).

D. Manner: How to Be Clear

"1. Avoid obscurity of expression.

2. Avoid ambiguity.

3. Be brief (avoid unnecessary prolixity).

4. Be orderly" (p. 46).

Various researchers have investigated communicative maturity during conversations. For example, Wiig (1982) found communicative maturity to be developed by age 13. At this time, youth can make the transition between an informal language code (i.e., peer register) and a more formal language code (i.e., adult register) of language. Moreover, Wiig found that by age 15, teenagers will use the more formal register, not only with adults but also with their own peer group, unless the peers are their very closest friends. Different surface structures of the speech act are appropriate for different situations depending upon the listener, setting, topic, and objectives (Wiig, 1983). Modification of the verb phrase is the most important aspect in making the surface structure changes from an informal code to a formal one (e.g., "Close the door" versus "Would you mind closing the door?"). A mature communicator will have many different structural forms to express the same intent.

As communicative maturity increases, inept communication acts should decrease. By third grade, students are able to recognize an inept communication act, but they cannot yet correct it (Johnson, Greenspan, and Brown, 1980). By sixth grade, students improve inept communication acts if those acts attempt to influence others' actions (e.g., "You're studying for a test at school. Lou calls you up and wants to come over to visit. You say, 'You picked a fine time to visit.' How would you correct your statement?"). Not until ninth

grade can students correct inept attempts to have others feel better (e.g., "Tom is sad because his dog died. You say, 'Cheer up, it's nothing to be upset about. Pretty soon you'll forget all about it.' How would you correct your statement?").

A possible explanation as to why inept communication acts decrease in late adolescence is that the person is capable of using more sophisticated communication strategies—for example, taking the perspective of the listener. Also, older adolescents have a greater range of interpersonal constructs that they apply to communication situations (Ritter, 1979).

We have completed the third year of a six-year longitudinal study in which we analyzed spontaneous conversational speech of eight normal adolescents, four boys and four girls, while they were in the seventh, eighth, and ninth grades, under two experimental conditions (McKinley and Larson, 1991). In one condition, adolescents talked with a familiar peer of their choice, while in the other condition they talked with an unfamiliar adult of the opposite sex. These two conditions were selected to represent bipolar situations.

The results of this study revealed that adolescents used more questions when with a peer than with an adult. They also initiated more topics and used more frequently the language functions of getting information and of entertaining. With an adult, they used more supportive gestures (e.g., head nodding "yes" while saying "yes"), positive verbal interruptions (e.g., saying "um-hm" during the adult's speaking turn), and the language function of giving information. The study found that boys, more so than girls, used a higher frequency of figurative language and the language function of entertaining. Girls used the language function of indicating readiness for further communication more frequently than boys. For all other language behaviors analyzed, boys and girls showed no differences in the frequency of use.

When grade levels were compared, there was a steady decrease in these language behaviors: vocalized pauses (i.e., any pause during which the speaker emits sounds such as "er," "um," and "ah" to initiate or maintain an utterance), verbal mazes, topic shifts in a new direction, abrupt topic shifts, and the language function of entertaining. In contrast, these language behaviors increased between seventh and ninth grades: positive verbal interruptions and the language function of indicating readiness for further communication.

Topic maintenance changes have been studied by Dorval (1980), who found significant differences between children and adolescents. The results of the study revealed the following:

1. Nonelaborated topic-related remarks increased in frequency during the elementary years but started to decrease during high school as more complex topic-related remarks increased.

2. More complex remarks such as factual and perspective-oriented evaluations/elaborations/questions were made during ninth grade and increased in frequency thereafter.

3. In ninth grade, but declining thereafter, there was a high proportion of evaluation comments relative to elaboration

comments and evaluations, elaborations, and questions that focused on people's perspectives or feelings. Thus, conversational quality (i.e., coordination associated with topic management) changes with age.

Topics of conversation have been indexed and classified using taped transcripts of 15-year-old adolescents (Rutherford, Freeth, and Mercer, 1969). While analyzing younger children, two broad topics surfaced: domestic and educational. Rutherford et al. (1969) found these to be insufficient when classifying topics of adolescents, and they added a third general topic, "philosophical." This added category absorbed topics that did not relate to the individual's immediate environment of school and home. Philosophical topics were discussed without immediate personal experience or knowledge and often reflected facts or opinions derived from television. Although these data were obtained from England, it is probable that the classification of the conversational topics of American youth would also require a philosophical category.

Rutherford (1976) made the astute observation that it is the way in which adolescents talk about certain topics, such as popular music videos, that causes adults to complain that adolescents "speak another language." The current system of beliefs and attitudes of adolescents can be seen through the medium of their conversations. Adolescents make remarks that allow peer group members to share the feeling expressed, but which intentionally prevent adult onlookers from understanding (e.g., "Well, just . . . [laugh] him" and "Well, not just his voice . . . but himself"

[Rutherford, 1976, p. 113]). Such utterances are not analyzable, according to Rutherford. They are part of normal adolescent secretiveness, a necessary mechanism that allows children to grow up and away from parents. Much of the secret nature of their lives is reflected through their language (Rutherford, 1976).

Narrations

Definition

Structurally, narrations are midway between oral and literate language (Westby, 1984, 1991). They form a transition from the language style of the home to the language style of the school. Personal narratives (on the oral end of the continuum) are either reports of "what happened," called personal experience narratives, or reports of the imagination, called stories (Lahey, 1988). Expository language (on the literary end of the continuum) is used for the planning and transmission of logic-based knowledge and involves comparisons, explanations, and opinions (McFadden, 1991). The discourse of instruction is closely tied to metalinguistic skills and the onset of formal operations in Piaget's (1970) view of cognition.

An important aspect of expository language is the requirement for explicitness (Wallach and Miller, 1988). In written exposition, explicitness is taken to an extreme, since punctuation must be used to map the meanings carried by gesture, facial expression, intonation, and prosody (McFadden, 1991).

Narrations may be viewed as suprasentential discourse units with underlying organizational rules, or *story grammars*; as conceptual units which reveal the speaker's expectations about event sequences, or *scripts*; as linguistic expressions requiring specific formal devices to bind them into coherent *texts*; and as *communication events* which demand thoughtful assessment of the listener's needs. (Johnston, 1982, p. 144)

Narrations can be viewed as extended monologues, in contrast with conversations, which are interactive dialogues.

Normal Development

Normal children have been found to produce true narratives by 5 to 7 years of age. Complex stories with multiple embedded narrative structures do not emerge until 11 to 12 years of age (Westby, 1984).

Applebee (1978) has summarized the normal development of narrative structure:

1. Initially, children use prenarrative structures starting with "heap stories." They talk about whatever attracts their attention, without regard for a relationship among the elements or a macrostructure.

2. A second prenarrative stage is "sequence stories," which have a macrostructure, but the storyteller does not actually have a temporal sequence in mind. Rather, characters, objects, or events are put together because they are perceptually associated with each other.

3. The next stage is "primitive narratives" in which characters, objects, or events are put together because they complement each other in some logical way. These narratives are the students' first

use of inference in stories. However, their inferences go in only one direction and they do not perceive the reciprocal causality between thoughts and events.

4. Another developmental stage in story grammars is the "unfocused chain." In unfocused chain stories, the elements are logically related to each other but not related to any macrostructure. Thus, the story has no theme or plot.

5. The next stage is the "focused chain," which has all the elements or events sequenced and related to the story's macrostructure. However, the story still lacks reciprocal relationships between characters' attributes and events, and among main events. Thus, the story does not have a strong plot.

6. The last stage of development is the "true narrative" that integrates logical cause-and-effect chaining of the macrostructure elements, which are linked to the macrostructure of the story. This results in the story having a strong, well-developed plot.

Normal children reach the true narrative stage by approximately 8 years of age. In fact, by age 5 or 6 years, children can begin to produce structurally complete fantasy narratives during oral storytelling (Botvin and Sutton-Smith, 1977). (Contrast this with Nelson [1988] and Nelson and Friedman's [1988] research on *written* personal narratives. Sixty-three percent of the regular seventh graders still produced primitive narratives. Of the tenth graders, 46 percent produced focused chains and only 39 percent produced true narratives. Of college freshmen, 25 percent produced focused chains and 75 percent produced true narratives.)

One way that narrations have been studied is through the use of story reformulation tasks. Several researchers have proposed that story schemata are used by listeners to guide comprehension and recall (Mandler and Johnson, 1977; Rumelhart, 1975; Stein and Glenn, 1979). Weaver and Dickinson (1982) summarized the way that efficient listeners maximize verbatim recall by using these processes:

1. recognition of verbal formulae (e.g., "Once upon a time there was . . .");

2. prediction of sentence structures based upon the constraining power of preceding sentences;

3. recognition and use of conjunctions and prepositions to mark relationships (i.e., temporal, causal, spatial) among propositions during encoding; and

4. integration of information gathered from these multiple sources.

Chappell (1980) found that early adolescents were pragmatically aware of what information needed to be retold, and they used appropriate syntactic structures. By adulthood, a story being retold is "filled in" if the original story does not follow a predictable story sequence (Johnston, 1985).

The amount of information recalled during story reformulation tasks showed developmental changes as age increased; however, basic organizational structure did not vary across ages (Mandler and Johnson, 1977). Young children tended to emphasize action sequence outcomes, but older children and adults emphasized the actions themselves or the internal events motivating them (Mandler and Johnson, 1977). Across all age levels, the most important units of a story were recalled most frequently (Brown and Smiley, 1977).

Thus, while some aspects of story reformulation differed with age (e.g., amount of information recalled, emphasis during recall), other aspects did not (e.g., organizational structure, judgment of importance of units). As Weaver and Dickinson (1982) pointed out, story grammar taxonomies such as Stein and Glenn's (1979) are relatively insensitive to developmental changes.

COMMUNICATION IN CULTURALLY AND LINGUISTICALLY DIVERSE POPULATIONS

The 1990 U.S. census projects the minority population will be more than 30 percent by the year 2000 (Carey, 1992a). Already in 23 out of 25 of the largest school systems in the United States, the "minority" is the majority (Willig and Greenberg, 1986). Within the next decade, as much as one-third of the speech-language pathology and audiology caseload in the schools will be children from Black, Hispanic, Asian, and Native American cultures (American Speech-Language-Hearing

Association, 1988; Crago, 1990). Put another way, the American Speech-Language-Hearing Association (1988) estimates that by the year 2000, 7 million people who are members of minority populations will have a communication disorder that warrants intervention.

Professionals cannot assume that all minority youths are linguistically diverse. Many are assimilated into the American mainstream culture and are monolingual English-speaking individuals. Others are bilingual, multilingual, or semilingual (i.e., neither the original language nor the new language is acquired satisfactorily). Anyone who speaks a language other than Standard American English is considered to be in the linguistic minority (Ratner and Harris, 1994). This does not mean the individual's language is disordered. As Taylor (1988) notes, " 'normal' for a given speaker is determined by his or her culture with the particular type of language used within these cultural constraints controlled by language interactions among several social factors" (p. 939).

Standard American English has many dialects. Competent language users can easily switch between Standard American English and their dialect in response to the communication situation. Dialects reflect only a difference in language use, not a pathology of language (Taylor, 1988).

One of the most common dialects in the United States is Black English. Taylor and Peters (1982) have presented an excellent description of Black English features by reviewing 29 linguistic rules. These 29 linguistic rules (e.g., invariant "be," negation, plurals, questions, and pronouns) have been analyzed to determine where there is overlap between Black English and several other dialects (i.e., Southern English, Southern White Nonstandard English, and Appalachian English). They also briefly reviewed Spanish-influenced English in terms of phonological and syntactic features.

A more extensive study by Mendelberg (1984) investigated the language of Mexican-American adolescents of migrant origin. The analysis of the data revealed distinctive language patterns used in different settings. Initially, it would seem that the language patterns chosen are determined as a matter of the subject's personal choice. However, upon further investigation, it appears that underlying the choice is the role played by language as a symbol of the group and the position the group occupies in the present social system. There is a relationship between language use and the development of a group identity. These findings concur with Taylor and Peters (1982), who concluded that major social and cultural factors influence language acquisition and behavior.

The pragmatic contrasts between Standard American English and common dialects (i.e., Black English, Hispanic English, and Asian English) are many (Taylor [in press] cited in Owens, 1991). Some features that distinguish Black English are these :

- Preference for indirect eye contact during listening and direct eye contact during speaking; preferences are opposite in Standard American English.

- Use of direct questions is sometimes seen as harassment. (E.g., "When will you be done?" is seen as rushing someone to finish something.)

- Asking personal questions of a person someone has met for the first time is seen as improper and intrusive; such inquiry is considered "friendly" in Standard American English.

Hispanic English has these pragmatic contrasts, to cite a few:

- Hissing to gain attention is acceptable; in Standard American English, it is impolite.

- Direct eye contact may be interpreted as a challenge to authority; it is a sign of respect in Standard American English.

- Business conversations are preceded by lengthy exchanges unrelated to the main point; getting quickly to the point is valued in Standard American English.

Asian English is distinguished by pragmatic contrasts such as the following:

- Interrupting a conversation is considered impolite; in Standard American English, interruptions are appropriate in certain circumstances.

- Kinship terms are very important in determining the relationship between two speakers and extend beyond the family; kinship terms have a less rigid effect on Standard American English speakers.

- Expressing affection publicly, especially between men and women, "looks ridiculous"; kissing and hugging in public are acceptable in Standard American English.

An excellent appendix that further delineates differences is provided by Owens (1991) called "Dialectal and Bilingual Considerations," which outlines major dialectal differences within Black English, Hispanic English, and Asian English. Selected portions of the appendix are reprinted with permission in Appendix A on pages 249–257. Readers should refer to this appendix for specific dialectal differences.

The level of proficiency a child has in his or her primary language when initially exposed to the second language (i.e., the dominant language of the community) will affect both languages' future development (Cummins, 1989). Regression in the primary language may occur from exposure to the second language at an unsuitable time. Cummins (1989) proposes that a threshold of competence in the primary language should be reached before a second language can be mastered; otherwise, semilingualism results. This threshold often does not occur until the mid-elementary years, and there are data to suggest that age 10 is the best time to introduce a second language (Skutnabb-Kangas and ToukoMoaa, 1976, cited in Pacheco, 1983). Even so, Duncan (1989) suggests the school-age child will take 18 to 36 months to function linguistically in the new language. Cummins (1989) cautions that academic language competence may take up to seven years to develop for normal children learning English after the age of 6.

NONVERBAL COMMUNICATION

DEFINITION

Nonverbal communication refers to communication that transcends spoken words and includes six categories (Knapp, 1978):

- kinesic behaviors;
- physical characteristics;
- touching behavior;
- paralanguage (including voice quality and vocalizations);
- proxemics; and
- artifacts (e.g., perfume, clothes).

While the discipline of communication sciences and disorders typically has not included paralanguage within nonverbal communication, we have selected to use Knapp's comprehensive definition of nonverbal communication. Edmondson (1981) defined *paralanguage features* as purposeful, directed, and controllable behaviors that may accompany or substitute for language and thus contribute to the development of a conversation.

Nonverbal factors are major determinants of meaning in the interpersonal context. Birdwhistell (1970) asserted that only 30 to 35 percent of the social meaning of a conversation is carried by words, while Mehrabian (1968) estimated that nonverbal factors are even more important. According to Knapp (1978), nonverbal communication serves these purposes: repetition, contradiction, substitution, complementation, accentuation, and regulation.

NORMAL DEVELOPMENT

Nonverbal patterns in today's adolescents may be quite different from those in the past (French, 1978). French (1978) has described several nonverbal behaviors now considered normal for adolescents that in the past would have been signs of hostility and rebellion. One such behavior is the blank stare, or focusing the eyes beyond the listener when engaging in a conversation. Another is the eye roll, once used as an expression of impudence. Now, the eye roll is used so extensively that the message it once conveyed has been weakened (French, 1978). Another behavior is the back turn, or shifting the body slightly, to expose the back to the receiver during the conversation. French believes the back turn has been influenced by the black culture, which views it as a sign of trust and of understanding what was said. He also described the "Black Walk," which is slower than the "White Walk." It is more of a stroll, with the head slightly elevated and casually tipped to one side. French (1978) analyzed the nonverbal message conveyed by the White Walk to be, "I am a strong [person], and I'm in a hurry to get somewhere" (p. 544). The nonverbal message conveyed by the Black Walk is, "I am strong. I am 'cool.' I can't be bothered by anything in this world" (p. 544). French has observed that both white and black youth have adopted nonverbal communication patterns of the black culture.

Some of the research in nonverbal communication during adolescence has analyzed recognition of facial expressions. In the 1920s, Gates (1923) conducted a facial expression recognition study and found that laughter was identified by age 3, pain by ages 5 to 6, anger by age 7, fear by ages 9 to 10, and surprise by age 11. None of the individuals studied had recognized scorn by age 14. The findings of this study have not been seriously challenged (Knapp, 1978). According to a report by Blanck and Rosenthal (1982), older children develop some degree of distrust toward facial expressions when accompanied by discrepant vocal cues. The researchers summarized the data on older children as evidence that these children put more weight on facial expressions under normal conditions of communication and less under conditions of discrepancy.

Age changes in deceiving and detecting deceit have been reported by DePaulo and Jordan (1982). Before adolescence, children's distinction of deception from truth by reading only facial expressions is by chance. When given both verbal and nonverbal cues, adolescents perceive feigned expressions of liking as less positive than sincere expressions of liking, and feigned expressions of disliking as less negative than honest expressions of disliking. Girls between 5 and 12 years of age are increasingly adept at masking their deceptions facially; the reverse tends to occur for boys. The strategy that seventh graders use to deceive a person is to convey the feigned affect with the same degree of intensity as when it occurs naturally when telling the truth, while college students deceive by exaggerating the dissimulated affect. Researchers speculated that students learn and practice deception by playing card games, board games, party games, and sports.

Two studies examining the development of eye contact, or gazing, disagree on whether there is a gradually increasing or decreasing trend in looking behavior up to adolescence (Ashear and Snortum, 1971; Levine and Sutton-Smith, 1973). Knapp (1978) reported that adolescence represents a low point for eye gazing. Such lack of eye contact noted in normal adolescents is important data for professionals to keep in mind when they are assessing gazing behavior during conversational speech.

Listener feedback, such as head nods and vocalizing "mm-hmm," has been found to be nearly absent through fifth grade (Dittman, 1972). Before junior high school, adults probably cannot expect much overt feedback, such as head nods, to indicate that children are listening to them. Our findings (McKinley and Larson, 1983, 1991) support Dittman's results. We found eighth grade students provided considerable nonverbal listener feedback during conversations, even more than they did while in seventh grade.

The decoding of nonverbal cues is a gradually increasing skill from kindergarten through ages 20 to 30, after which time a leveling off occurs (Dimitrovsky, 1964). On tests of nonverbal sensitivity, females consistently outperformed males from grade school through the middle 20s (Knapp, 1978). Nonverbal ability was not found to be significantly related to intelligence quotients, class rank, *Scholastic Aptitude Test* scores, or vocabulary test scores (Knapp, 1978). The findings show that, in general, if persons were good senders of nonverbal communication, they were also good receivers (Knapp, 1978).

The empirical research reported in this section underlines the continuing development of nonverbal communication during adolescence. Developmental changes in both encoding and decoding nonverbal cues occur in normal preadolescents and adolescents.

WRITTEN LANGUAGE

Language, whether oral or written, has the same components (i.e., two people are needed for communication to occur—speakers need listeners and writers need readers; also needed are a reason to communicate [pragmatics], meaning [semantics], and structure [syntax], which is coded phonetically or graphically) (Westby, 1990). However, two differences should be noted: contextualization and immediacy of the audience (Nelson, 1988). "Although it is not altogether clear how knowledge of specific differences between spoken and written language emerges, it is clear that children apply their realizations about modality differences relatively late in the language development process" (Gillam and Johnston, 1992, p. 1304).

REQUIREMENTS OF WRITTEN LANGUAGE

Written language requires that the meaning of the message be clear, independent of an immediate reference (i.e., it is decontextualized), whereas spoken language is thought to be context dependent since it usually relies on the immediate context to convey the communication message. In oral communication, the audience is generally physically present or on the phone and the communication is a shared turn-taking dialogue in which speaker and listener may share common information. In written communication, the audience may be unknown or must be imagined by the writer. The writer does not get immediate feedback as does the speaker, and thus the writer must anticipate the degree to which the written message must be made explicit (Nelson, 1988).

"Whole language" advocates adhere to the idea that all areas of language are important and each area assists the others. They maintain that listening, speaking, reading, and writing abilities develop concurrently and interrelatedly, rather than sequentially (Schory, 1990; Teale and Sulzby, 1986; Westby, 1990). Perera (1986), while discussing later language development, suggested that complex linguistic structures are encountered first in reading and then are practiced in writing. She called writing "a potent agent in the process of language development" (p. 518). Writing is also an ideal medium for the acquisition of complex structures, "because it allows the language user to deliberate, to review and to correct, without pressure from conversational partners" (Perera, 1986, p. 518).

NORMAL DEVELOPMENT

Students who have developed adequate writing skills meet the demands of written communication in four domains (Rubin, 1987):

1. They invent subject matter in an internally cohesive fashion, without the benefit of shared understandings with their communication partners that are inherent in dialogue.

2. They address remote and indeterminate audiences, without the benefit of environmental or nonverbal cues.

3. They engage in cooperative discourse (i.e., they tailor their writing to contribute to an ongoing knowledge base, yet also conform to certain conventions expected by the anticipated audiences).

4. They monitor their messages constantly, while engaged in ongoing revision.

Competent writers use three major processes while writing: planning, sentence generation, and revising (Hayes and Flower, 1987). *Planning* involves information retrieval and the shaping of that knowledge to match the audience. *Sentence generation* translates the plan into formal prose. Even the most extensive outline is expanded on the average by a factor of eight in the final essay (Kaufer, Hayes, and Flower, 1986).

Revising involves rewriting the generated sentences with the goal of improving the text. Unfortunately, revisions are not always beneficial. One study found that fourth graders hardly revise at all, eighth graders' revisions hurt more than they help, and twelfth graders' revisions that are helpful narrowly outnumber harmful ones (Bracewell, Scardamalia, and Bereiter, 1978). One possible explanation is that students are not usually expected to write a revised paper and the teacher's comments on a paper may or may not teach a student how to write better.

However detailed and constructive a teacher's comments may be, their effectiveness depends upon the extent to which the students read the comments and upon whether simply reading them is enough to teach a student how to correct the errors. Since students rarely are asked to write another draft, they have few chances to learn how to use an editor's suggestions and revisions to produce a better manuscript. (Applebee, 1981, p. 103)

Specific parameters of written language were examined during Loban's (1976) classic study of language development. (See the normal language development highlights reported on pages 48–51 of this chapter.) For all groups in Loban's study, an upward spurt in the use of noun clauses occurred at grade 8 (rather than at grade 7 as in oral language). When examining the average number of words per communication unit, Loban found an erratic pattern, not the smooth development pattern found in oral language. Large upward trends in average number of words were followed by downward shifts. Despite the erratic pattern, the high language group in Loban's study was approximately four or five years ahead in written language development compared with the low group— roughly the same margin found in oral language. All groups showed a rapid growth in writing from grades 9 to 10.

Writing skills continue to develop throughout late adolescent and adult years. Particularly for individuals whose vocations depend on writing talent, development of additional skills may become a lifelong pursuit. For other adults, research suggests that writing is the language art least used (Werner, 1975); the average adult spends only 12 percent of his or her communication time engaged in writing.

SUMMARY

The physical and psychological changes occurring during adolescence affect how youth perceive themselves and communicate with others. Professionals working with preadolescents and adolescents need to be cognizant of the interrelationships among physical, psychological, and language development. The language development that occurs during preadolescence and adolescence is often subtle, yet it is critical to the student's academic, social, and eventual vocational success. Unlike early language, later language is more individualized as youth become diverse in their curricular and social experiences. Learning how to distinguish between normal and disordered language behaviors during preadolescence and adolescence is paramount for professionals working with these age groups.

The underlying cognitive development that parallels language development is also crucial for professionals to consider. Whether a Piagetian approach or an information processing approach is used, cognitive development is marked by quantitative and qualitative changes during preadolescence and adolescence.

Researchers have only recently begun to map the changes that occur in older students' comprehension and production of linguistic features and in their discourse skills. Perhaps not surprisingly, language continues to develop throughout adolescence and into the adult years.

Nonverbal language development also continues throughout the teen years. Given the potential miscommunication that can occur when adults wrongly interpret acts like the "eye roll," it behooves professionals to observe the nonverbal behaviors of normal adolescents before making judgments about "disordered" behavior.

Linguistically diverse populations are on the increase. Major social and cultural factors influence language acquisition and behavior. Students with language differences must not be mistaken as having language disorders.

Knowledge of the normal development of written communication is also critical for professionals to have. Like oral language skills, written language skills continue to emerge throughout the middle grades and high school.

DISCUSSION QUESTIONS

1. Discuss the relevance that the physical and psychological development data have on the older student's communication behaviors.

2. Critique the language development data presented in this chapter. Describe several research topics that would significantly add to our database on normal language development in older students.

SUGGESTED READINGS

Nippold, M. (Ed.). (1988). *Later language development: Ages nine through nineteen.* Boston, MA: Little, Brown and Company.

Wiig, E., and Secord, W. (1992). From word knowledge to world knowledge. *The Clinical Connection, 6*(3), 12–14.

DISORDERS OF LANGUAGE IN OLDER STUDENTS

4

GOALS:

To present cognitive, language, and social characteristics of preadolescents and adolescents with language disorders

To summarize major communication expectations and problems

As the demands of school curricula at each grade level increase, language skills in preadolescents and adolescents must become increasingly sharpened and refined. Thus, language disorders have a profound effect on school performance and frequently exist concomitantly with other disabilities (e.g., learning disabilities, behavioral disorders). Unfortunately, children who were language impaired during their early years experience a "continuum of failure" as they mature into adolescents (Aram, Ekelman, and Nation, 1984; Aram and Hall, 1989; DeAjuriaguerra, Jaeggi, Guignard, Kocher, Maguard, Roch, and Schmid, 1976; Garvey and Gordon, 1973; Griffiths, 1969; King, Jones, and Lasky, 1982; Strominger and Bashir, 1977; Weiss, Hansen, and Heubelein, 1979).

A 15-year follow-up study of 50 speech-language students ranging in age from 13 years, 10 months to 20 years, 5 months was conducted by King et al. (1982). At the time of the investigation, 42 percent of the students still had some form of a communication problem. These students' spoken language disabilities frequently underlie and interact with reading failures that persist into adolescence and adulthood (Allington and Fleming, 1978; Johnson, 1985; Lewis and Freebairn, 1992; Rees, 1974; Snyder and Downey, 1991; Velluntino, 1978). Lewis and Freebairn (1992), using a cross-sectional study, suggest that remnants of preschool phonology disorders are detectable past grade school age and into adulthood; and subjects with a history of language problems in addition to the phonology disorder performed more poorly on reading and spelling measures than subjects with a history of preschool phonology disorders alone.

Byers Brown and Edwards (1989) reinforced the notion of a "continuum of failure." They responded to questions first posed by Byers Brown and Beveridge (1979):

1. "Is there a continuum of language disturbances seen initially in the acquisition of the spoken word and later revealed as deficits in the secondary systems of reading and writing" (p. 19)? Authorities are inclined to answer yes to this first question, according to Byers Brown and Edwards (1989).

2. "Can we assume that all children with initial disorders of language must be at risk educationally" (p. 19)? The answer to this second question is yes if the initial disorder was correctly diagnosed as affecting language.

3. "Is there an underlying factor which is causal and thereby links all language manifestations? Or, are the skills all related by factors in the child's disposition, neurological, emotional, or environmental but not causally linked" (p. 19)? The answers to these questions are not readily available. Nonetheless, the questions are important to consider.

4. "Are different language and learning problems occurring independently in vulnerable children rather than being bound together by one definable disability" (p. 19)? Likewise, the answer to this question is not yet available. The complexity and diversity of conditions cast under the broad heading of "language disorder" suggest a homogeneity that does not exist. The same can be said of "learning disability."

Lahey (1990) spoke to the diversity of procedures for identifying children with language disorders and the resultant confusion about the meaning of the term *language disorder*. The clinical forum on specific language impairment as a clinical category (Kamhi, 1991; Leonard, 1991) also stressed that *language disorder* is not a homogenous category and debated the nature of specific language impairment. Leonard (1991) argued that "children with language limitations are not simply late in reaching early language milestones, but have limitations that are long standing, at least in the absence of intervention" (p. 67) and he proposed the concept of a continuum of language ability.

Limited English proficiency (LEP) students are considered communicatively handicapped when limited competency exists in both the primary language and the second (i.e., English) language (American Speech-Language-Hearing Association, 1985). Difficulty in learning the primary language delays reaching the threshold of competence described by Cummins (1989) and fails to facilitate the acquisition of English. The result is likely to be confusion and frustration. Another result may be inappropriate placement in special education classrooms.

THE LABEL OF "LANGUAGE DISORDER"

Who should be called language disordered as preadolescents and adolescents is a perplexing question. Language development charts tend to end around age 10, and development past that point is less universal and more individual, depending upon the youth's interests and experiences. Language ability and/or disability needs to be judged in the context of how it impacts the student's academic, social, and vocational environments. The language of preadolescents and adolescents can be viewed as disordered when it negatively interferes with academic success, social acceptance, and vocational potential.

Nelson (1993) posits three main groups of older students with language disabilities:

- An "ABNQ" group, i.e., the students who "almost but not quite" fit into the mainstream; they are characterized by relatively normal cognitive ability but with specific disabilities in language and learning. This group is somewhat competitive in participation with same-age peers.

- A group that is more severely impaired with moderate to severe cognitive limitations related, for example, to autism or mental retardation. This group will probably always need somewhat protected environments and may remain at early- or middle-stage levels of language ability, which need to be used for later stage activities such as job interviewing.

- A group that has peripheral physical or sensory impairments that interfere with the acquisition of language and social interaction skills. This group is diverse; some individuals may be fully competitive across settings with only occasional consultation from a speech-language pathologist, and others may require extensive support and augmentative communication.

Of the three groups of older students cited by Nelson (1993) who have communication, learning, and social problems, this book addresses primarily the first group.

A classification system for learning disabilities was compiled by Weller and Strawser (1987) and expanded in detail by Weller, Crelly, Watteyne, and Herbert (1992). They identify five subtypes, which can range from mild to severe:

- *Production Deficit Disorder*—This group exhibits problems with sustained attention, which limits the students' abilities in adaptive behaviors of production and social coping. The majority of their language is equivalent to that of the mainstream and few difficulties with linguistic application, organization of space and time, or social cognition are noted (unless sustained attention is involved).

- *Verbal Organizational Disorder*—This group exhibits difficulties in mathetic language (i.e., morphology, syntax, and semantics), verbal reasoning, and figurative application of language. These students find it difficult to give straightforward and logical verbal explanations or to follow oral instructions. Their language difficulties depress their knowledge base, and they lack the ability to produce any kind of work that requires high-level verbal understanding and communication skills.

- *Nonverbal Organizational Disorder*— Members of this group also lack adaptive language ability, but their problems stem from difficulties in organizing time, space, and paralinguistic communication (e.g., tone of voice, rate of speech). They tend to get lost easily and are frequently late getting to or are absent from where they are supposed to be. They tend to lack understanding of their own adaptive abilities, perceiving themselves as using appropriate verbal reasoning and figurative language. Meanwhile, "significant others perceive their use of language as being excessive, boring, rambling, or circuitous" (Weller et al., 1992, p. 32).

- *Global Functional Disorder*—This group tends to exhibit poor social cognition. These students have difficulties with understanding cause and effect, with information processing, and with comprehension and use of humor. Memory tasks usually cause them difficulty. They often speak and act without thinking and incorrectly interpret the feelings of others. One of the most distinctive characteristics is their individual pattern of strong and weak abilities in adaptive language. The pattern is inconsistent and individuals display profiles that are uneven in terms of adaptive language performance.

- *Non-Learning Disabled*—This group exhibits academic achievement levels or intelligence quotients that fall almost one standard deviation below the mean. These students struggle with higher-order cognition and lack problem-solving strategies. They do not follow through on tasks and need to be shown, not just told orally, how to do tasks. Overall, their adaptive language abilities are similar to those of individuals without learning disabilities, except the pace of their adaptation is slower.

Of these five subtypes of learning disabilities, Weller (1989) reported that students with verbal organizational disorder are the most likely to receive speech-language services. They receive approximately six years of speech-language intervention during their school careers. (No information was available concerning the most typical grade levels at which services were provided.) The other subtypes tend to be served primarily through other services. For example, individuals with production deficit disorder and those within the non-learning disabled subtype tend to receive approximately seven years of resource room or special class placement. Students with nonverbal organizational disorder receive approximately four years of either special physical education, general special education, or treatment in private clinics. Students with global functional disorder receive approximately five years of assistance from general special education, private tutors, medical facilities, or special clinics. Thus, while all of the subtypes present specific language patterns that might warrant speech-language intervention, only the students with verbal organizational disorder tend to be placed on caseloads with any consistency. Additional research is needed to verify that this is the group of students most often referred to as "language-learning disabled," but the probability appears strong.

Most significant to this discussion are the ongoing language disabilities and concomitant cognitive deficits that can be anticipated when young children advance to middle grades and beyond. These deficits are summarized in the next sections.

DEFICITS IN COGNITION

Many researchers have found that preadolescents and adolescents with cognitive deficits often fail to attain higher levels of abstract reasoning (Ellsworth and Sindt, 1991; Feuerstein, 1980; Hains and Miller, 1980; Havertape and Kass, 1978; Neimark, 1980; Seidenberg, 1988). In other words, these adolescents remain concrete thinkers and do not use organized, efficient strategies for solving problems.

Referring back to Table 3.2 (see page 43), which summarized the cognitive levels found in each grade level, the range of ability is apparent (Ellsworth and Sindt, 1991). Secondary-level teachers are faced with many students who remain at the concrete level. Relatively few, however, are at the onset level (i.e., just transitioning into the concrete period) or below. These students would have particular difficulty with school curricula and

would be at risk for concomitant language disorders.

Students with low cognitive levels struggle with conceptual development. Wiig and Secord (1992) summarized two categories of concepts important for learning: spontaneous (intuitive) and scientific (scholastic, disciplinary). The latter category is especially at risk among students with language disabilities, according to Wiig and Secord (1992). Scientific concepts are constantly being added throughout each grade level and often build upon one another.

Patterns of task approach were studied by Stone and Forman (1988). Preadolescents and adolescents with learning disabilities showed patterns of general conceptual disorders, specific developmental delays, and poor awareness of the implicit demands of the research situation. Learning disabled adolescents tend to blame "inadequate ability" more for their failure than nondisabled students; they tend to believe that intelligence is fixed and static, thus promoting their negativeness when faced with obstacles to their achievement (Golumbia and Hillman, 1990).

While it might be tempting to blame hereditary or environmental factors, Feuerstein (1980) argues that errors in methods of teaching are frequently the cause of low levels of abstraction in adolescents. He cites a lack of mediated learning experiences as the primary cause of cognitive deficiencies and sees all other potential causes (e.g., poverty of stimulation, low functioning level of parents) as secondary reasons for the deficit. His teaching methods designed to combat low levels of abstraction are summarized in Chapter 7, "Language Intervention with Older Students."

METALINGUISTIC DEFICITS

Three stages occur in metalinguistic development: intuitive use of linguistic knowledge, awareness and executive use of the knowledge in tasks that require such awareness, and automatic use of the knowledge (Menyuk, 1991). Youth with language disorders do progress in language development and, therefore, gradually and intuitively acquire knowledge of language, but they have great difficulty in achieving conscious awareness of that knowledge (Menyuk, 1991).

When the firm establishment of linguistic representations and automatic retrieval are delayed, language development is delayed (Menyuk, 1991). Children who have language impairments have difficulty bringing to awareness categories and relations in all aspects of language. Menyuk (1991) argues that language delay might be "caused by metaprocessing difficulties since awareness of structures precedes and is necessary for comparison of what is known to what is still to be learned and for automatic use of structures" (p. 395).

Kamhi (1987) summarized research that has examined the meta-abilities in language-impaired children across six areas:

1. repairing communicative breakdowns;
2. making listener judgments;
3. making judgments of language content;
4. analyzing language into linguistic units;
5. understanding and producing rhymes, puns, and riddles; and
6. understanding and producing figurative language.

A synthesis of the studies indicates that metalinguistic deficits exist in children with language disorders but are not all-pervasive (Kamhi, 1987). For example, 9- to 14-year-old students with language impairments have been found to have more difficulty than language-age matched peers in identifying, revising, and justifying revisions of morphological errors, but they produce the same types of clarification requests.

In general, youth with language impairments have difficulty acquiring various linguistic forms and, once acquired, also have difficulty reflecting on these forms (i.e., metalinguistics). Nelson (1993) underscores the importance of older students' ability to reflect consciously on language, to process it on more than one level simultaneously, and to know the labels and to talk about language during formal education. Students with language disorders often have deficits that surface when engaging in such metalinguistic tasks.

LINGUISTIC FEATURE DEFICITS

COMPREHENSION

Comprehension deficits during adolescence are often marked by less understanding of the figurative uses of language when students are matched with same-age peers (Blackwell, Engen, Fischgrund, and Zarcadoolas, 1978; Jones and Stone, 1989; Nippold, 1991). For example, late adolescent males (16 to 18 years of age) with learning disabilities provide significantly fewer correct metaphor interpretations than do normally achieving peers (Jones and Stone, 1989). Even after instruction has raised students' levels of literal language comprehension to within normal limits, individuals with histories of language disorder may demonstrate significant deficits in metaphor comprehension ability (Nippold and Fey, 1983).

Riedlinger-Ryan and Shewan (1984), using a series of standardized tests, investigated the auditory comprehension of linguistic features by learning disabled and academically achieving adolescents. This study supported the findings presented in previous studies that documented the persistence of auditory language comprehension deficits in adolescents with learning disabilities. While some deficits in auditory comprehension were clearly demonstrated, deficits in comprehension of supersegmental features remain controversial. For example, evidence conflicts regarding the ability of adolescents with learning disabilities to comprehend stress and intonation patterns (Vogel, 1974; Wiig, Kutner, Florence, Sherman, and Semel, 1977). Indeed, Cruttenden (1985) concluded that even normal 10-year-olds are still very limited in interpreting utterances whose intonations are critical for comprehension to occur.

Little information exists on comprehension monitoring by youth with language impairments (Dollaghan, 1987). Some evidence suggests that they produce fewer spontaneous requests for clarification than their normal peers (Donahue, 1984; Donahue, Pearl, and Bryan, 1980). Even when given instruction in making clarification requests, Donahue (1984) found that students with learning disabilities perform less well than their peers. This is in contrast to Kamhi's (1987) summation.

Interest in listening comprehension deficits has also been sparked by examining the differences between those who become poor readers and those who become skilled readers (Wong, 1991). A growing body of evidence indicates that poor readers do not comprehend sentences as well as good readers do (Mann, Cowin, and Schoenheimer, 1989). They perform less well on spoken instructions such as those in DiSimoni's (1978) *Token Test for Children* (e.g., touch the small red square and the large blue triangle) (Smith, Mann, and Shankweiler, 1986). Wong (1991) stresses that poor readers do not have trouble with the grammatical structures involved in comprehension tasks so much as a short-term memory problem. "It seems as if poor readers are just as sensitive to syntactic structure as good readers; they fail to understand sentences because they cannot hold an adequate representation of the sentence in short-term memory" (Wong, 1991, p. 146).

PRODUCTION

Production deficits during adolescence may be evident in agrammatical sentences (Wiig and Semel, 1975), sentences of shorter length (Donahue, Pearl, and Bryan, 1982; Wiig and Semel, 1975), sentences with insufficient cohesion (Lapadat, 1991), and sentences that are less syntactically complex than those of normal peers (Donahue, Pearl, and Bryan, 1982; Geers and Moog, 1978). Word-retrieval problems, the inability to call up an intended word from memory, are common (Blalock, 1981; Wiig and Becker-Caplan, 1984; Wiig and Semel, 1975). Wiig and Semel (1975) noted longer response lags in producing sentences.

Lapadat (1991) analyzed the results of 33 studies that have investigated the language of students with language disorders and learning disabilities. Some of these studies involved children between the ages of 3 and 8 years, while others involved middle-grade students, ages 9 to 12. Results indicated that students' difficulty with using sufficient cohesion to communicate intention led to problems that involved misunderstandings, confusion, and incomplete discourse (Lapadat, 1991).

Asking questions may be difficult (Bryan, Donahue, and Pearl, 1981) and may occur with low frequency in specific situations. Donahue (1984) found that teaching students to ask questions did not improve their use of questions when clarification was needed; students need to be taught *how* and *when* to ask for appropriate clarification. In addition, adolescents with language disorders often have problems expressing themselves concisely (Wiig and Semel, 1976), and they tend to overuse a limited and concrete vocabulary (Wiig and Semel, 1975, 1976).

During referential communication tasks, oral descriptions of an item or activity by adolescents with learning disabilities tend to be less informative for listeners than those provided by normal adolescents (Knight-Arest, 1984; Noel, 1980; Spekman, 1981). Knight-Arest (1984) found that boys with learning disabilities talked more but conveyed less information than their normal peers. The boys with learning disabilities appeared more comfortable when doing than when describing a task to a listener. Furthermore, they were less effective at adapting messages to the needs of the listener than their normally achieving peers (e.g., repeating rather than reformulating what they said). They often appeared to be oblivious to the listener's needs.

On the plus side, Bunce (1989) concluded that students with learning disabilities can benefit from training on referential communication tasks. Her trained subjects learned to provide specific information needed by the listener to complete a particular task, to generalize their newly learned skills to a different referential communication task, and to retain most of their skills when a follow-up check was completed seven months later.

In Loban's (1976) classic study, differences between more effective and less effective oral language production were summarized (i.e., high language skills group versus low language skills group). The less effective subjects did not appear to have a plan for their talking that showed coherence and unity. Their vocabulary was meager and they were not flexible in expressing their ideas. Speaking style was hesitant, faltering, and/or labored.

DISCOURSE DEFICITS

CONVERSATION

Production deficits during conversational speech may include a lack of sustaining and monitoring conversations (Bryan, Donahue, and Pearl, 1981); a lack of requesting clarification of inadequate or ambiguous messages (Donahue, Pearl, and Bryan, 1980); an inability to keep abreast of the verbal exchange (Donahue and Bryan, 1984); and a lack of arguing for or against a position (Bryan et al., 1981). No significant differences have been found between normal adolescents and those with learning disabilities regarding the number of conversational turns (Bryan et al., 1981), the number of times they engaged in conversations with peers (Schumaker, Sheldon-Wildgen, and Sherman, 1980), or the number of times they were targets of peer initiation (Schumaker et al., 1980). Furthermore, some studies have found a lack of evidence that these adolescents, despite their social communication hindrances, are any more withdrawn, rejected, or isolated than normal adolescents (Bryan et al., 1981; Deshler and Schumaker, 1983).

Donahue and Bryan (1984) have suggested that there is a strong relationship between the knowledge and use of slang by adolescents with learning disabilities and their amount of interaction with and acceptance from the normal peer group. Thus, for students with learning disabilities, "failure to conform to peer group norms for appropriate language use may have increasingly negative consequences"

(p. 18); establishing and maintaining friendships and enhancing self-esteem may be difficult. Their misunderstanding of metaphors, jokes, puns, and sarcastic remarks, and their inadequate skills for rapid humorous verbal exchanges place older students with language disorders at a disadvantage when interacting with their peers.

Students with learning disabilities may lack basic social skills (e.g., they don't know how to use an appropriate tone of voice) or they may have knowledge of social skill strategies but fail to generalize them for a variety of reasons (Ellis and Friend, 1991). Other students are under *inappropriate stimulus control* (i.e., it is more reinforcing to act in a socially incompetent manner than to act competently) (Kerr and Nelson, 1989). Some adolescents avoid participating in class to avoid the risk of being humiliated for giving an inept answer (Ellis, 1989).

Blalock (1981) argued that the adolescent's oral language deficits and social imperceptions prevent quality interactions with others and impede close friendships. Nisbet, Zanella, and Miller (1984) found that adolescents with moderate handicaps are less talkative when conversing with nonhandicapped peers than with fellow handicapped peers. Their speech is typically "simple, direct, imperative, and informal, rather than subtle, complex, elaborate, or polite" (Bergman, 1987, p. 162).

Schumaker and Hazel (1984) reported students with learning disabilities who are in the speaker role are less likely to adapt their behaviors to meet the needs of their listeners and exhibit a lower occurrence of appropriate verbal/nonverbal skills than their nonhandicapped peers. Bergman (1987) was even more direct in her observations of adolescents with language-learning disabilities, noting that these individuals typically are not adaptive to their listeners and rarely express support, compliment them, or consider the feelings of others. For some adolescents, listening to conversational speech may also be impaired. Blalock (1981) observed that listening to fast-paced conversations is difficult for older students with learning disabilities and language disorders.

Adolescents with learning disabilities who have disturbed visual spatial functioning also present conversational deficits (Bergman, 1987; Ratner and Harris, 1994). Unlike adolescents with language disorders, this group appears to have relatively intact language skills during early childhood and the elementary years. However, by adolescence, these individuals may exhibit speech and affect that is flat and stereotyped (Bergman, 1987). "Language emerges as grammatically precise, but also as loquacious, superficial, inappropriate, and tangential . . . nodes of relating are similarly automatized, perseverative, and meaningless" (Bergman, 1987, p. 164). This group of adolescents functions with extreme inconsistency during conversational exchanges in social situations.

NARRATION

Studies investigating story recall in children and adults with language disorders and learning disabilities have revealed that these individuals tend to preserve the order of events in a story and recall the patterns of story organization with the same degree of accuracy as their normally achieving counterparts; but they tend to recall significantly less information from stories (Weaver and Dickinson, 1982; Worden, Malmgren, and Gabourie, 1982). Researchers found these same differences in quantity of information within spontaneous story production by learning disabled students (Roth and Spekman, 1986). Although some studies report no differences in storytelling or retelling between normal and learning disabled students, these findings may be the result of applying story grammar analysis procedures that are insensitive to subtle developmental changes (Weaver and Dickinson, 1982).

Merritt and Liles (1987) investigated 9- to 11-year-olds and found differences between story retelling and telling in both normal children and those with language disorders. The retelling task was less difficult for both groups than the story generation task. In both groups of children, the retold stories were longer and contained more story grammar components and complete episodes. In the story retelling task, the children with language disorders had shorter clause length and fewer complete episodes than did the normal children.

Differences have also been found when rating stories on the importance of their idea units (Worden and Nakamura, 1982). Older students with a learning disability had more difficulty rating stories on the importance of their idea units than did their normal counterparts. Worden and Nakamura (1982) suggested that the lower agreement on the ratings by students with learning disabilities may reflect a deficit in comprehension of the story or in remembering it. Older students also have difficulty comprehending expository language such as classroom lectures (Blalock, 1981; Nelson, 1993).

Using another approach, MacLachlan and Chapman (1988) studied the communication breakdowns in children's conversations and narrations. They found that children with language-learning disabilities (LLD) between 9 years, 10 months and 11 years, 1 month incurred a significantly greater rate of communication breakdowns per communication unit in narrations than conversations compared to the normal control group. Also, they found that the mean length of the communication unit was significantly greater in narrations than conversations for the LLD group compared to the control group.

Blalock (1982), summarizing persistent auditory language deficits, reported that young adults have difficulty in conveying extended explanations and narratives, in relating experiences, in explaining ideas or problems, in retelling stories, and in organizing the narrative.

DEFICITS IN NONVERBAL COMMUNICATION

Although our clinical experiences indicate that many adolescents with language disorders have deficits in nonverbal behavior, little formal research confirms or refutes these observations. Wiig and Harris (1974) found that students with learning disabilities may have an inability to recognize nonverbal

emotional expressions. Bryan (1977) also found that students with learning disabilities were less skillful at understanding nonverbal behavior when compared with their normal counterparts. Blalock (1981) documented inappropriate use of proxemics (i.e., social distance) during conversational speech.

Adolescents (from ages 13 to 16 years) with emotional disturbance have been found to be significantly poorer at nonverbal encoding than normal adolescents (Feldman, White, and Lobato, 1982). Likewise, they are less accurate in decoding nonverbal communication than normal adolescents. Still, adolescents with emotional disturbances have some nonverbal encoding and decoding skills in that they have been found to perform at levels greater than chance.

Our own observations of adolescents with language disorders have indicated these nonverbal communication problems:

1. frequent failure to interpret accurately the facial expression accompanying a spoken message;

2. inconsistent understanding of gestures used by others;

3. occasional failure to inhibit socially unacceptable gestures;

4. significantly less eye contact (not related to cultural issues) than that of normal adolescent communicators; and

5. inappropriate maintenance of distance (not related to cultural issues) during various conversational situations.

DEFICITS IN WRITTEN LANGUAGE

Students with oral language disorders almost always display written language deficits during preadolescent and adolescent years. Children with speech and language impairment encounter reading problems at least six times more often than controls do (Mason, 1976). Children with reading problems have concomitant writing disorders.

Children with a reading disability show a significant lag in their development of grammatical sensitivity (i.e., the ability to correct grammatically incorrect sentences, the understanding of acceptable word order, control over regular and irregular morphological features of English, and the ability to remember sentences with varied grammatical structures) (Siegel and Ryan, 1988). They also show deficits in short-term memory and an even greater deficit in phonological skills (Siegel and Ryan, 1988).

Hull (1987) summarized this error taxonomy for written language:

1. *Production errors*—errors that are traceable to the demands of writing a sentence, such as lost or abandoned patterns. (Example: "Tom's judgment, impaired by his lack of motivation, his fatigue, and his failure to remember directions.")

2. *Rhetorical errors*—errors arising from the requirements of producing discourse rather than sentences, such as topic/comment structure mistakes. (Example: "His response to this story he felt he was talked into a different viewpoint.")

3. *Accidental errors*—errors resulting from "slips of the pen" (or of the fingers on the keyboard). (Example: "Many people of our generations [sic] want to interact will [sic] older people.")

4. *Interference errors*—errors caused by interference from a second register, dialect, or language. (Example: "We be at the dance.")

5. *Systematic errors*—errors signifying an idiosyncratic or unstable rule system. (Example: "They had to designed everything they made.")

Inexperienced writers do not integrate their writing plans like competent writers do (Hayes and Flower, 1987). They write significantly shorter essays with fewer words per sentence part (7.3 words per part versus 11.2 words per part) (Hayes and Flower, 1987). Also, novices see revision largely as a sentence-level task in which the goal is to improve individual words and phrases without modification of the text structure (Hayes and Flower, 1987). Experts detect about 1.6 times as many problems in a faulty text than do novices (Hayes, Flower, Schriver, Stratman, and Carey, 1985). Abundant evidence exists that those identified as learning disabled have difficulty with editing (Gregg, 1983).

When Gillam and Johnston (1992) compared the written and spoken narratives of 9- to 12-year-old children who were language and learning impaired with three groups matched for age, or spoken language, or reading, they found that spoken narratives were superior to written narratives in the organization of textual form for all groups. Conversely, written narratives were superior to spoken narratives in the organization of textual content. Sentences were longer in spoken narratives than in written narratives, but not necessarily more complex. The group with language and learning impairments in particular performed appreciably worse on a measure of complex sentence usage. They also produced a large percentage of grammatically unacceptable sentences, especially in their written narratives, making errors on both simple and complex sentences.

SUMMATION OF CHARACTERISTICS

Using data from studies presented, extrapolating from curricular materials for youth, and drawing upon our clinical experiences with preadolescents and adolescents, we have constructed Table 4.1, "Characteristic Problems of Older School-Age Students with Language Disorders." We have listed language expectations within each of seven areas (cognition, metalinguistics, comprehension and production of linguistic features, discourse, nonverbal communication, survival language, and written language), followed by a summary of the data describing problems observed when expectations are not met. The expectations are derived from the type of communication demands that educators, parents, and peers place upon preadolescents and adolescents. The problems are derived from the review of the literature just presented and from our clinical experiences with older students who have language disorders.

Note when reviewing Table 4.1 that typically a single problem would not result in a student being placed on the caseload, although there may be exceptions (e.g., a severe word-retrieval problem). Usually, a number of concomitant problems would exist before a preadolescent or adolescent would become a candidate for speech-language services. Candidates for services have communication deficits that interfere with achieving academic progress, developing personal-social skills, or reaching vocational potential.

This book focuses on preadolescents and adolescents who display the problems listed in Table 4.1, regardless of etiology or setting. When professionals examine the multitude of problems that can interfere with the academic, social, and vocational well-being of the student, they realize that they cannot afford to ignore youth with communication disorders after the elementary years. Special compensatory programs for elementary grades only might make sense if sixth-grade-level skills were the end goal of intervention. Early childhood and elementary speech-language programs have not failed, but by themselves they perform only a portion of the task. Some students, without continued intervention, will regress to previous levels of functioning by the time they enter junior high school (Larson and Dittman, 1975). Other adolescents need continued assistance to learn the language skills demanded for higher grade levels. Still other students surface for the first time during preadolescence when they have not acquired the necessary communication skills to survive the verbal and social demands of higher grade levels.

TABLE 4.1

CHARACTERISTIC PROBLEMS OF OLDER SCHOOL-AGE STUDENTS WITH LANGUAGE DISORDERS

CATEGORY	EXPECTATIONS	PROBLEMS
COGNITION	To be at the formal operational level	They often remain concrete operational thinkers.
	To observe, organize, and categorize data from an experience	They make chaos out of order.
	To identify problems, suggest possible causes and solutions, and predict consequences	They may not recognize the problem when it exists; if they do, they do not know how to develop alternative solutions.
	To place concepts into hierarchical order	They often cannot place concepts in a hierarchy.
	To find, select, and utilize data on a given topic	They have limited strategies for finding, selecting, and utilizing data.
METALINGUISTICS	To demonstrate conscious awareness of linguistic knowledge	They have difficulty bringing to awareness categories and relations in all aspects of language.
	To talk about and reflect on various linguistic forms	They do not know the labels for talking about language during formal education.
	To assess communication breakdowns and revise them	They do not have awareness of breakdowns and, if they do, they lack repair strategies.
COMPREHENSION AND PRODUCTION OF LINGUISTIC FEATURES	To comprehend all linguistic features and structures	They misunderstand advanced syntactical forms.
	To follow oral directions of three steps or more after listening to them one time	They may not realize that they are being given directions and/or have difficulty following them.
	To use grammatically intact utterances	They often use sentences that are fragmented and that do not convey their messages.
	To have a vocabulary sufficient for expressing ideas and experiences	They have word-retrieval problems as well as a high frequency of low-information words.
	To give directions with clarity and accuracy	They often leave their listeners confused.
	To get information or assistance by asking questions and to respond appropriately to questions asked of them	They may know what questions or answers to give, but they do not know how to do so tactfully.
	To comprehend and produce the slang and jargon of the hour	They do not comprehend or produce slang/jargon, thus they are ostracized from the group to which they most desire to belong.

(continued)

CATEGORY	EXPECTATIONS	PROBLEMS
TABLE 4.1—*Continued*		
DISCOURSE	To produce language that is organized, coherent, and intelligible to their listeners	They use many false starts and verbal mazes.
	To follow adult conversational rules for speakers (e.g., maintaining a topic, initiating a topic)	They consistently violate the rules.
	To be effective listeners during conversation without displaying incorrect listening habits	They often have poor listening skills.
	To make a report, tell or retell a story, and explain a process in detail	They often leave their listeners confused.
	To listen to lectures and to select main ideas and supporting details	They often do not grasp the essential message of a lecture.
	To analyze critically other speakers	Their judgments are arbitrary, illogical, and impulsive.
	To express their own attitudes, moods, and feelings and to disagree appropriately	They have abrasive conversational speech.
NONVERBAL COMMUNICATION	To follow nonverbal rules for kinesics	They violate the rules and misinterpret body movements and facial expressions.
	To follow nonverbal rules for proxemics	They violate the rules for social distance.
SURVIVAL LANGUAGE	To comprehend and produce situational phrases and vocabulary required for survival in our society	They do not have the necessary concepts and vocabulary needed in places such as banks, grocery stores, and employment agencies.
	To comprehend and produce concepts and vocabulary required across daily living situations	They do not have the necessary concepts and vocabulary needed across daily living situations such as telling time, using money, and understanding warning signs.
WRITTEN LANGUAGE	To comprehend written language required in various academic, social, and vocational situations	They do not consistently and/or efficiently process information obtained through reading.
	To produce cohesive written language required in various academic, social, and vocational situations	They do not consistently and/or efficiently generate written language that conveys their messages.

By using the expectations and problems listed in Table 4.1, professionals can begin to determine where a given preadolescent or adolescent matches or mismatches with educators', parents', and peers' expectations. Based on this information, appropriate assessment protocols and intervention programs can be built.

SUMMARY

Much evidence exists that older school-age children do not "outgrow" their language deficits. Rather, they display a continuum of failure that negatively impacts their performance in academic and social settings. Deficits in cognition, metalinguistics, language comprehension and production, discourse, nonverbal communication, and written language may all contribute to the failure.

When cognitive, metalinguistic, linguistic, and nonlinguistic expectations are not met, concomitant problems arise. Young people who fall short of the expectations have communication problems that put them at risk academically, socially, and vocationally.

DISCUSSION QUESTIONS

1. Study the list of expectations and problems in Table 4.1. Which have you observed? Should any be added? If so, which ones?

2. What advantages and disadvantages do you see in labeling an older student as having a "language disorder"?

SUGGESTED READINGS

Lahey, M. (1990). Who shall be called language disordered? Some reflections and one perspective. *Journal of Speech and Hearing Disorders, 55*(4), 612–620.

Weller, C., Crelly, C., Watteyre, L., and Herbert, M. (1992). *Adaptive language disorders of young adults with learning disabilities.* San Diego, CA: Singular.

ASSESSMENT: A DYNAMIC PROCESS 5

GOALS:

To define the assessment process

To describe a comprehensive/holistic model of assessment

To explain the factors involved in multidimensional assessment

To present multicultural issues in assessment

Assessment is a dynamic process in which the examiner selects and administers appropriate measurement instruments (formal tests and informal procedures) and observes and records the student's communication behaviors, as well as those of the members of the student's environment, to determine the existence, type, nature, and severity of a communication disorder. Before beginning the process, the exact purpose for completing the assessment must be considered. For example, is the purpose to determine the existence of a problem, to establish appropriate intervention goals, or to decide if dismissal is warranted? Questions such as these must be answered first to select procedures and subsequently to obtain the information needed.

This chapter provides a comprehensive assessment model for evaluating the preadolescent and adolescent (9 to 20 years of age) during an initial speech-language evaluation or periodic retesting. Rather than presenting procedures that test isolated behaviors, a comprehensive assessment approach is described.

COMPREHENSIVE/HOLISTIC ASSESSMENT MODEL

When using a comprehensive/holistic model for assessment, a number of paradigm shifts are occurring, thus changing what behaviors we assess and how we assess them. A

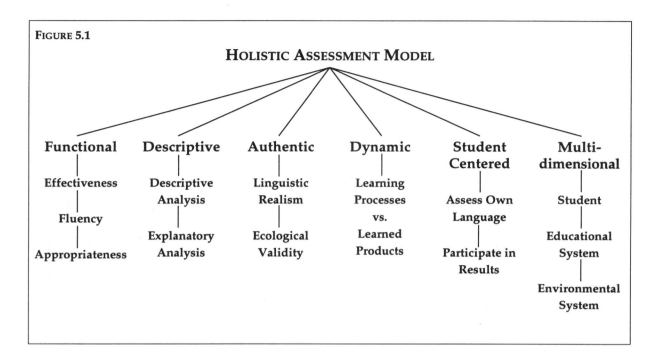

FIGURE 5.1

HOLISTIC ASSESSMENT MODEL

Functional	Descriptive	Authentic	Dynamic	Student Centered	Multi-dimensional
Effectiveness	Descriptive Analysis	Linguistic Realism	Learning Processes vs.	Assess Own Language	Student
Fluency			Learned Products		Educational System
Appropriateness	Explanatory Analysis	Ecological Validity		Participate in Results	Environmental System

paradigm, according to Kuhn's (1970) text, *The Structure of Scientific Revolutions,* is a set of beliefs for viewing the world. A paradigm affects decision making by influencing perceptions and interpretations of a given problem and its potential solutions (Westby and Erickson, 1992). The following shifts in assessment paradigms are changing the way we assess behaviors (Westby and Erickson, 1992):

1. Away from discrete point, decontextualized, standardized tests to authentic, functional, descriptive, naturalistic assessment.

2. Away from a totally client-centered approach to a more multidimensional approach that takes into account the student's social systems.

3. Away from exclusively assessing spoken communication to including written communication and problem-solving

skills. The interaction between spoken and written language in older students is acknowledged.

4. Away from a focus on student similarities to an awareness of cultural and linguistic diversity among students.

5. Away from exclusively using quantitative data and procedures to including qualitative data and procedures.

To achieve a comprehensive assessment of the student's communication performance, the assessment process must be functional, descriptive, authentic, dynamic, student centered, and multidimensional (see Figure 5.1). These six facets of a comprehensive assessment model are not mutually exclusive and interact to create a holistic approach to determine whether the student is an effective communicator across and within a variety of communication situations.

FUNCTIONAL ASSESSMENT

According to Damico (1993), examiners need to be concerned about how the older student's performance is evaluated. Previously, the focus has been on structural components and particularly on the surface level of grammatical features. Instead, the focus should be on the student's ability to communicate effectively.

Damico (1993) goes on to state that how effectively a student communicates depends on three criteria: "the effectiveness of meaning transmission, the fluency of meaning transmission, and the appropriateness of meaning transmission" (p. 29). Obviously, the primary goal of communication is the transmission of meaning between two or more individuals. However, it is also important that the communicators formulate, speak, or understand the message within the time constraints of the communicative interaction/situation. If a student is interrupted or delayed when communicating, that interruption may in fact devaluate the individual's role as a communicator.

To assess a student's functional communication behaviors, the evaluation must be holistic in nature and not consist solely of discrete point testing. Functional communication assessment demands that the student's ability to communicate be evaluated in a wide array of realistic situations.

DESCRIPTIVE ASSESSMENT

In descriptive assessment, the evaluation must document and describe the student's communication problem and determine the underlying causes, if possible. A bilevel analysis paradigm is required (Damico, 1993) to accomplish descriptive assessment. A bilevel analysis paradigm suggests that there be both a *descriptive analysis* of the communicative performance and a detailed *explanatory analysis* of language proficiency.

A *descriptive analysis* would focus on directly observing and recording behaviors that (1) have been found to be necessary for successful communication in selected contexts in which the student is likely to communicate and in selected modalities that the student is likely to use, and (2) are believed to be valid indices of communicative difficulty.

An *explanatory analysis* would determine the causal factors for the communication disorder that was observed during the descriptive analysis. The explanatory phase does not involve more data collection, according to Damico (1993), but is a deeper interpretation of the data collected in the descriptive phase. The examiner needs to sort out the communication behaviors that were successful and those that were not under the descriptive analysis.

For those communication behaviors that were not successful, it is important to ask, "Why not?" Was it because of the student's social/cultural experiences, cognitive abilities, emotional abilities, physical abilities (e.g., hearing or fine motor abilities), or a combination of the above?

Damico (1993) has generated a set of questions that should be used in systematically analyzing those variables that might have contributed to the communicative difficulties. These two general sets of questions (i.e.,

TABLE 5.1	EXTRINSIC AND INTRINSIC EXPLANATORY FACTORS

EXTRINSIC EXPLANATORY FACTORS

1. Are there any overt variables that immediately explain the observed communicative difficulties? Among the potential considerations:

    • Are the documented problematic behaviors occurring at a frequency that would be considered within normal limits or in random variation?

    • Were there any procedural mistakes in the descriptive analysis phase that account for the problematic behaviors?

    • Is there an indication of extreme test anxiety during the observational assessment in one context but not in subsequent ones?

    • Is there significant performance inconsistency between different contexts within the targeted manifestation?

2. Is there evidence that the problematic behaviors noted in the descriptive analysis phase can be explained according to normal second language acquisition or dialectal phenomena?

3. Is there any evidence that the problematic behaviors noted in the descriptive analysis phase can be explained according to cross-cultural interference or related cultural phenomena?

4. Is there any evidence that the problematic behaviors noted in the descriptive analysis phase can be explained according to differences in the student's past history or experience?

5. Is there any evidence that the problematic behaviors noted in the descriptive analysis phase can be explained according to any bias effect that was in operation before, during, or after the assessment?

    • Is the student in a subtractive language learning environment?

    • Is the student a member of a disempowered community?

    • Are negative or lowered expectations for this student held by the student, the student's family, or the educational staff?

    • Were specific indications of bias evident in the referral, administrative, scoring, or interpretative phases of the evaluation?

If the communicative difficulty cannot be accounted for by asking the first five questions, then the final question aimed at intrinsic explanatory factors should be conducted.

INTRINSIC EXPLANATORY FACTORS

6. Is there any underlying linguistic systematicity to the problematic behaviors noted during the descriptive analysis phase? This can be determined by completion of the following steps:

    • ensure that no overt factors account for the problematic behaviors (first five questions);

    • isolate the turns or utterances that contain the problematic behaviors; and

    • perform a systematic linguistic analysis on these data points, looking for consistency in the appearance of problematic behaviors.

From "Language Assessment in Adolescents: Addressing Critical Issues," by J. Damico, 1993, *Language, Speech, and Hearing Services in Schools, 24*(1), p. 33. © 1993 by the American Speech-Language-Hearing Association. Adapted with permission.

extrinsic explanatory factors and intrinsic explanatory factors) are listed in Table 5.1.

AUTHENTIC ASSESSMENT

Authentic assessment has been of major interest to classroom teachers and administrators who are concerned about standardized measures and feel there is a need to develop new kinds of testing measures based on performances. Zessoules and Gardner (1991) define authentic assessment as follows:

> Currently, taking the form chiefly of portfolios and performance-based tasks, these measures are often referred to as authentic assessment, and they are designed to present a broader, more genuine picture of student learning. . . . Authentic assessment is fast becoming the buzzword of hope among educators who value more expansive descriptions of learning. (p. 49)

The move toward authentic assessment in general education is equivalent to the move toward functional communication and pragmatics in communication sciences and disorders. Both movements are attempting to establish a more realistic assessment of the student's communication as opposed to isolated language elements in standardized testing that may or may not add up to the whole picture of how the student can and does perform in various communication situations.

Authentic assessment evaluates the actual behaviors we want students to be able to do. If we judge "students to be deficient in writing, speaking, listening, artistic creation, research, thoughtful analysis, problem posing, and prob-

lem solving" (Wiggins, 1989, pp. 41–42), then the tests should measure how students "write, speak, listen, create, do original research, analyze, pose, and solve problems" (Wiggins, 1989, pp. 41–42). According to Wiggins (1989), authentic tests have four basic characteristics:

1. They are designed to be representative of performance in the field; problems of scoring reliability and logistics of testing are considered after that.

2. Attention is paid to the teaching and learning of the criteria to be used in the assessment.

3. Self-assessment plays a much greater role than in conventional testing.

4. Students frequently are "expected to present their work and defend themselves publicly and orally to ensure that their apparent mastery is genuine" (p. 45).

Table 5.2 presents a more thorough list of characteristics of authentic tests.

According to Damico (1993), the data collected for assessment should be actual utterances that serve to transmit ideas or intentions as a speaker/writer to a listener/reader in real communication situations. He states that authentic assessment possesses both *linguistic realism* and *ecological validity. Linguistic realism* means assessment must be meaning based and integrative as opposed to fragmenting language into discrete components. *Ecological validity* means that assessment must be accomplished in naturalistic/realistic settings (Damico, 1993).

Language data gathered that are contrived (e.g., in a testing situation with discrete point

TABLE 5.2

CHARACTERISTICS OF AUTHENTIC TESTS

STRUCTURE AND LOGISTICS	GRADING AND SCORING STANDARDS
• Are more appropriately public; involve an audience, a panel, and so on.	• Involve criteria that assess essentials, not easily counted (but relatively unimportant) errors.
• Do not rely on unrealistic and arbitrary time constraints.	• Are not graded on a "curve" but in reference to performance standards (criterion-referenced, not norm-referenced).
• Offer known, not secret, questions or tasks.	
• Are more like portfolios or a season of games (not one-shot).	• Involve demystified criteria of success that appear to students as inherent in successful activity.
• Require some collaboration with others.	• Make self-assessment a part of the assessment.
• Recur—and are worth practicing for, rehearsing, and retaking.	• Use a multifaceted scoring system instead of one aggregate grade.
• Make assessment and feedback to students so central that school schedules, structures, and policies are modified to support them.	• Exhibit harmony with shared schoolwide aims a standard.

INTELLECTUAL DESIGN FEATURES	FAIRNESS AND EQUITY
• Are "essential"—not needlessly intrusive, arbitrary, or contrived to "shake out" a grade.	• Ferret out and identify (perhaps hidden) strengths.
• Are "enabling"—constructed to point the student toward more sophisticated use of the skills or knowledge.	• Strike a constantly examined balance between honoring achievement and native skill or fortunate prior training.
• Are contextualized, complex intellectual challenges, not "atomized" tasks, corresponding to isolated "outcomes."	• Minimize needless, unfair, and demoralizing comparisons.
• Involve the student's own research or use of knowledge, for which "content" is a means.	• Allow appropriate room for student learning styles, aptitudes, and interests.
• Assess student habits and repertoires, not mere recall or plug-in skills.	• Can be—should be—attempted by all students, with the test "scaffolded up," not "dumbed down," as necessary.
• Are representative challenges—designed to emphasize depth more than breadth.	• Reverse typical test-design procedures: they make "accountability" serve student learning. (Attention is primarily paid to "face" and "ecological" validity of tests.)
• Are engaging and educational.	
• Involve somewhat ambiguous ("ill-structured") tasks or problems.	

From "Teaching to the (Authentic) Test," by G. Wiggins, 1989, *Educational Leadership, 46*(7), p. 45. © 1989 by the Association for Supervision and Curriculum Development. Reprinted with permission.

testing) will be of little value in determining what type of communicator the student is in actual communication situations. The examiner should evaluate the preadolescent or adolescent across and within a variety of natural communication situations (e.g., in the classroom, at home, in sports activities) and with familiar and unfamiliar listeners. Communication styles change as a function of the situation and the listener. These changes must be taken into account during the assessment process.

DYNAMIC ASSESSMENT

Dynamic assessment, sometimes referred to as *learning potential assessment*, focuses on learning processes rather than learned products, which are the focus of traditional assessment procedures (Lidz, 1991). When the focus of assessment is on the product, no information is gathered regarding the reason(s) for failure or the individual's ability to achieve (e.g., profit from instruction and intervention).

According to Lidz (1991), there are variations in the interpretation of the dynamic assessment model. However, there are defining characteristics on which all proponents appear to agree:

1. following a test-intervene-retest format;

2. focusing on learner modifiability (i.e., assessing the amount of learner change as a response to the intervention and the learner's increased implementation of relevant metacognitive processes in problem solving);

3. providing useful information for developing intervention; and

4. documenting the intensity of intervention needed to produce change.

Examiners using dynamic assessment procedures are interested in the metacognitive processes of problem solving, as well as in the extent to which the learner's metacognitive abilities can be enhanced. However, dynamic assessment is more than a model with procedures; it also represents an attitude. According to Lidz (1991), dynamic assessors are

> convinced that children can learn if sufficient time and effort is expended to discover the means by which they can profit from intervention. Dynamic assessors are also more interested in spending this time to derive ideas for intervention rather than for placement or classification decisions. (p. 9)

Lidz (1991) goes on to summarize, "The focus of dynamic assessment is on the assessor's ability to discover the means of facilitating the learning of the child, not on the child's demonstration of ability to the assessor" (p. 9).

The theoretical underpinnings for dynamic assessment go back to Vygotsky's (1962) concept of the zone of proximal development (ZPD). "The ZPD is the difference between the child's level of performance when functioning independently and the child's level of performance when functioning in collaboration with a more knowledgeable partner. This can also be viewed as a definition of potential" (Lidz, 1991, p. 7). Three prevailing models dominate the dynamic assessment literature in English:

1. Feuerstein's (1979) *The Dynamic Assessment of Retarded Performers: The Learning*

Potential Assessment Device, Theory, Instruments, and Techniques and its intervention component *Instrumental Enrichment* (1980);

2. Campione and Brown's (1987) research approach, which attempts to standardize and quantify data and embeds assessment into academic content; and

3. Budoff's (1987) approach, which explicitly uses procedures to serve as an alternative to IQ tests in classifying children for special education.

"Like Feuerstein, and in contrast to Campione and Brown, Budoff chooses to emphasize tasks that are minimally related to academic content, preferring to assess the child's ability to profit from experience rather than demonstrate the already apparent school failure" (Lidz, 1991, p. 22). Budoff refers to his approach as *learning potential assessment.*

We have elected to use Feuerstein's (1979) *Learning Potential Assessment Device* (LPAD) approach because it is based on a theory of "structural cognitive modifiability," which involves three core concepts:

1. The learner's behavior may be characterized by a series of cognitive functions and deficiencies that are organized according to an input-elaboration-output model of the mental act.

2. The assessor's behavior is characterized in terms of the components of the mediated learning experience (e.g., the assessor might bridge a current experience to a previous experience or might attribute value and highlight the importance of

the content through voice modulation and affect).

3. The task is conceptualized in terms of a cognitive map that reveals the features that distinguish one task from another. The cognitive map comprises seven dimensions on which the mental act can be described. These dimensions are content, modality, phase of the mental act, cognitive operations, level of complexity, level of abstraction, and level of efficiency; all dimensions are part of the LPAD.

STUDENT-CENTERED ASSESSMENT

In student-centered assessment, the student directs and assesses the language/communication process along with the diagnostician. Many times, adolescents provide insights into their problems that no one else has. Many students are engaging in meta-awareness tasks such as thinking about their thinking (metacognition), using language to analyze their language (metalinguistics), and revising communication breakdowns (metacommunication), which provide important information about how students perceive their own performance. Other preadolescents and adolescents may be oblivious to their own communication disorders.

By asking for an explanation of the problem, the examiner can determine whether there are discrepancies among examination results, the adolescent's perspective, and the perspectives of persons within the educational and environmental systems. If a discrepancy exists among any of these dimensions, it may suggest the need for further evaluation, educational inservice, or family counseling.

In a student-centered assessment process, the student has the right to know about the assessment procedures to be used. The examiner should explain to the adolescent, before the evaluation procedure, what behaviors are to be assessed, how they are to be assessed, and the reason for the various procedures. By doing this, the examiner will usually find the adolescent is a more cooperative and active participant. The adolescent should be encouraged to challenge and to question what is being done. After all, who should be more interested in what is happening than the person to whom it is happening?

Likewise, in a student-centered assessment process, we strongly recommend that adolescents, in conjunction with the professionals and parents present, participate in the evaluation results and recommendations. If that is too threatening or otherwise undesirable, then separate meetings could be held with adolescents to discuss evaluation performance and its implications for their academic, social, and vocational goals.

Adolescents should be told about their strengths as well as their weaknesses. Whenever possible, examiners should illustrate how they may use strengths to overcome weaknesses. If intervention is not indicated, this interaction will provide insight into the inconsistencies in performance that the older student has probably been experiencing. If the student is scheduled for intervention, these comments can prepare him or her for such an experience.

MULTIDIMENSIONAL ASSESSMENT

Multidimensional assessment means that all aspects of the preadolescent's or adolescent's environment are assessed. The student is evaluated, but so are the school, home, and community settings.

An analysis of the student's educational and environmental systems may reveal:

- that one or both systems may be contributing to the student's language disorder;

- that one or both systems may be supportive of the student with a language disorder; or

- that one or both systems, not the student, may be the primary "problem" (i.e., the student does not have a language disorder).

To determine precisely the relationships among students and their educational and environmental systems, careful assessment procedures are needed. The next sections highlight critical factors to consider during multidimensional assessment.

Educational System

The educational system consists of a variety of professionals, but for the purpose of this chapter, the assumption is made that teachers are involved in the majority of professional interactions with older students. Five major areas of assessment need to be considered: structure of the educational system, teacher language, the teachers' and administrators' attitudes toward preadolescents and adolescents with language disorders, curriculum variables, and postsecondary education.

Structure of the Educational System

The structure of the educational system is important to assess because it indicates how flexible administrators and teachers might be when modifications to the system are proposed. Using a checklist of the following questions allows for quickly assessing the structure of the educational system. This information is helpful in pinpointing the amount of openness to change. (Some educational systems will be ready for change, while others will be resistant.)

1. Is there a willingness to implement new programs or alternative programs for older students with communication disorders?

2. Are there concerted efforts to find ways to reduce the dropout rate?

3. Are minimum competency tests required of all adolescents to graduate?

4. Is the organizational framework the same as it has been for decades (i.e., teachers teach as they were taught [lecturing, monitoring, and quizzing]; high schools continue to be horizontally structured by age group [freshmen, sophomores, juniors, seniors] and vertically organized by program track [e.g., college-bound, vocational education, special education])?

5. Is the educational system aware of the speech-language pathologist and the role this professional plays in the interdisciplinary evaluation team?

6. What are the state's and region's entrance and exit criteria for speech-language programs?

7. Do these criteria need to be revised and, if so, is there a willingness on the part of administrators to do so?

This checklist of questions will allow for better insight into the history of speech-language programs within the educational system in question; history influences planning for future changes. Likewise, those speech-language pathologists who have initiated programs in the past, and who are now in the maintenance phase, may use the checklist of questions as a summary of the current status of the educational system.

Responses to the questions should be analyzed to determine what variables within the educational system might be changed (e.g., modification of criteria for entrance and exit; an increase in the number of interdisciplinary teams to which speech-language pathologists are assigned). When armed with this information, speech-language pathologists are better able to engage in program planning and to initiate modifications in the educational system that are beneficial to older students.

Teacher Language

Assessment of teacher language in the classroom is essential to determine if modifications are necessary to meet the needs of students. The language of the classroom teacher directly and indirectly influences students' responses (Gruenewald and Pollak, 1984). Teacher language is comprised of an instructional mode (explanations/directions and questions), a syntactical mode (word order and sentence complexity), and a speaking mode (length, rate, and intonation) (Gruenewald and Pollak, 1984).

Some adolescents may find rapid speech, lengthy directions, or complex questions too difficult to process. Therefore, failure in that teacher's classroom continues until modifications are made. Assessment of the teacher's rate of speech, tone of voice, length of directions, complexity of directions, level of vocabulary, and organization of ideas, as well as the ease of listening by others, should be documented to determine where communication breakdowns occur. Is the breakdown in the teacher's messages or in the student's comprehension of those messages?

One method for evaluating the teacher's language is to use a self-evaluation technique. While teacher language might be analyzed best by speech-language pathologists, we have found that teachers who welcome such professionals into their classrooms for the purpose of evaluating their language during instruction are rare. More common reactions have been feelings of anxiety, fear, and invasion of privacy or academic freedom. Yet most teachers are interested in improving their classroom instruction, and many are receptive to self-evaluating their language if data remain confidential.

A self-evaluation form designed for use in the classroom is provided in Appendix B. Speech-language pathologists should train teachers in this technique of self-evaluation. Each student is given a response form by the teacher immediately following a 10- to 15-minute lecture or some detailed instructional situation. Teachers may also wish to complete the form from their own perspective.

Students should be assured that there are no "wrong" answers and that their answers will not influence their grade(s) for the course. The request for the student's name on the form is to encourage taking the test seriously and to discourage "silly" responses. The requirement of names is, however, at the discretion of the teacher. If there are a number of poor readers in the classroom, the teacher should read aloud the response form for all students before, or during, their completion of the form. Explanations of the characteristics of the teacher's language to be rated should be provided, whether or not students ask for them. Honesty of answers should be stressed.

Teachers should collect the forms and compute means for each item on the response form. Forms containing responses that are on the extreme low end of the rating scale should be analyzed carefully. For example, is only one student evaluating level of vocabulary as too difficult, or are a number of students reacting negatively to the difficulty level? Teachers who notice a number of students (e.g., 20 percent) assessing various aspects of their language of instruction negatively might wish to consider modifications in their language.

It is particularly helpful for a teacher to use the self-evaluation technique when a student in his or her classroom has been referred for testing for a suspected communication disorder. This self-evaluation will allow a comparison of that student's perception of the teacher's language with the perceptions of peers in the classroom. Is the referred student unique in responses on the form? Were the responses primarily negative? If they were, the teacher's language within that particular course may be problematic for the student.

Teachers' and Administrators' Attitudes

Assessment of teachers' and administrators' attitudes toward speech-language services, and especially toward preadolescents and adolescents with communication disorders, is important. Specifically, attitudes should be assessed regarding the speech-language delivery models for middle-grade and secondary students; communication disorders within adolescents; and teacher and curriculum modifications for students with disabilities. When the attitudes of a teacher or an administrator are consistently and resoundingly negative, speech-language pathologists could select from any or all of these alternatives:

1. attempt to change educators' attitudes through information dissemination activities;

2. advocate placing students with teachers who have expressed positive attitudes; and/or

3. counsel students to cope with educators holding negative attitudes.

Assessment data on attitudes are useful when determining the course of intervention for a particular student. If the identified problem is within the preadolescent or adolescent, then the speech-language pathologist should advocate, whenever possible, to schedule the student with teachers who have the best attitudes toward disabilities and toward appropriate modifications that might be needed in their classrooms. If the identified problem is not within the adolescent but lies within the

educational system, attitudinal data may help to document why the problem has its roots in the system.

Measurement of teachers' and administrators' attitudes toward adolescents with communication disorders may be accomplished through an attitudinal scale. Several attitudinal scales toward disabilities have been developed previously; these scales are designed to be used at the university level by faculty (Fonosch and Schwab, 1981; Morris, Leuenberger, and Aksamit, 1985). In 1987, Larson and McKinley designed an attitudinal scale to be used by speech-language pathologists in junior and senior high schools. This scale is included in Appendix C.

Curriculum Variables

The types of curriculum variables that might be interfering with a student's academic success constitute another area to be assessed within the educational system. Several of the curriculum variables to be considered are these:

1. **Comprehension of spoken information:** Is the older student having difficulty understanding what is said in many different situations or primarily in one course? What is the nature of the comprehension problem?

2. **Organization of the course:** Is the course organized sequentially (i.e., little interaction among units [e.g., one topic is "geology" and the next is "electricity"]) or in a spiral fashion (major interaction among units [e.g., parts of speech are taught to provide the background for

sentence diagramming])? If the course is organized sequentially, have all units been problematic for the preadolescent or adolescent, or only some?

3. **Requirements in the course:** Does the course demand significantly different requirements than other courses in which the student is not struggling (e.g., excessive reading, lengthy term papers, or public speaking)?

4. **Textbook and tests in the course:** Is the readability of the textbook appropriate for the preadolescent or adolescent? Is it organized like other texts that the student is using? Are the course tests significantly different from those in other courses (e.g., essay questions or objective questions that demand synthesis of information)?

Examiners should keep in mind that it is plausible that several problems will be identified. The student might be having difficulty in a course because of an underlying language disorder, but at the same time there may be problems in the curriculum (e.g., the readability of the text is not at grade level; the course has spiral organization and the student has been "lost" for months, even years). It should also be considered whether negative attitude and poor motivation are contributing factors to the student's failure in the course.

One method of assessing the curriculum is through the use of a curriculum analysis form (see Appendix D). The intent of the curriculum analysis form is not that it be completed for every student undergoing assessment for every content area. Rather, the form should

be completed whenever one or two subject or content areas are particularly troublesome to the student undergoing an initial assessment. Completion of the curriculum analysis form would help to locate the problem (i.e., within the adolescent and/or educational system). This is necessary for appropriate program planning.

The curriculum analysis form may be especially helpful once older students with language disorders begin intervention. The form then serves as an organized, coherent approach to studying the older student's abilities within existing curricula. The form may also serve as a referent for needed modifications in the classroom if a consultation model is used.

Alternative procedures for curriculum assessment are these:

- *Handbook for Evaluating and Selecting Curricula Materials* (Gall, 1981);

- *Language Interaction in Teaching and Learning* (Gruenewald and Pollak, 1984);

- curriculum-based language assessment and intervention (Nelson, 1989, 1992);

- *Classroom Script Analysis* (Creaghead, 1992); and

- *Descriptive Assessment of Writing* (Scott and Erwin, 1992).

Postsecondary Education

Measuring the academic performance of the postsecondary student with a language disorder is an essential component of the educational process in universities and colleges including vocational technical colleges. It is true that taking a test under typical standard conditions (usually written timed tests) requires certain skills apart from those areas being assessed on the test (Heath Resource Center, 1985). The speech-language pathologist should simulate the assessment situations in which the student is likely to be placed within the postsecondary environment. Students need to be assessed under "typical" conditions likely to be found in postsecondary settings; then an analysis should be conducted and interpretation presented so that students understand what their strengths and weaknesses are within a standard test-taking format.

Students whose situations fall under Section 504 of the Rehabilitation Act of 1973 have the right to request adaptations to the testing situation. For example, if the student has a severe speech disorder, written examinations might be substituted for oral recitation exams. The student may write responses for oral recitation and have that presentation read by an interpreter. If the student has a language disorder and is easily distracted, then the student may request that the test be given individually in a quiet room without distractions. If writing is difficult, then the student may arrange for alternate methods of recording answers, such as taping the responses or typing them.

Thus, the student may need a different test environment, the presence of exam proctors, and/or additional test time. Whatever the adaptation needed based upon analysis of the situation, it is critical that the student and educators know that adaptation does not mean changing or lowering standards for the course or admission requirements.

Environmental System

Evaluating the environmental system consists of assessing the family system, the peer group to which the older student belongs, and the employment setting. Examination of all these areas is critical to determine if the preadolescent or adolescent has a language disability.

Family System

Examiners assessing the environmental system should realize that the American "family" has changed dramatically over the past decades. Before the 19th century, most activities revolved around the family, and parents were responsible for educating their own children. The economy was agrarian, and all family members (which usually included extended family members) worked to sustain the unit.

The Industrial Revolution brought profound changes, such as families moving from farms to cities, and women entering the workforce (Simpson, 1982). As a result of these two changes, urban families, unlike rural families, decreased their contacts with extended family members. Attitudes, values, and beliefs about the family unit changed. Also, with women in the workforce, less of their time was spent with family members. As a result, children began to spend more time without parental supervision; thus, the peer group and the educational system began to assume a stronger role in attitude and value formation.

Since World War II, monumental changes in the American family have occurred. The American family of father and mother and 2.5 children, more than ever, does not exist. It is important for the examiner to know about the preadolescent's or adolescent's family situation because it provides the foundation for language and communication. Major purposes for assessing the family unit are these:

1. to understand the family members' perceptions of the older student's communication disorder, or suspected disorder, including past history and future goals;

2. to gather information on feelings and attitudes of family members toward the preadolescent or adolescent with a communication disorder and toward the educational system; this may indicate how supportive and tolerant the environment is of disabilities and how amiable the relationship has been between the environmental and educational systems; and

3. to obtain information about the family's communication style; this permits speech-language pathologists to determine if a language difference exists.

Data obtained from the family regarding previous speech-language services and the importance of improving speaking, listening, and thinking should be compared with the preadolescent's or adolescent's responses for agreement. Data should also be gathered from families to address these issues:

1. Do the family members feel that a problem exists, or do they feel that the school or someone else is fabricating the problem?

2. If the family members feel a communication disorder exists, is it a primary or secondary concern?

3. If they feel that a problem exists, do they feel frustrated, embarrassed, guilty, and ashamed, or are they accepting of the adolescent's communication?

4. How does or doesn't the family attempt to cope with the child with a communication disorder (e.g., by talking for the adolescent, by excluding the preadolescent from the mainstream of family life and decision making, by ignoring the disorder)?

5. What are the goals and expectations of the family for the preadolescent or adolescent with a communication disorder or a suspected disorder? Are they realistic?

In addition, the examiner should investigate the family's attitudes toward students with communication disorders, and toward educational services and professionals providing services. By evaluating the parents' attitudes toward issues such as the value of good communication, the examiner can determine if there is a mismatch between familial or cultural expectations and professional or educational system expectations.

Attitudes and feelings of families may change over time. Family members of adolescents being assessed may have experienced many years of professionals trying to help, and still the youth may have problems. As adolescents grow older, parental involvement usually lessens, but not parental concern. For example, parental pressures may not result in the adolescent's willingness to be evaluated, even though the parents are concerned about their child's progress. Parents may become frustrated, anxious, guilty, exhausted, and more negative toward their child and/or the educational system. Parents/caregivers may need to sort through their feelings toward the educational system or professionals with whom they have interacted.

Particularly if the interaction has not been pleasant, family members should be given the opportunity to express their feelings and attitudes during the assessment process without value judgments from involved professionals. Families may be resentful of the educational system if they have experienced frustration in getting necessary services in the past, or if professionals have not followed through with their commitments. These feelings should be allowed to be freely expressed, and in addition, families should be assured that the educational system's goal is to provide the most appropriate services for their children.

Determining the family's communication style/behaviors is important in evaluating whether the older student has a communication disorder or difference. If the older student's communication style is similar to that of other family members, probably a communication difference, and not a disorder, is present. This decision is complicated when English is not the primary language spoken in the preadolescent's or adolescent's home. Communication style must be assessed from the perspective of the first language in the family, even if that language is not English. Through the use of an interpreter, the examiner should determine whether the older student understands and produces the primary language similarly to other family members who are approximately the same age or older.

Peer Group Members

It is important to obtain the peer group members' perceptions of the preadolescent's or adolescent's communication behavior and to determine whether they have difficulty understanding the individual. Peers' feelings and attitudes toward the preadolescent's or adolescent's communication should also be evaluated. If they feel a problem exists, are they teasing, rejecting, or accepting the person as a friend or a member of the group? Do they avoid talking or listening to the individual with a communication disorder? What is most disturbing to them about their peer's communication? Answers to these questions will help to document the amount of social isolation the student being assessed may or may not be experiencing.

In addition, the peers' communication styles should be assessed to determine the normal communication behaviors for this age group. By analyzing the peers' communication styles, the examiner can determine how the peers may be requiring the youth being assessed to comprehend or produce social-interactive language (e.g., idiomatic expressions, slang).

The procedures used to assess the family and peer members' perceptions of the preadolescent or adolescent, their feelings and attitudes, and their communication styles involve a combination of interviewing, observing, and recording behaviors (Larson and McKinley, 1987). Interviewing is a directed conversation in which the examiner seeks to get information and to give information that will be helpful to the student and others in the student's environment in solving or preventing problems. The observing and recording of behaviors should document communication styles of family members and peers. As discussed previously, if family members or peers and the youth being assessed speak similarly, the problem may not be a communication disorder but a communication difference, and should be evaluated accordingly.

Employment Setting

As older students with language disorders graduate from school and plan to enter the workforce, the transition could be easier on everyone if students are assessed to determine whether they have the ability to enter the workplace. Table 5.3 summarizes a series of employability skills that were found to be needed for an individual to be successful within the workplace. Stemmer, Brown, and Smith (1992) have developed a portfolio assessment model using the skills in Table 5.3 as indicators to recognize successes, to seek opportunities to fill gaps in skill areas needed for employment, and to assist the student in gaining confidence in preparing for work.

Of the employability skills listed in Table 5.3, the speech-language pathologist should carefully assess the student's ability to speak and write in the language needed for the business setting in which the student desires employment. Can the student engage in basic problem-solving skills? Can the student follow written and oral instructions? Can the student listen to other employees and attempt to accommodate their suggestions? This means that the speech-language pathologist will need to talk with the human resource person or personnel director in the company to determine the communication and problem-solving skills required to do the job. At the same time, accommodations under the Americans with Disabilities Act that might be made for the youth can be discussed.

MULTICULTURAL ISSUES IN ASSESSMENT

As cited in Chapter 3, there will be ever-increasing numbers of bilingual and multicultural children in the United States by the year 2000 and beyond. Changing demographics must be taken into account when establishing assessment procedures. Speech-language pathologists must be sensitive to related legal issues, and the cultural and linguistic factors require that a wide array of assessment procedures be used when assessing minority students.

The speech-language pathologist must be aware of the legal mandates for service to linguistically and culturally different students. The legal bases for assessment of linguistically and culturally different clients "reside in Section 504 of the Rehabilitation Act of 1973 (29 USC 794 et seq.), in Title VI of the Civil Rights Act of 1964 (20 USC 200d et seq.), and in PL 94-142 (20 USC 1401 et seq.)" (Carpenter, 1990, p. 72). Collectively, these legal mandates require nondiscriminatory practices. The examiner cannot discriminate on the basis of race, national origin, or handicap if receiving federal funds. Furthermore, assessment materials and procedures must

TABLE 5.3

EMPLOYMENT SKILLS PROFILE

ACADEMIC SKILLS	PERSONAL MANAGEMENT SKILLS	TEAMWORK SKILLS
• Read and understand written materials	• Attend school/work daily and on time	• Actively participate in a group
• Understand charts and graphs	• Meet school/work deadlines	• Know the group's rules and values
• Understand basic math	• Develop career plans	• Listen to other group members
• Use mathematics to solve problems	• Know personal strengths and weaknesses	• Express ideas to other group members
• Use research and library skills	• Demonstrate self-control	• Be sensitive to the group members' ideas and views
• Use specialized knowledge and skills to get a job done	• Pay attention to details	• Be willing to compromise if necessary to best accomplish the goal
• Use tools and equipment	• Follow written and oral instructions	
• Speak in the language in which business is conducted	• Follow written and oral directions	• Be a leader or a follower to best accomplish the goal
• Write in the language in which business is conducted	• Work without supervision	• Work in changing settings and with people of differing backgrounds
• Use scientific method to solve problems	• Learn new skills	
	• Identify and suggest new ways to get the job done	

From "The Employability Skills Profile," by P. Stemmer, B. Brown, and C. Smith, 1992, *Educational Leadership, 49,* p. 33. © 1992 by the Association for Supervision and Curriculum Development. Reprinted with permission.

not be racially and culturally discriminatory and must be administered in the language or mode of communication in which the client is most proficient.

The Committee on the Status of Racial Minorities (1983) has stated, "no dialectal variety of English is a disorder or a pathological form of speech or language" (p. 23). Thus, some students will have communication differences and not disorders. *Communication differences* are defined as communication behaviors that meet the norms of the primary linguistic community but that do not meet the norms of standard English. It is possible, though, for dialectal speakers to have speech and language disorders within the native language. To determine if the adolescent has a dialectal difference or a communication disorder, speech-language pathologists must have the following competencies (Cole, 1983):

1. knowledge of the particular dialect as a rule-governed linguistic system;

2. knowledge of nondiscriminatory testing procedures;

3. knowledge of the phonological and grammatical features of the dialect;

4. knowledge of contrastive analysis procedures;

5. knowledge of the effects of attitudes toward dialects; and

6. thorough understanding and appreciation for the community and culture of the nonstandard speaker. (p. 25)

The purposes of assessment with linguistically and culturally different children are (1) to determine if academic difficulties, inappropriate personal-social interactions, or limited vocational potential are due to a language disorder or a language difference, and (2) to determine if instructional programming is needed and, if so, what programming is the most appropriate. To accomplish these two purposes, examiners must engage in bias-free assessment (Chamberlain and Medinos-Landurand, 1991) by:

• increasing their knowledge and awareness about students with different cultural and linguistic backgrounds;

• determining the student's level of acculturation;

• determining how to control for cultural variables that interfere with testing outcomes;

• determining the language to be used in testing;

• knowing when an interpreter is needed and whom to use as an interpreter; and

• being aware of problems resulting from the examiner's cultural insensitivity, such as miscommunication attempts, cross-cultural stereotyping, misperceptions, and not understanding that some cultures are based on cooperation and collaboration, not competition.

According to Bernstein (1989), "appropriate identification and assessment of bilingual/bicultural children require: (1) the use of appropriate assessment instruments and techniques, and (2) the use of appropriate personnel in the assessment process" (p. 16). She goes on to note that when using standardized tests with these students, the tests need to have certain characteristics (i.e., they should have a solid theoretical underpinning, be valid and reliable, and be standardized on the population for which the test will be used). These are also appropriate criteria for monolingual students. Whenever possible, the examiner should use a naturalistic assessment approach (i.e., informal procedures that allow the speech-language pathologist to describe specifically the communication behaviors of the student across and within a wide array of communication situations).

Bernstein (1989) also confronts the need to use appropriate personnel in the assessment process. Federal law mandates that the abilities of limited English proficient (LEP) children be assessed in their native tongue. Since very few speech-language pathologists are bilingual, and even those who are may not be proficient in the language of a particular student, it is necessary to implement this federal mandate by applying several alternative approaches to using linguistically qualified personnel. Bernstein recommends using a trained interpreter/native speaker during the assessment process so that the assessment materials and procedures are as culturally and linguistically relevant as possible.

Another approach recommended by Bernstein (1989) is to use bilingual teacher aides. The advantage to this approach is, again, that the aide is familiar with the student's cultural/linguistic background. The disadvantage is that it takes the aide away from instructional tasks that he or she has been hired to do, and thus some educators may resist the aide being used in this way. Likewise, some aides may find it difficult to shift roles between being part of the assessment process and assisting with intervention procedures.

Another approach, recommended by Bernstein (1989) when trained interpreters and bilingual aides are not available, is to use a family member (i.e., parent or sibling) to act as the interpreter. The approach appears to work best when using a more informal assessment procedure and in a more naturalistic setting than when using standardized procedures (i.e., formal tests).

In summary, Bernstein (1989) captured it well when she said:

> Until such time as skilled speech-language pathologists and audiologists who are competent foreign language users become available, the needs of the estimated 3.5 million linguistic minority persons in the United States who have speech, language, and hearing disorders must be met by culturally sensitive professionals who can train and integrate others into the assessment process. (p. 20)

SUMMARY

This chapter presented a definition of the assessment process. It outlined a comprehensive, six-faceted model of assessment as a functional, descriptive, authentic, dynamic, student-centered, and multidimensional process. The multidimensional aspect of assessment encompasses the evaluation of the older student's educational and environmental systems. This broad-based approach to assessment is important, because students with suspected language disorders must function in school, home, and community settings. In some instances, the primary problem may lie not within the student but within an educational system that is disorganized or inflexible in adapting to students' needs. In other cases, the primary "problem" may be a language difference, which is observed in the family, and not a language disorder.

Students who have been identified as having language disorders may have their communication difficulties exacerbated by factors within their educational and environmental systems. For example, teacher directions might be too long and complex to comprehend and, thus, the student is at even greater risk for academic failure. Maybe the youth's peers interact only by teasing or withdrawing. Perhaps an older youth has difficulty getting employed because of poor verbal interaction skills. Ultimately, these factors, noted during the assessment process, will enter into the overall intervention plan for the preadolescent or adolescent.

Various multicultural issues need to be considered throughout the assessment process. Examiners must be alert to language differences and aware of culturally biased assessment procedures. Trained interpreters are frequently necessary when English is not the student's primary language.

DISCUSSION QUESTIONS

1. Discuss the holistic assessment model proposed and how you would implement this assessment model in evaluating older students.

2. What multicultural issues arise when assessing the communication behaviors of bilingual students versus students with dialectal differences?

SUGGESTED READINGS

Damico, J. (1993). Language assessment in adolescents: Addressing critical issues. *Language, Speech, and Hearing Services in Schools*, 24(1), pp. 29–35.

Lidz, C. (1991). *Practitioner's guide to dynamic assessment*. New York: Guilford Press.

ASSESSMENT: SPECIFIC BEHAVIORS AND PROCEDURES

6

GOALS:

To list what behaviors to assess

To discuss how to assess cognitive-communication behaviors using informal procedures

To summarize formal assessment instruments that might be used with older students

This chapter focuses on the following aspects within the preadolescent or adolescent who is in an early, middle, or late stage of development: history, learning style, cognition, comprehension and production of linguistic features, discourse (conversations and narrations), written communication, meta-abilities, nonverbal communication, and survival language skills. Assessment of these aspects can be accomplished through use of a case history form and through formal and informal testing procedures.

Before describing how to assess the preadolescent or adolescent, a description of what to evaluate is presented. An overview of the direct assessment of the preadolescent and adolescent is illustrated in Table 6.1.

WHAT TO ASSESS

HISTORY

Relevant data on the older student's history, current status, and future goals should be obtained during the initial part of the evaluation process. Only in this way can an accurate assessment battery be planned.

The examiner should obtain information about the student's environmental, educational, vocational, and health histories. As previously stated, an environmental history should be accumulated on family members and peers. An educational and vocational history should

TABLE 6.1	DIRECT ASSESSMENT	
WHO?	**WHAT?**	**HOW?**

Preadolescents
Adolescents
    Early
    Middle
    Late
	History
	Learning style
	Cognition
	Comprehension and
	    production of linguistic
	    features
	Discourse
	Written communication
	Meta-abilities
	Nonverbal communication
	Survival language skills
		INFORMAL ASSESSMENT PROCEDURES
		(administration, analysis,
		interpretation)
		  A. Case history form
		  B. Learning style questionnaire
		  C. Portfolios
		  D. Discourse samples
		     1. Conversations
		     2. Narrations
		  E. Directed tasks
		
		FORMAL ASSESSMENT INSTRUMENTS
		(administration, analysis,
		interpretation)

be gathered to document specific strengths and weaknesses in academic subject areas and current and future vocational goals. Relevant health data that might affect performance should be collected (e.g., past and present medications, allergies, seizures). Irrelevant data collection should be avoided (e.g., the age the student first walked, the age at which the student was toilet trained, etc.). However, any records of past speech, hearing, and language services should be reviewed, regardless of the age of the student when services were received.

Another critical area to investigate is feelings and attitudes toward current thinking, listening, and speaking abilities, and the willingness to modify these abilities. This investigation will reveal the student's perspective of the suspected communication problem. It will also assist in documenting metacognition, metalinguistic, and metacommunication awareness.

Feelings and Attitudes Toward Thinking

Feuerstein (1980) emphasized that adverse affective-motivational factors can result in deficient cognitive functioning. Furthermore, negative attitude may affect general involvement with cognitive tasks that are demanded in academic and real-life situations.

Learned helplessness describes the phenomenon of individuals who, when faced with a problem, act helplessly. Youth with learned helplessness view outcomes as uncontrollable. Other effects of learned helplessness are passivity, negative beliefs about oneself, severe reduction in persistence, and depression (Greer and Wethered, 1984). Older students with learned helplessness have no strategies, or ineffective ones, for solving problems, and they perceive few alternatives. By high school, they have made so many mistakes and have failed so often that they mistrust their own thinking. Thus, students who could have intact cognitive functions believe they cannot think and, therefore, they do not.

Feelings and Attitudes Toward Listening

Feelings and attitudes toward listening may be influenced by the following barriers: calling the subject dull; criticizing the speaker's looks, actions, or speaking style; getting over-stimulated and emotionally involved; listening for isolated facts; outlining everything; wasting the extra time available between normal speaking speed (175 wpm) and thinking speed (450 wpm); listening only to what is easy to understand; allowing personal prejudices and biases to impair understanding; letting emotionally laden words get in the way; and allowing distractions to interfere (Nichols and Stevens, 1957).

In addition to asking older students about their listening, the examiner should investigate whether they have any misconceptions about listening that may interfere with their learning to be a better listener. Wolff et al. (1983) summarized 10 major misconceptions about listening:

1. *Listening is a matter of intelligence.* Intelligence is not a criterion for listening, and there appears to be no strong relationship between intelligence and efficient listening. Efficient listening is more a result of training.

2. *Good hearing and good listening are closely related.* Although there is a relationship between hearing and listening, good hearing does not guarantee good listening. Hearing is a physical activity, whereas listening is a mental activity.

3. *Listening is an automatic reflex.* Listening is not an innate skill, but one that is learned.

4. *Daily practice eliminates the need for training in listening.* Practice does not necessarily mean a skill becomes better, especially if it is not practiced correctly. Therefore, to be a better listener, one must be trained to practice the skill correctly.

5. *Learning to read will automatically improve listening.* This is a false assumption, since the two activities place different demands on the individual. Listening may actually be a more difficult activity because a listener cannot reread a passage and thus cannot control the rate of the message as one can in reading.

6. *Learning to read is more important than learning to listen.* Wolff et al. (1983) argue that this is not true, since most people listen three times more than they read.

7. *The speaker is totally responsible for success in oral communication.* Successful communication is a 50/50 proposition. Equal importance must be given to the role of listening, and listeners should not assume that the speaker is 100 percent responsible for successful oral communication.

8. *Listening is essentially a passive activity.* This is an erroneous assumption, since

the only way successful communication can occur is if the listener is actively engaged in the process.

9. *Listening means agreement.* Good listeners do not necessarily agree with the speaker, but they listen first and then agree or disagree as a result of listening to what the speaker has to say.

10. *Consequences of careless listening are minimal.* This is a misconception, since careless listening can be time consuming, costly, and socially destructive.

Professionals must examine the student's listening habits and determine whether the adolescent holds any of these misconceptions about listening. By realizing that these beliefs are erroneous, more efficient and effective listening abilities can be developed.

Feelings and Attitudes Toward Speaking

The feelings and attitudes of older students toward their oral language production can reveal their awareness of communication, their ability to take another's perspective, and their motivation to change behaviors. Preadolescents and adolescents may be marginal communicators who have a "defective" attitude toward communication, but who may not qualify for speech-language services (Blue, 1975). Marginal communicators do not initiate conversation; they respond with minimal, faint but intelligible utterances in a one-to-one situation. For these students, the assessment procedure will need to determine if it is their attitude toward communication that is defective, or their communication system, or both.

Attitudes and feelings about speaking may differ, contingent upon the listener (e.g., a friend, a group of peers, a teacher) and upon the setting (e.g., school, home). Therefore, the professional should explore both the student's general feelings and attitudes toward his or her own communication, as well as variations that occur during specific communicative contexts.

LEARNING STYLE

It is important to obtain data on how preadolescents and adolescents learn certain tasks best. These data can then assist them to use their strengths to overcome their weaknesses and thus be more successful in school or on a job. Some of the factors to investigate that might affect how the student learns a new or difficult subject are:

1. the best time of day to learn a task (e.g., morning, afternoon, evening);

2. the level of noise in the room (e.g., quiet, music, radio or TV, conversation);

3. the level of light in the room (e.g., dim, moderate, or bright);

4. the temperature in the room (e.g., cold, warm, or very warm);

5. the presence or absence of food or drink intake;

6. the best place to learn (e.g., home, school, library);

7. the best location to learn (e.g., desk, floor, sitting, reclining);

8. the reasons that motivate the adolescent to complete a task (e.g., I want to;

My parents expect/want me to; I get money); and

9. the desire to work alone or with other people.

In addition to these factors, the professional should investigate the student's strategy for learning materials presented via lectures or textbooks, inside the classroom as well as outside the classroom. Collectively, this information can be analyzed to determine how the individual learns best in school and home, and it should be shared with teachers and parents. Obtaining this information may also provide older students with some insight into their own behaviors, and thus increase their awareness levels and their willingness to change their attitudes toward learning new tasks.

COGNITION

While literature on teaching cognitive strategies and thinking skills is rapidly expanding (Greenberg, 1990; Hallahan, 1980; Hayes, 1981; Kriegler and van Niekerk, 1993; Lochhead and Clement, 1979; Maxwell, 1983; Parrill-Burnstein, 1981), there has been no corresponding surge in literature addressing the assessment of cognition. Although most speech-language pathologists would agree that it is important to assess cognition, the specific behaviors evaluated remain dictated, in large part, by the few commercial tests available. Therefore, it is important to have a clear idea of what to assess about cognition, and then to select a method by which that information can be obtained (e.g., observation, informal assessment, standardized testing). Too often in cognitive assessment, this proce-

dure has been reversed. In other words, a test is administered and then analyzed for the cognitive functions that were required. This method can result in piecemeal information regarding cognition.

As with any assessment, examiners can look for functions that are present and intact, or they can look for functions that are weak, deficient, or absent. Ideally, both methods are used, and a pattern of strengths and weaknesses surfaces. The cognitive functions in the input, output, and elaboration phases have proven to be an effective guide for what to assess during preadolescence and adolescence (Feuerstein, 1979). The input phase involves gathering needed information; the elaboration phase involves using the information that was gathered; the output phase involves expressing the solution to a problem.

A cognitive function that is consistently applied across a variety of contexts is a strength for that adolescent. Cognitive functions may be deficient if they do not appear spontaneously, regularly, and predictably in an individual's behavior. Deficient cognitive functions can provide a method for profiling weaknesses within adolescents.

Cognitive functions that should be assessed are taken from Feuerstein (1979) and are listed in Table 6.2. The interaction of language and cognition becomes obvious when the list of cognitive functions is examined. Many language disorders present during adolescence have underlying cognitive deficits. Professionals should be concerned not only with which cognitive functions are intact or deficient during assessment, but also with the student's awareness of these functions (i.e.,

TABLE 6.2	COGNITIVE FUNCTIONS	
INPUT PHASE	**ELABORATION PHASE**	**OUTPUT PHASE**
CLEAR PERCEPTION Is the student using senses (e.g., hearing, seeing) to gather clear and complete information?	**ANALYZING DISEQUILIBRIUM** Can the student define problems and determine what needs to be done?	**OVERCOMING EGOCENTRIC COMMUNICATION** Is the student being clear and precise in language so that the listener understands the message?
SYSTEMATIC EXPLORATION Is a plan being used so that important information is not being skipped or missed?	**RELEVANCE** Is the student using only the information that is relevant to the problem and ignoring the rest?	**OVERCOMING TRIAL AND ERROR** Is the student thinking through the response instead of immediately trying to answer and making a mistake?
LABELING Is the student consistently naming objects and events so that they can be remembered and talked about clearly?	**INTERIORIZATION** Does the student form "good pictures in the mind" about what must be done to solve the problem?	**RESTRAINING IMPULSIVE BEHAVIOR** Is restraint being used before saying or doing something that will be regretted later?
TEMPORAL AND SPATIAL REFERENTS Are events and objects being described in terms of where and when they occur?	**PLANNING BEHAVIOR** Is the student making a plan that includes steps needed to reach a goal?	**OVERCOMING BLOCKING** Is a strategy being used to help find answers rather than panicking when stuck on a problem?
CONSERVATION/OBJECT PERMANENCY Are characteristics of objects and events recognized as the same even when changes take place? (E.g., Is a square tilted onto its corner still recognized as a square?)	**BROADENING THE MENTAL FIELD** Are the various pieces of information needed to solve the problem being remembered?	
USING TWO SOURCES OF INFORMATION Can the student organize information by several characteristics simultaneously (e.g., by date and time of day; by size and by shape)?	**PROJECTING RELATIONSHIPS** Is the student looking for relationships by which separate objects, events, and experiences can be tied together? (E.g., A flat tire, a sick child, and an overdrawn checkbook have made my mother very upset today; therefore, this is not the time to ask for a new jacket.)	
NEED FOR PRECISION Does the student know when and how to be precise and accurate (e.g., when reporting data about an emergency to the appropriate authorities)?	**COMPARATIVE BEHAVIOR** Are objects and experiences being compared to others to determine what is similar and what is different?	
	CATEGORIZATION Is the student finding the class or set to which new objects or experiences belong?	
	HYPOTHETICAL THINKING Is the student thinking about different alternatives and what would happen if one or another were chosen?	
	LOGICAL EVIDENCE Is logic being used to prove answers and to defend opinions?	

metacognition). Feuerstein (1980) contends that a greater awareness of cognitive functions produces more control over applying those functions when appropriate situations present themselves.

COMPREHENSION AND PRODUCTION OF LINGUISTIC FEATURES

A select number of linguistic features should be assessed in the older student with a suspected language disorder. In addition, the examiner should assess the student's ability to engage in a variety of informational listening tasks (Boyce and Larson, 1983). Informational listening requires the ability to listen for main ideas and significant details, and to listen for oral directions or a sequence of events. This type of listening also assumes the ability to identify and to recall main ideas, and to take notes on orally presented information. Table 6.3 presents questions to be answered concerning linguistic features and informational listening abilities.

Arwood (1983) argued against looking at comprehension of linguistic features in isolation from the speech act, because professionals

---

TABLE 6.3

COMPREHENSION AND PRODUCTION OF LINGUISTIC FEATURES

COMPREHENSION OF LINGUISTIC FEATURES

LINGUISTIC FEATURES	INFORMATIONAL LISTENING
• Can the student identify morphological structures, such as compound words, prefixes, and suffixes?	• Does the student comprehend factual information (e.g., directions and dates)?
• Can the student differentiate grammatical phrases, clauses, and sentences as incorrect or incomplete?	• Does the student concentrate attention on the speaker?
• Can the student comprehend various sentence trans-formations?	• Does the student use advantageously the time differential between thinking and speaking speed (i.e., people think) 2½ times faster than they listen)?
• Can the student comprehend sentences of various lengths and complexity?	• Does the student understand and differentiate between main ideas and supportive details?
• Can the student comprehend various semantic features (e.g., multiple-meaning words, verbal analogies, inclusion-exclusion, idioms)?	• Does the student formulate questions of clarification?

PRODUCTION OF LINGUISTIC FEATURES

• Does the student use simple and complex sentences?	• Does the student use figurative language such as slang, jargon, idioms, metaphors, similes, and language for the purpose of entertainment or humor?
• Does the student use appropriate sentence fragments (e.g., a response of "eleven o'clock" to the question, "What time will you be home tonight?")?	• Does the student avoid overuse of nonspecific language such as low-information words (e.g., *things, stuff, everybody*)? When requested to do so, can the student rephrase, using more specific language?
• Does the student avoid an excessive number of run-on sentences that are strung together with *and* or *and then*?	• Does the student display few, if any, word-retrieval problems?
• Does the student use a variety of question forms, such as wh-questions, tag questions, interrogative reversals, and questions marked by rising intonation?	

may end up assessing products rather than processes. To determine, for example, that a student does not understand comparative adjectives tells the examiner nothing about why comprehension is absent or what effect this has on the speech act. While it is important to assess the student's ability to comprehend language features, examiners cannot lose sight of the reason for doing so (i.e., to determine the impact upon communication). In the second half of this chapter, authentic and functional directed tasks are provided for assessing linguistic features.

Production of linguistic features must also be considered during assessment. Unlike younger children who may have extremely limited output, older students generally have a production repertoire, albeit inefficient and often redundant. For example, they may start the majority of their question forms with "what," using a variety of forms (e.g., "What time" rather than "when"). Thus, when assessing production features, focus is on the flexibility of the language system. How much variation is used? Are complex sentences used, or just simple sentences? Is figurative language used? Can the student clarify the meaning of nonspecific words?

DISCOURSE

During assessment of discourse, specific aspects of conversations and narrations need to be analyzed: cohesion devices, critical listening, communication functions, and verbal mazes. Table 6.4 summarizes the discourse parameters that should be assessed in the older student and they are also described next:

1. *Cohesion Devices*—Cohesion devices should be analyzed to determine whether they contribute to or disrupt the continuity of meaning in the conversation or narration. Cohesive devices that contribute to continuity are the referent (i.e., a word whose meaning is apparent from the context), the conjunction (i.e., a linking word whose meaning is appropriate to the words being linked), and the ellipsis (i.e., a redundant word or words that are eliminated from the context but can be determined). Disruptive cohesion devices are referent errors (i.e., using a word to refer to elements that are absent from the context), conjunction errors (i.e., using linking words that are inappropriate to the context), and ellipsis errors (i.e., eliminating elements whose referents cannot be determined from the context).

2. *Critical Listening*—Critical listening is essential to the older student's comprehension during discourse. A critical listener must be a critical thinker (i.e., capable of engaging in higher-level thought when required by the situation).

3. *Communication Functions*—Communication functions have been described by a variety of taxonomies (Austin, 1962; Chapman, 1972, 1981; Dore, 1974, 1975; Greenfield and Smith, 1976; Halliday, 1975; Hymes, 1972; Searle, 1965). The system for the older student population to which we adhere was extrapolated from the work of Austin (1962), Searle (1965), and Hymes (1972).

TABLE 6.4

DISCOURSE PARAMETERS THAT APPLY TO CONVERSATIONS AND NARRATIONS

COHESION DEVICES	COMMUNICATION FUNCTIONS
• Does the student use cohesion devices that contribute to the continuity of meaning in the conversation or narration? • Does the student use cohesion devices in a way that avoids the disruption of continuity?	• To what extent does the student give information? • To what extent does the student get information (i.e., ask questions)? • To what extent does the student describe an ongoing event? • To what extent does the student get the listener to do, believe, or feel something (i.e., persuade)? • To what extent does the student express his or her own intentions, beliefs, and feelings (i.e., practice self-disclosure)? • To what extent does the student indicate a readiness for further communication? • To what extent does the student use language to solve problems? • To what extent does the student use language to entertain?
CRITICAL LISTENING	
• Does the student identify and recognize the credibility of the source or speaker? • Does the student recognize and use inductive and deductive reasoning? • Does the student detect false reasoning (e.g., does he or she discriminate between fact and opinion)? • Does the student recognize propaganda devices (e.g., loaded words)? • Does the student draw inferences and judge statements heard?	**VERBAL MAZES**
	• Does the student avoid an excessive amount of verbal mazes that interfere with communication? • Does the student avoid an excessive amount of false starts that interfere with communication?

The taxonomies developed by Austin (1962) and Searle (1965) were primarily designed to analyze adult speech acts, whereas the taxonomies developed by Halliday (1975) and Dore (1974) were created to analyze child-based speech acts. Searle (1965) refined Austin's (1962) classification system and proposed this taxonomy: representatives (i.e., statements that convey a belief or disbelief in an idea), directives (i.e., attempts to influence the listener to do something), commissives (i.e., commitments of self to some future course of action), expressives (i.e., expression of a psychological state, such as "thank you"), and declaratives (i.e., statements of facts that presume to alter a state of affairs, such as "I confer upon you").

Our extrapolated taxonomy includes eight functions (Boyce and Larson, 1983). All eight functions should be present within the language of the preadolescent and adolescent. The eight functions are listed as part of Table 6.4. Missing functions limit the communicative intents that can be expressed.

4. *Verbal Mazes*—Verbal mazes can impair communicative intent. While all speakers engage in some verbal mazes (i.e., words or unattached fragments not necessary to the message), the expectation is not to exceed significantly what is normal for a given grade level (Loban, 1976). Some students use verbal mazes with such high frequency that it is impossible to comprehend their spoken message. Along with verbal mazes, the speech-language pathologist should assess the presence of false starts at the beginnings of utterances (e.g., "You know," "Guess what?"). Both verbal mazes and false starts during conversations and narrations can be distracting to listeners and can interfere with the clarity of the speaker's message.

Conversations

Numerous rules govern conversational exchanges. In conversation, one person selects a topic that is maintained until a topic shift is initiated. When assessing students' use of conversational rules, speech-language pathologists should observe the behaviors listed in Table 6.5.

Switching topics can be accomplished abruptly with no warning provided for the listener, or it can be cued directly (e.g., "Can I talk with you about something else for a minute?") or indirectly (e.g., "That reminds me of . . ."). During conversation, the speaker and listener take turns. Turn-taking should occur with a minimum of interruption; repairs and revisions should be made when necessary (Rees and Wollner, 1982).

TABLE 6.5 CONVERSATIONS
• Does the student know the rules of conversation?
• Does the student initiate conversations in a variety of situations?
• Does the student select appropriate topics?
• Does the student maintain a topic over a number of speaker-listener exchanges?
• Does the student switch topics in an appropriate and orderly manner?
• Does the student terminate conversations in a timely manner?

As stated in Chapter 3, Grice (1975) proposed four fundamental rules of conversations that summarize expectations held by speakers and listeners. We are hypothesizing that these rules are intact by late adolescence, but they may emerge even earlier and therefore should be evaluated to determine the student's knowledge and application of the rules.

Wiig (1983) has stressed the importance of the adolescent's ability to switch registers, or codes, during conversational speech. While talking with peers, an informal register is acceptable. However, when talking with adults, a more formal register is used. A formal register contains more noun phrase elaborations and verb phrase complexity, and it assumes that the speaker and listener do not share mutual information; thus, it necessitates more precise descriptions and explanations. A formal register also uses more polite forms than an informal register. Failure to discriminate which register to use for each communicative situation is a major problem for some adolescents.

Narrations

The student's ability to comprehend and to produce narratives should be investigated, because this task demonstrates whether the information can be integrated. Also, "narratives are structurally midway between the language of the oral tradition and the language of the essayist literary tradition" (Westby, 1984, p. 124). Thus, knowing the student's ability to generate narratives should allow the examiner to determine readiness to develop a more literary language structure and to learn the written form of language.

When analyzing story grammar units, the speech-language pathologist can use either a developmental approach (Applebee, 1978) or a story grammar taxonomy (Roth and Spekman, 1986). When using a developmental approach during assessment, the professional should keep in mind the developmental hierarchy leading up to the true narrative as explained in detail in Chapter 3 (Applebee, 1978). Table 6.6 lists the questions that should be answered and, therefore, the narrative behaviors to be assessed in the preadolescent and adolescent.

TABLE 6.6 NARRATIONS	
DEVELOPMENTAL ASSESSMENT QUESTIONS	**STORY GRAMMAR TAXONOMY**

• At what stage of narration is the student functioning:
   • heap stories?   • unfocused chains?
   • sequence stories/ macrostructure?   • focused chains?
   • primitive narratives?   • true narratives? (5–7 years of age)
 	
• Is the student capable of summarizing stories? (7–11 years of age)
 	
• Is the student capable of categorizing stories both subjectively and objectively? (7–11 years of age)
 	
• Does the student understand and produce complex stories with multiple embedded narratives? (11–12 years of age)
 	
• Is the student capable of analyzing stories? (13–15 years of age)
 	
• Is the student capable of generalizing from the meaning of the story, formulating abstract statements about the theme or message, and focusing on reactions to the story? (16 years–adulthood)
	• Is a setting provided?
	
	• Are the characters identified and described?
	
	• Are the events of the story presented sequentially?
	
	• Is a goal present?
	
	• Is there an initiating event?
	
	• Is there a causal relationship between events?
	
	• Is an internal response present?
	
	• Is there an attempt to attain the goal?
	
	• Is there a consequence?
	
	• Are multiple plans used to meet the goal?
	
	• Is a partial or complete episode embedded in the episode?
	
	• Are there two characters with separate goals and actions that influence each other's actions?

The other type of story grammar analysis is that of using a taxonomy that identifies the elements common to stories and specifies a formal set of rules underlying the construction of any story (Mandler and Johnson, 1977; Rumelhart, 1975; Stein and Glenn, 1979; Thorndyke, 1977). All story grammars have a setting in which the main character is introduced, and/or a description of the social, physical, or temporal context of the story. All story grammars have a goal that is met in an episode system. Episodes have a beginning, which is an initiating event; a reaction of the characters to the initiating event; an action, or attempt by the characters to deal with the initiating event; an outcome, or consequence of the attempt; and an ending. All the elements of a story grammar taxonomy should be present in the student's narration.

Written Communication

As the student becomes older, there is an interaction between oral and written communication. It appears that oral communication can enhance written communication skills and vice versa.

According to Stewart (1991), "The complex task of writing involves three major stages: planning, translating, and reviewing" (p. 420). These stages are equivalent to the planning, sentence generation, and revising stages noted by Hayes and Flowers (1987).

Table 6.7 lists the questions that need to be answered about each stage. Stewart (1991) has noted that those who are poor writers tend not to plan (i.e., not to gather and organize data before writing), but just begin writing; dwell on mechanical concerns such as spelling and punctuation, which stifles their writing process; and frequently do not see their own errors and revise passages appropriately.

Meta-abilities

Van Kleeck (1987) defines students' various *meta-abilities,* or their abilities to "know that they know" as "awareness of strategies

TABLE 6.7	WRITTEN COMMUNICATION	
PLANNING	**TRANSLATING**	**REVIEWING**
• Can the student develop ideas in written form? • Can the student gather information about a topic? • Can the student organize content? • Does the student take the reader (audience) into consideration? • Has the student considered the purpose for writing (e.g., to tell a story, to explain a process, to give directions)?	• Does the student use appropriate syntax and semantics to write a passage? • Does the student spell and punctuate appropriately?	• Does the student edit the written product? • Does the student find errors and make revisions?

and mental activities while carrying out various cognitive processes such as memory, comprehension, learning, and attention" (p. vi). She further defines metalinguistic ability as "being able to consciously reflect on the nature of language—that it is meaningful, arbitrary, conventional, and made up of elements (words, sounds, and bound morphemes) that are combined by rules (grammar)" (p. vi). Furthermore, metapragmatic skill, according to van Kleeck (1987), "consists of the child's conscious awareness of the cultural rules for using language effectively in various social contexts" (p. vi).

Developing meta-abilities is critical to students being able to reflect on the effectiveness of their current communication behaviors (i.e., to determine current communication breakdowns and correct them by adapting to the needs of the listener) and to incorporate consciously new

---

TABLE 6.8

META-ABILITIES

- Does the student show evidence of metalinguistic skills (e.g., the ability to assess communication breakdowns and revise them)?

- Does the student show metacognitive skills (i.e., the ability to assess thinking or to think about thinking)?

- Does the student show metapragmatic skills (i.e., the ability to be aware of cultural rules for using language appropriately across and within various social contexts)?

- Does the student show metanarrative skills (i.e., the awareness of story elements and structure so as to manipulate intentionally the various story elements)?

---

communication behaviors. Therefore, as part of the assessment process, determination of the adolescent's or young adult's ability to engage in metalinguistic, metacognitive, metapragmatic, metanarrative, and meta-communication behaviors is important (Schuele and van Kleeck, 1987). Table 6.8 lists the types of questions to ask when assessing the student's meta-abilities.

NONVERBAL COMMUNICATION

Research indicates that people will believe nonverbal messages over verbal messages; when the two may contradict each other, it is frequently the nonverbal communication behavior that creates first impressions (Samovar and Porter, 1991a). Research in communication has revealed that as much as 90 percent of the social intent of a message is transmitted paralinguistically, or nonverbally (Samovar and Porter, 1991b). According to Samovar and Porter (1991a), "Nonverbal communication involves all those stimuli (except verbal stimuli) within a communication setting, generated by both the individual and the individual's use of the environment, that have potential message value for the sender or receiver" (p. 179).

Nonverbal communication serves these basic functions: to repeat, complement, or contradict what one has said; to substitute for a verbal action; to regulate a communication event; and to accentuate a message. Nonverbal messages are communicated by various means: body movements (kinesics and posture), proxemics (space and distance), dress, facial expressions, eye contact, touch, smell, and paralanguage.

French (1978) noted expectations for appropriate kinesic and proxemic behaviors. The expected kinesic behaviors include the use of gestures that match the spoken message, avoidance of adaptor behaviors that detract from the message (e.g., constantly pushing hair off one's forehead), communication of emotion through facial expression, and appropriate eye contact.

Proxemic behaviors include the maintenance of socially acceptable space or distance while conversing. One's age makes a difference in how one communicates nonverbally. For example, proxemically, children interact the closest, adolescents at an intermediary distance, and adults at the greatest distance. Dolphin (1991) noted that there are cultural differences in how children use space by age 7. Black children require less personal space than white children, and mixed-sex dyads need more space than same-sex dyads.

Paralanguage features that should be observed while assessing older students include the rate of speech, tone of voice, use of inflection, and unfilled pause time (i.e., silence) within and between utterances. Also, the presence of filled pauses (e.g., "ah," "um," "er") should be noted. Are pauses occurring so often that the message being communicated is significantly impaired? Abnormal paralanguage features impair communication as much as restricted language features do, and thus they become critical variables to evaluate during assessment. Table 6.9 lists some characteristics to assess.

SURVIVAL LANGUAGE SKILLS

Preadolescents and adolescents with more severely impaired thinking, listening, and speaking often have accompanying survival language deficits (i.e., difficulty functioning in one or more environments because of their

TABLE 6.9	
NONVERBAL COMMUNICATION SKILLS	
KINESIC AND PROXEMIC BEHAVIOR	**PARALANGUAGE FEATURES**
• Does the student use facial expressions appropriately? • Does the student have appropriate eye contact when speaking and listening? • Does the student stand at a distance from the speaker/listener that seems appropriate and comfortable? • Does the student use body movements to enhance communication rather than detract from it?	• Does the student use an appropriate rate of speech? • Does the student use an appropriate tone of voice? • Does the student use a variety of vocal inflections? • Does the student pause appropriately between utterances? Between speaker-listener turns? • Does the student avoid overuse of filled pauses (e.g., "ah," "um," "er")?

language disorder). Valletutti and Bender (1982) have identified six major environments in which the adolescent must function:

1. at home, as a family member;

2. at school, as a student;

3. in the community, as a citizen;

4. in the marketplace, as a consumer of goods and services;

5. in society, as a participant of leisure; and

6. in the workplace, as a producer of goods or services.

Each of these settings demands appropriate and varying cognitive, language, and communication behaviors.

Assessment of survival language skills is not always a concern during the speech-language pathologist's initial assessment of an adolescent, but exceptions to this are possible. If an adolescent is in a secondary-school setting and has only a year or two of instructional time remaining, survival language skills may be a primary emphasis for both assessment and intervention. If an adolescent is spending only a few months at a juvenile detention center, assessment of survival language skills necessary for integration and survival in the home community would be an extremely legitimate concern. Speech-language pathologists conducting the assessment of adolescents must use their best clinical judgment in determining whether to evaluate survival language skills, and if so, which ones.

Frequently, survival language skills can be assessed better after beginning speech-language services, as part of an ongoing

diagnostic intervention paradigm. For example, within the role of consumer of goods and services, students would be expected to comprehend and produce language needed in a fast-food restaurant. An initial baseline assessment would determine what vocabulary and communication skills were already in the student's repertoire and which ones were absent. If sufficient communication skills needed for survival in a fast-food restaurant were present, then no further work would be done. However, if deficiencies were noted, then intervention would begin to focus on development of appropriate restaurant language.

In addition to completing the type of situational analysis just described, multi-situational skills can be assessed. For example, the language of money, time, space, warning labels, and signs can be evaluated. The vocabulary for these areas crosses a number of settings and roles in which the student functions.

HOW TO ASSESS

An individual's behaviors are "relative, conditional, complex, and dynamic. Accordingly, clinical assessment must be relative, contextual, process oriented, and dynamic" (Muma, 1978, p. 211). This type of clinical assessment can best be accomplished by using informal assessment procedures that are holistic, modifiable, and accommodating to the individual within a natural setting rather than by conforming the individual to the test methodology. Not only is the test situation artificial, but the language of formal tests is often characteristically different from daily communicative exchanges (Lund and Duchan, 1983).

Frequently, professionals say they cannot use informal procedures because these procedures are not objective (i.e., they provide no quantitative scores). Also, they say it is too time consuming to obtain and to analyze spontaneous communication samples across relevant situations and listeners. Both of these issues are examined next.

OBJECTIVITY VERSUS RELEVANCE

Objectivity is assumed when formal (i.e., standardized) tests are administered. Assume for a moment that a standardized test is more objective than an informal procedure of obtaining, observing, recording, and analyzing communication behaviors in a natural context. This objectivity should not be construed as more important than relevance (Muma, 1978). A standardized test that is supposedly objective cannot be considered worthwhile and valid if it is not assessing relevant behaviors in relevant situations.

Quantitative scores may not be as advantageous as professionals have been led to believe. Muma (1978) stated that scores may work against both the examiner and student, because when complex dynamic behaviors are reduced to numbers, essential information about the individual is lost, thus making it difficult or impossible to generate appropriate intervention goals and procedures. As Lund and Duchan (1983) have noted, "Scores are of little value for the purposes of describing language

and planning therapy, so clinicians must analyze performance on each item" (p. 299).

THE TIME FACTOR

A second argument for not obtaining and analyzing spontaneous language samples is that they are too time consuming. What has allowed speech-language pathologists to conclude that assessment must be quick and easy? Perhaps it has been large caseloads or administrative number games. Whatever the reasons, those variables that force professionals to conclude that language sampling is too time consuming should be changed, and the sampling procedure should be retained. Quick and easy assessment procedures may lose more than is gained by neglecting the responsibility to assess an individual's needs appropriately (Muma, 1978). None of us would want ourselves or our loved ones to be assessed in a "quick and easy" fashion by a physician or psychologist or speech-language pathologist. The consequences may be far too severe.

At some time during the assessment procedure, the examiner must obtain from the student several spontaneous conversational samples, which in turn can be analyzed for phonological, morphological, syntactic, semantic, and pragmatic features. If such samples are not gathered and only formal tests are administered, isolated aspects of communication may be obtained. These isolated aspects do not constitute the total communication process and could lead to false conclusions. Using both selected formal tests and informal procedures, the examiner can more effectively evaluate the total communication process and thus implement the comprehensive model discussed in Chapter 5.

Suggestions in the remainder of this section will emphasize the integration of the assessment process and how to evaluate *simultaneously* cognitive, language, and communication behaviors. Five informal assessment procedures are proposed: a case history form, a learning style questionnaire, portfolios, discourse samples, and directed tasks. In addition, formal tests are listed. Regardless of whether informal and/or formal testing procedures are used, the examiner must be aware of the variables that affect the administration of procedures, analysis of data, and interpretation of the student's performance.

INFORMAL ASSESSMENT

Case History Form

A general case history form for obtaining information on the preadolescent's or adolescent's health, education, and environmental history is printed in Appendix E. Information can be obtained by interviewing the youth or a parent/caregiver. Some of the information may be derived from cumulative records. In most instances, the case history form should not be given to the student to complete, but should be retained by the examiner who asks questions and records responses.

If students have the necessary skills, another alternative would be to have them write or audiotape an autobiography. These options can provide insight into their perspective of the past, present, and future.

A supplemental case history form is printed in Appendix F. A questionnaire devised by Schwartz and McKinley (1984) has also been included for assessment of the student's misconceptions about listening.

The general case history form should be reviewed to determine whether the student has had previous speech-language services. If so, is the student willing to receive additional services? Also, the case history should be analyzed to determine a need to refer for additional professional services. The supplemental case history form should be reviewed to see if the student is aware of his or her own thinking, listening, and speaking abilities. The student who displays some meta-abilities may be more motivated to change these behaviors and therefore may be a good candidate for speech-language services.

Learning Style Questionnaire

A learning style questionnaire has been developed to determine when, where, what, why, and how the older student learns best. (See Appendix G.) The student should not be expected to read the form independently, but should be given a form to follow along with the examiner. The examiner should systematically go through the form, asking the questions and recording responses. This gives the examiner the opportunity to explain any unfamiliar terms or to ask additional questions to clarify responses.

During field testing, the form has not been useful with all students; it appears to be most useful with those who already possess a good deal of insight and self-confidence. Students who are less secure are more likely to give answers that they think the examiner wants to hear, or that they think are correct, than they are to report how they actually learn best.

Portfolios

According to Paulson, Paulson, and Meyer (1991):

> A portfolio is a purposeful collection of student work that exhibits the student's efforts, progress, and achievements in one or more areas. The collection must include student participation in selecting contents, the criteria for selection, the criteria for judging merit, and evidence of student self-reflection. (p.60)

In portfolio assessment, the student and/or classroom teacher places samples of the student's work in a file or portfolio. The artifacts placed in the portfolio involve generalized comparisons rather than detailed analyses of the student's work. This procedure allows for a comparison of the student's current performance with his or her past performance and helps to determine the student's progress over time. If the materials that are put into a student's portfolio are chosen wisely and are representative of meaningful and ecologically valid situations, then this procedure would be very effective in the academic evaluation of students (Damico, 1993).

A portfolio can be particularly helpful in assessing written language skills. Why have student portfolios? According to Wolf (1989):

- They help students to take responsibility for their work and for evaluating their progress.

- They help students to enlarge their view of what's learned because portfolios contain a range of work (e.g., fiction, poems, essays, journal entries).

- They help students to understand that learning is a process and not a product (e.g., writing is a process of planning, writing, rewriting, revising, and completing numerous drafts, not just the finished product on paper).

- They help students to take a developmental point of view of how their work has progressed and how to objectively evaluate their own work.

Paulson et al. (1991) offer the following guidelines for realizing the power of portfolio assessment:

1. The portfolio should demonstrate that the student is learning about learning and engaged in self-reflection.

2. The portfolio is something the student does, not something done to the student.

3. The portfolio is not the same as the cumulative folder.

4. The portfolio should represent the student's activities.

5. The portfolio may serve a different purpose during the year than at the end of the year.

6. The portfolio may have multiple purposes, but they should not conflict with each other.

7. The portfolio should illustrate the student's growth.

8. The portfolio should not happen by chance but should deliberately enhance skills and techniques useful to the student.

In summary, Paulson et al. (1991) stated it best when they said:

A portfolio, then, is a portfolio when it provides a complex and comprehensive view of student performance in context. . . . Above all, a portfolio is a portfolio when it provides a forum that encourages students to develop the abilities needed to become independent, self-directed learners. (p. 63)

When using portfolios, the student becomes a participant in, rather than the object of, assessment.

Discourse Samples: Conversations

Conversational samples are a critical part of informal assessment of older students. These samples have been a major recommended source of information for decades, and they are the preferred method of language elicitation from "toddler to adult" (Atkins and Cartwright, 1982). We concur with this position. While a disadvantage of spontaneous conversational samples is the risk of not eliciting all the language behaviors in the individual's repertoire, a powerful advantage of conversational samples is the more realistic picture of the student's communication that is gained.

Arwood (1983), who advocates unstructured conversational sampling, commented that to determine level of functioning rapidly, professionals have only to listen to the individual talk. What can be detected about the way the student organizes ideas, expresses communicative intents, and uses a variety of structures? To the recommendation to listen, we would add, "Watch the student communicate." What can be noted about eye contact, gestures, body space, and facial expressions?

A partial transcript is reprinted in Table 6.10. This unstructured language sample was obtained by a speech-language clinician evaluating a 14-year-old boy. This boy successfully passed tests that measured isolated aspects of language (i.e., discrete point tests), and yet his conversational sample revealed problems in communicating messages to listeners. The excessive number of verbal mazes, lack of message cohesiveness, and high incidence of low-information words frequently left his listeners confused.

Administration

Procedures for obtaining language samples have changed very little since first recommended by McCarthy (1930). Speech-language pathologists should:

1. establish good rapport with the individual being sampled;

2. keep their remarks to a minimum; and

3. use open-ended questions or comments that will facilitate longer responses.

Usually, older students should select their own topics of conversation. The goal of obtaining a sample is that it be "representative" of the individual's communication. However, "representative" has held different meanings in the literature, including "comprehensive," "idealized," and "typical" (Gallagher, 1983).

TABLE 6.10	
	TRANSCRIPT OF A 14-YEAR-OLD BOY
Adolescent:	What do we talk on? No. Oh, I got a good one. You should see my . . . um, Uncle Boos had to move and they're in this really cool house. It's, it's like, it's round. It's sort of li . . . okay, it's, it's peaked at the top and then it gets round or somethin' . . . no, it goes . . . it's . . .
Clinician:	It goes down and then (demonstrates)
Adolescent:	Yeah! And then inside they, they have this bedroom . . . They're going . . . Okay, there's the living room and their bedroom is . . . ya go up the, the st . . . and three stairs, and then you go up there and then they're gonna block it that off from the . . . so people can't see them in the living room and in the kitchen. They're gonna put a door there and plus they got this neat bar and it's real cool. They have it . . . um, in the living room. It's real cool. They don't have much furniture though.
Clinician:	They should get some.
Adolescent:	Uh-hum. They'll have a couch and two chairs. You should see. Oh, it's really awesome. You know, like in a restaurant. They have the table and it's like in the kitchen and it's hitched to the wall. It's real cool!
Clinician:	(Laughs)
Adolescent:	And then . . . okay, there's . . . they have about eight kids and there's one downst in the living room but two down in . . . Wait a minute! They have six, but counting the parents it's eight. And they . . . okay, upstairs they have . . . it's like a closet . . . like it's about maybe this big. About from this square and that's their bedroom. And it's, okay, from there to there. That's their bedroom. Their mom and dad's bedroom. And there's this kind of like closet thing that closes.
Clinician:	How can they get into it?

To be comprehensive, a conversational sample has to be large enough to be reliable, but small enough to be efficient. McCarthy (1930) originally proposed a 50-utterance sample; others have recommended 100 utterances (Crystal, Fletcher, and Garman, 1991; Engler, Hannah, and Longhurst, 1973; Tyack and Gottsleben, 1974). Bloom and Lahey (1978) and Miller (1981) recommended a minimum of 30 minutes of sampling time. Bloom and Lahey (1978) also suggested that 200 or more utterances be obtained within the recommended sampling time.

To be a representative conversational sample, the sample should evoke the best possible range of abilities (McLean and Snyder-McLean, 1978). The conversational analysis should neither underestimate nor overestimate the student's communication abilities, since "a language sample is considered unrepresentative if it leads to an analysis that results in either one of these errors" (Gallagher, 1983, p. 3). The notion that an "idealized" sample should be collected is contradictory to the notion that it also be "typical," or representative of daily communication performances. When assessing older students, we have been most concerned with collecting samples that represent "usual" language performances, rather than optimal samples.

In addition to considering what is a *representative* sample, speech-language pathologists must consider how language use varies with context (Gallagher, 1983). Many clinicians have responded by obtaining language samples in more than one context, using a variety of stimuli, conversational partners, and settings (McLean and Snyder-McLean, 1978; Miller, 1981; Muma, 1978). The problem is that the "number of possible combinations of stimulus materials, conversational partners, and settings is infinite" (Gallagher, 1983, p. 4). The selection of combinations is either arbitrary or the result of trial-and-error sampling. Therefore, whether sampling in multiple contexts solves the assessment problems arising from language use variability is questionable (Gallagher, 1983).

There is little available data to describe how adolescents' communication varies as a function of changes in stimuli, conversational partners, or settings. Our own longitudinal study (which utilizes a school setting, and no stimulus materials, to gather data while adolescents converse with peers of their choice and with unfamiliar adults of the opposite sex) is some of the first research that describes how language use varies in these contexts (McKinley and Larson, 1983). Clearly, more information is needed.

In the meantime, we recommend, at the minimum, that two 10-minute conversational samples be collected, one while the student is conversing with the speech-language pathologist (usually an unfamiliar adult during initial assessment) and one with a

peer of the youth's choice. Additional samples might be collected using other partners. The conversational samples should require the student to switch from an informal to a formal register. The speech-language pathologist should keep in mind that after age 15, adolescents begin to use a more formal register even with their peers, unless they are the best of friends (Wiig, 1982a).

Analysis

Both partners' turns should be transcribed in order to analyze certain pragmatic features. Rather than delineating utterances, as would be done for young children, conversational units should be marked when transcribing preadolescent and adolescent language. A conversational unit is defined as "the utterance(s) of one conversational partner that continue(s) until the other conversational partner initiates an independent utterance" (Boyce and Larson, 1983, p. 221). A phonetic transcription may or may not be necessary. If phonological errors are evident, it may be desirable to complete a phonetic transcription. In all cases, the transcription should reflect what was actually said and include all false starts, verbal mazes, and filled pauses.

Perhaps the greatest difficulty with conversational samples is how to analyze them once they are transcribed. One reason for the difficulty is that calculation of the mean length of utterance in morphemes (MLU-M) for the purpose of comparing it with Brown's (1973) stages of psycholinguistic development is not appropriate for the older school-age population.

How can professionals determine that an adolescent's language system is different from what might be expected? Loban (1976) has described an analysis procedure that allows the quantification of a variety of linguistic characteristics (e.g., maze words, words per communication unit). (See Tables 3.3, 3.4, and 3.5 in Chapter 3.) This quantification begins to give a sense of an individual's functioning, but the focus is on products of communication rather than on processes. Thus, adopting analysis procedures that attempt to quantify developmental changes during preadolescence and adolescence should not be the only method used, since the desired outcome is a description of the adolescent's communication, sufficiently detailed to suggest whether intervention is needed. When quantitative analysis procedures are used, they should still be combined with descriptive data that discuss how the youth's language system differs from the norm.

Several procedures that emphasize descriptive data have been suggested in the literature and are adaptable for the preadolescent and adolescent population. Arwood (1983) described her system in detail and developed appropriate summary forms. Prutting and Kirchner (1983) developed a "pragmatic protocol" organized around the utterance, propositional, elocutionary, and perlocutionary acts. Readers are urged to consult the original sources for more information on these analysis procedures.

We have found that the chart of competent and incompetent language features (Simon, 1979; Simon and Holway, 1991) provides a useful guide when analyzing the student's language. The chart provides a gestalt of the student's communication, not just isolated features. By noting competent features that are present, absent, or inconsistent, and describing typical utterances as evidence, the speech-language pathologist can begin to develop a sense of the total effectiveness and efficiency of a student's communication. *Evaluating Communicative Competence—Revised Second Edition* (Simon, 1994) is a language sample procedure that gathers observational data on 21 performance tasks, which analyze a student's listening and speaking behaviors. According to Simon (1994), as the student is observed performing these tasks, "it is possible to obtain a systematic description of language processing, metalinguistics, and expressive language proficiencies and deficits" (p. xi).

Damico (1991) has developed a procedure, titled *Clinical Discourse Analysis*, that assesses functions of language in school-age students. It is an excellent tool for identifying students who are language impaired. A description of the procedure reveals that it is organized according to the four categories described by Grice (1975). The categories and the problem behaviors pertinent to each category are described in Table 6.11. For more information about the procedure, the original source should be consulted.

Drawing from a variety of sources (Duncan and Fiske, 1977; Grice, 1975; Hymes, 1972; Rees and Wollner, 1982; Simon, 1979; Wiig and Semel, 1980), we have constructed a form called "Adolescent Conversational Analysis." This form may be reproduced from Appendix H. It is unique from other analyses in that it examines the student's role both as a listener and a speaker, not simply as a speaker, during conversation.

TABLE 6.11
CLINICAL DISCOURSE ANALYSIS
THE ORGANIZATION OF PROBLEM BEHAVIORS UNDER GRICE'S CATEGORIES IN CLINICAL DISCOURSE ANALYSIS
QUANTITY CATEGORY
• Failure to provide significant information to listeners • Use of nonspecific vocabulary • Informational redundancy • Need for repetition
QUALITY CATEGORY
• Message inaccuracy
RELATION CATEGORY
• Poor topic maintenance • Inappropriate response • Failure to ask relevant questions • Situational inappropriateness • Inappropriate speech style
MANNER CATEGORY
• Linguistic nonfluency • Revision • Delays before responding • Failure to structure discourse • Turn-taking difficulty • Gaze inefficiency • Inappropriate intonational contour

From "Clinical Discourse Analysis: A Functional Approach to Language Assessment," by J. Damico. In *Communication Skills and Classroom Success: Assessment and Therapy Methodologies for Language and Learning Disabled Students* (p. 131), by C. Simon (Ed.), 1991, Eau Claire, WI: Thinking Publications. © 1991 by Thinking Publications. Reprinted with permission.

The microcomputer can also be used for analyzing language samples. Language assessment software programs such as *Lingquest 1: Language Sample Analysis* by Mordecai, Palin, and Palmer (1985), *Systematic Analysis of Language Transcripts (SALT)* by Miller and Chapman (1983, 1991), *Computerized Language Sample Analysis* by Weiner (1984), *Pye Analysis of Language* by Pye (1987), and *Computerized Profiling* by Long and Fey (1993) allow for the sorting, calculating, and tabulating of data from language samples.

Lingquest 1: Language Sample Analysis (Mordecai et al., 1985) uses concepts from Lee (1974), Tyack and Gottsleben (1974), Crystal et al. (1991), and Miller (1981). *Lingquest 1* provides for an analysis of lexical items including a type-token ratio (TTR) and eight grammatical forms (i.e., nouns, verbs, modifiers, prepositions, conjunctions, negations, interjections, and wh-question words), mean length of utterance in words and morphemes, and an analysis of 81 subcategories of parts of speech. To accomplish this analysis, the speech-language pathologist must transcribe and code the utterances to be analyzed. This process may be difficult and time consuming, with resulting summaries that are valuable but that provide no developmental information (Retherford, 1993).

SALT (Miller and Chapman, 1983, 1991) is based on the principles and procedures described by Miller (1981). *SALT* has five major features for analyzing a language sample: transcript entry, transcript utility, standard analysis, search, and wizard word lists. The standard analysis procedures conducted by *SALT* are number and percentage of complete and incomplete utterances, the TTR, mean length of utterance in morphemes, a distributional analysis of the number of utterances by word or morpheme and speaker turns, the frequency of usage of structures designated by the speech-language pathologist, and an analysis of morpheme usage. This software is one of the most flexible and complicated. It allows for the examiner to have some flexibility in what features can be analyzed. Likewise, because of the sophistication, considerable practice is needed to use the program (Retherford, 1993). A reference database has been developed up through early adolescence but is not included with the software.

Computerized Language Sample Analysis by Weiner (1984) summarizes the frequency of occurrence and accuracy of use for 14 grammatical categories. In addition, analysis of nouns, verbs, sentence types, length of utterance, and word usage can be accomplished. A tutorial is provided that assists the examiner in learning to code utterances and to use this program. An updated version of this program is available under the title *Parrot Easy Language Sample Analysis* (Weiner, 1988).

Pye Analysis of Language by Pye (1987) permits morphologic, syntactic, and phonologic analyses using procedures described by Ingram (1981). Other analyses can be done manually by coding the transcript.

Computerized Profiling, developed by Long and Fey (1993), contains several analysis systems such as LARSP (Crystal et al., 1991), PRISM+ (Crystal, 1982), and "Developmental Sentence Score" found within *Developmental Sentence Analysis* (Lee, 1974). Pragmatic and phonological analyses are possible as well.

The brief description of these software programs illustrates that they offer a range of analysis features and varying degrees of flexibility. How time consuming a particular analysis system will be is contingent upon the type of analysis chosen, the amount of information processed, and the skills of the speech-language pathologist in coding utterances (Schwartz, 1985). Although these software packages should ultimately allow clinicians to be more efficient, the software should also assist them to become more effective in determining the type and severity of a language disorder and in establishing appropriate intervention programs. Regardless of the software language analysis system used, the speech-language pathologist must obtain an accurate and representative language sample, transcribe the sample accurately, and code the language structures correctly.

Long and Masterson (1993) discuss what computerized language analysis (CLA) software can and cannot do. They conclude that CLA software can: (1) conduct language analysis more quickly than when it is done by hand; and (2) allow for detailed analyses that, due to time constraints, would rarely be done by hand. They conclude that CLA software cannot: (1) assist in the orthographic or phonetic transcription of a student's language, (2) assure that the transcript is being transcribed correctly, (3) yield irrefutable truth, or (4) tell us the answers to diagnosis and intervention. This last item may be possible someday when "expert systems" become available.

Interpretation

Quantitative data may be compared to those presented on existing developmental charts such as Loban's (1976). Caution is advised, however, because Loban's results were obtained in a contrived conversational situation. Quantitative data in the form of TTR should not be compared with existing data for children's utterances or with adult norms. We recommend that local normative data be obtained on the TTR of preadolescents or adolescents. With the use of the computer, this is a realistic goal.

The adolescent conversational analysis that we recommend could be interpreted with the use of the profile summary provided in Appendix H. Conversational behaviors are determined to be either appropriate or inappropriate. Determination of the appropriateness or inappropriateness of a behavior is made by judging whether it is penalizing to the student; a behavior perceived by the clinician as penalizing is marked as inappropriate (Prutting and Kirchner, 1983). Our clinical experiences have been that the student probably has conversational deficits in need of intervention if a significant number of conversational behaviors are indicated as inappropriate (i.e., 30 percent or more, disregarding items marked "not observed," which approximates two standard deviations below the mean on standardized tests). Certain items should carry more weight during interpretation because they may carry more negative consequences during communication exchanges than other items do (i.e., main ideas, word-retrieval skills, fluency, intelligibility, turn-taking). If consistent problems are evident on any one of these items, then direct or indirect intervention should be considered even if most of the other items are judged to be appropriate.

Discourse Samples: Narrations

The use of narratives can be an excellent assessment procedure (Arwood, 1983). Narrative tasks are more structured than conversational speech, but they are less structured than the directed tasks that will be discussed in the section that follows.

Administration

The way examiners obtain a narrative language sample can result in different types of samples. For example, if preadolescents or adolescents are asked to relate a personal experience, they will produce a more orally structured narrative. If asked to tell a story, they will use a more literary style. However, if they are asked to tell a story like it is written in a book, they will use the most literary style.

When both the examiner and the student can see the stimulus picture and share in the pictorial situation, there is a tendency to resort to a more oral style and to make the narrative less explicit. Also, what is depicted in a picture may make a difference. Pictures that display an action may lead a student to describe only the action, whereas pictures that display a setting often yield a more complex story. Telling a story from a wordless picture book requires that the student recognize the scenarios depicted, whereas telling a story from a single picture requires that the student formulate and organize the story, not simply recognize it.

Some students show minimal differences based upon how the instructions are given or how the stimuli are depicted. However, others tend to switch from a more oral to a more literary mode, depending on the task. Perhaps this demonstrates that these latter individuals have a metalinguistic awareness toward story grammars.

Story reformulation has also been used as an assessment procedure (Chappell, 1980; Culatta, Page, and Ellis, 1983). In story reformulation tasks, preadolescents and adolescents have to comprehend, retain and recall information, understand sequences, and express themselves precisely when retelling the story.

We recommend that at least two samples of narration be obtained, one being a formulated and the other a reformulated task. The type of story selected for the reformulation task should be sensitive to the student's social-emotional level and to memory capacity. The specific type of formulated task selected would be contingent upon whether a more oral or more literary sample was desired. Generally, we first choose a formulated task that requires the student to relate a personal experience, since the recounting of a personal story and a story reformulation task are the most distant tasks on the oral-literary style continuum. If relating a personal experience is a much stronger ability for the student than reformulating a story, then additional formulated narration tasks requiring a more literary style may be necessary to determine where the individual falls on the continuum.

After each narrative sample is collected, the examiner should ask questions that require the student to summarize the story, categorize it, analyze it, and generalize it. For example, these types of questions or directives might be given:

- Now tell me in one sentence what your story was about.

- What would be a good title for this story?

- In what category would you put this story (e.g., drama, mystery, comedy)?

- How else could you categorize this story (e.g., short, long, exciting, boring)?

- How did this story make you feel?

- Why do you think [main character] acted like he (she) did?

- What was the moral of this story?

Analysis

Once a student has formulated or reformulated a story, the speech-language pathologist should transcribe it. Recall that there are two primary ways in which narratives can be analyzed once transcribed—through a developmental hierarchy and through a story grammar taxonomy. We advocate analysis primarily through the developmental stage progression (Applebee, 1978) because of its underlying theoretical premises (Piaget, 1959; Vygotsky, 1962). Story grammar taxonomies appear to be independent of theoretical constructs. Nonetheless, they provide a glimpse of organizational style, and questions provided in Table 6.6 (see page 113) can be used as an analysis guide.

Using Applebee's (1978) developmental hierarchy, we have developed a narration analysis form. (See Appendix I.) Applebee (1978) noted that stories do not always fit precisely into one of the first six categories. Thus, judgments will need to be made on the basis of the predominant mode of organization. Based on the student's response to the examiner's questions about summarization, categorization, analysis, and generalization, the rest of the form in Appendix I can be completed.

For a very detailed analysis of storytelling skills, professionals can also consult Hedberg and Westby (1993), who provide a variety of practical ways to analyze and interpret narrative structure and content. Along with a review of the literature, their approach is illustrated using normal students and students with language disorders.

Interpretation

Once the speech-language pathologist has analyzed the student's story to determine the predominant mode of organization in the developmental hierarchy, then it is possible to interpret these data in terms of the underlying cognitive level and the chronological age at which most youths learn this aspect of narration. Preadolescents or adolescents whose narration skills are consistently three or more years delayed, compared with their chronological age, may be candidates for language intervention.

Directed Tasks

Directed tasks are any structured procedures that require thinking, listening, and/or speaking. These tasks share commonalities:

1. Focus is directed toward the process through which the older student goes to perform the directed task. The correct product is frequently irrelevant.

2. Each directed task should be followed with appropriate metacognitive, metalinguistic, and/or metacommunication questions. For example, examiners would want to consider questions such as:

   a. What did you have to think about to solve that problem? What went on in your mind?

   b. How did you figure out what was important to listen to?

   c. Was that direction difficult for you to understand? Why? What words were unfamiliar to you?

   d. What made that story (message, direction) difficult to tell?

   e. Do you think that was a clear message? Do you think I understood what you meant?

   f. Why didn't I understand what you meant?

   These types of questions help to determine what the individual knows about cognitive functions, language, and communication. A youth who has little "meta" awareness is likely to be more impaired than one who has awareness but inconsistent application.

3. Directed tasks that are difficult for preadolescents and adolescents should be administered again, with slight variations, following metacognitive, metalinguistic, and/or metacommunication questions. This will permit the examiner to comment on the adolescent's prognosis for modification, given a

structured learning experience. For example, one of the directed tasks presented later in this discussion is organization. If the adolescent fails to handle the grocery store task suggested in that section (see page 131), the examiner should question the adolescent about knowledge of cognitive functions, such as categorization (e.g., "Do you know what some grocery store categories are?") and systematic exploration (e.g., "Do you know how you would systematically look for an item in a grocery store?"). Following these metacognitive questions, once they are successfully discussed, the examiner should present a new problem slightly different from the first. For example, "If I send you to a drug store to buy aspirin, cotton balls, and toothpaste, how would you find those items?" Students who can transfer cognitive functions such as categorization and systematic exploration to this new situation would be viewed as having greater potential for learning and a more promising prognosis than those who fail to benefit from the metacognitive, metalinguistic, and metacommunication discussions.

Problem Solving

Areas Assessed

The informal assessment task for problem solving provides information primarily on cognition, but it also provides data on conversational abilities when the problem-solving task involves dialogue. Survival language skills may or may not receive focus, depending upon the content of the problems solved.

Administration

During this task, the examiner will want to ascertain whether the student can apply a problem-solving model (summarized in the next section, "Analysis"). A variety of common problems that relate to academic, social, and/or vocational concerns should be presented. Problems to be solved may range from common daily occurrences (e.g., "Which of four homework assignments should be tackled first?") to novel situations (e.g., "How would you find a doctor to go to if you moved to a new city?"). A number of excellent computer programs (e.g., see *Solutions Unlimited* [Agency for Instructional Technology, 1984]) focus on the student's ability to apply a problem-solving model, and these programs could be adapted for use during informal assessment procedures. Guiding questions may be asked by the examiner to determine application of the problem-solving model (e.g., "How do you know if you've made the best decision?").

Analysis

The student's responses to the various problems presented should be recorded and analyzed as to whether he or she could usually respond to the various steps of the problem-solving model (with or without guiding questions) delineated below:

1. identify the problem;

2. propose alternative solutions;

3. choose the best alternative;

4. make a plan to implement the alternative; and

5. evaluate the decision.

The steps of the model that were often problematic to the preadolescent or adolescent should be noted.

Interpretation

Older students have deficits in the area of problem solving that warrant intervention if they do not identify the problem to be solved, propose only one or two alternative solutions, or choose a solution that is not the best one. When requested to justify the "best alternative," if they provide a weak rationale, or none at all, they may be candidates for intervention. If preadolescents or adolescents have difficulty primarily with steps 4 and 5 (i.e., making plans and evaluating decisions), this is generally a less severe deficit.

Organization

Areas Assessed

The informal assessment task for organization provides information primarily on cognition. However, because the task involves a dialogue between the examiner and the preadolescent or adolescent, the task may also provide discourse and "meta" data. Depending upon the content of the dialogue, information may be obtained on survival language skills.

Administration

During the assessment process, the examiner should obtain information about the preadolescent's or adolescent's perceptions of organization. A familiar task should be proposed, such as, "Suppose I sent you into a grocery store to buy carrots, milk, and ice cream. You have never been in the store before. What is your strategy for finding these food items?"

Students should be able to describe a number of strategies, such as asking someone, looking for the signs that hang above the aisles, or walking around the outer perimeter of the store and then the aisles (i.e., systematic exploration). If they do not describe all of the possible strategies, discuss additional approaches they could use to find the named grocery items. From grocery store organization, the examiner can bridge to other situations by asking questions such as, "What other stores are organized? How are they organized? What is organized besides stores (e.g., schools, hospitals, houses)? How are they organized? Does everything you can think of have some sort of organization? Why do we organize?"

An alternative task to assess organization is to use a computer program such as *The Factory* (Kosel and Fish, 1984), which requires the older student to "manufacture" a model product by subjecting raw material to the correct sequence of production steps. Consistent organizational strategies must be applied to be successful at running *The Factory*. As with the grocery store procedure, the student should verbalize a number of strategies for determining the rules for constructing the model products.

Analysis

Record responses to the questions posed during administration. Analyze how many different strategies for finding items (e.g., in the grocery store) the student could report. Determine if any strategies discussed during the grocery store example were generalized to other situations presented. Note whether the youth recognized that organization differs among settings (e.g., "One way that schools are organized is by grade level. This is not an organizational system used in stores"). Finally, analyze whether the student has any awareness of the importance of organization.

Interpretation

An individual who has no strategies, or only one or two, for finding an item (person) in an organized setting may need focused intervention for organization. This finding should match reports from related professionals and/or family members that the student is disorganized (e.g., frequently loses assignments, forgets to bring requested items). If the disorganization is accompanied by lack of awareness of the importance and utility of being organized, it is likely that structured intervention is needed to improve organizational skills.

Giving Directions

Areas Assessed

The informal assessment task for giving directions provides information on comprehension and production of linguistic features. It is expected that older students can give directions. This task can also provide data on cognition, conversation, and survival language.

Administration

A directed task suggested by Arwood (1983) is that of giving directions for a game or sport. For example, the student might describe how a favorite video game is played, or how the sport of football is played. Completing such a task requires organizing the main ideas, sequencing the description, and communicating messages clearly enough for another person to understand them. During this assessment

procedure, it is best that the adult examiner demonstrate little or no prior knowledge of the game or sport. Students will feel little need to communicate the information if they perceive that the adult already knows it. Prompting should be used by the examiner when the student deletes essential information. Also, the examiner should request clarification of low-information words.

Having the older student describe how to go from one location to another is also an appropriate directed verbalization task (Boyce and Larson, 1983). An agreed-upon referent point (e.g., one's house) is needed from which directives (e.g., left, right) can be given to arrive at an ending destination (e.g., one's school). Locations should be familiar to the student (e.g., describing how to get from one's house to the nearest grocery store). If the examiner has prior knowledge of the directions, the task can be restructured to have the student pretend to explain to strangers how he or she would travel between the two points.

Analysis

The directions given by the student should be analyzed for organization, clarity, and precision. Analysis should determine if a listener could follow the direction or would be left confused. Were essential elements consistently omitted that were necessary in the direction? Was the student able to include those essential elements when prompted by the examiner? Directions should neither be contaminated with low-information words (e.g., *junk, thing, stuff*) nor filled with verbal mazes that obscure the intended message.

Interpretation

Older students who consistently leave their listeners confused when giving directions may have a deficit in this area. Whether the confusion is caused by low-information words, verbal mazes, or deletion of essential message elements, the student is at a disadvantage when direction giving is lacking. When the student does not clarify the direction even with examiner prompting and after requests to define low-information words, intervention might be warranted.

Referential Communication Activities

Areas Assessed

The informal assessment task involving referential communication activities provides information on comprehension and production of linguistic features. This task, like the preceding one (giving directions), can also provide data on cognition, conversation, and survival language (Schwartz and McKinley, 1984). Nonverbal communication, especially gestures, can be observed. Referential communication activities can also be completed with written language, thus offering another assessment option.

Administration

A related procedure to giving directions is to immerse the student in referential communication activities, also known as barrier games. A referential communication activity involves a speaker who relays messages to a listener across a barrier, or screen. The listener then responds to the message. Activities may range from reproducing three-dimensional patterns to describing

how to draw an identical two-dimensional design. Messages may be delivered "step by step" from the speaker to the listener, or with a number of steps at the same time. When the examiner is giving directions for the student to follow, rate of speech should be varied to determine its effect upon comprehension. The individual undergoing assessment should be observed in both the role of speaker and listener during this activity. Excellent opportunities will be afforded the examiner to observe when and why communication breakdowns occur and whether repair takes place.

Analysis

The student's productions should be analyzed when he or she is in the role of speaker, as indicated in the preceding task giving directions. Likewise, the student's ability to comprehend messages when in the role of listener should be analyzed by determining how lengthy, and how rapid, the speaker's message can be before the student has difficulty following it. Any responses to messages that break down because of examiner error should be disqualified.

Interpretation

Speakers who consistently leave their listeners confused may have a deficit in this area. Listeners who do not comprehend adequate speaker messages, or who follow directions only when delivered one step at a time, or who need directions stated with an abnormally slow rate of speech have a deficit that warrants intervention.

Informational Listening

Areas Assessed

The informal assessment task for informational listening provides information on comprehension and production of linguistic features. This task may also assess narration if the task is structured to do so (i.e., when retelling of the information is requested).

Administration

To determine informational listening ability, a 5- to 10-minute lecture appropriate to the student's current grade level should be played, preferably on videotape. A substitute activity would have the examiner present main ideas and relevant details about a given topic informally to the student (i.e., do not read the information). After listening to the information, questions are asked of the student to ascertain what factual information was retained, whether the main idea was comprehended, and so forth. The syntactical level of the questions should be simple enough so as not to obstruct comprehension. To assess narration skills, the student could be asked to reformulate the lecture in lieu of, or in addition to, extensive questioning by the examiner.

Next, a second taped lecture, or topic expounded upon by the examiner, should be presented that is equal in difficulty to the first activity. The second oral presentation should be accompanied by a printed outline that guides the student's listening. This will allow a comparison between listening comprehension ability with and without accompanying visual input. The majority of students should listen better when following along with a printed outline. Improved performance with a printed outline will be important to document if teachers are to be convinced during indirect intervention that listening guides are important.

A third taped lecture might be on a topic of great interest to the student. If the student listens better to a lecture of interest than one in which the student doesn't hold an interest, this would indicate the student can listen but does so selectively.

Analysis

The examiner should record main ideas and relevant details of the information presented to the student and compare this information with the responses to questions about main ideas and relevant details. The examiner can then compute the percentage of questions answered accurately, given the total number asked for each of the listening conditions (with and without listening guides) and when using a topic of great interest to the student. The percentages should then be compared.

Interpretation

A student who consistently answers questions incorrectly is likely to have difficulty with informational listening in a classroom setting. If the number of questions answered accurately increases when the preadolescent or adolescent is given a written listening guide, then teachers who expect classroom listening should be informed of the testing results and should be encouraged to supply such guides to their students. When students perform noticeably better while listening to a topic of great interest, the student might need counseling about selective listening and how choosing not to listen may be harmful in classroom situations.

Critical Listening

Areas Assessed

The informal assessment task for critical listening provides information on discourse. The task also provides data on cognition, since critical listening strongly parallels critical thinking.

Administration

Taped advertisements and political speeches may be good stimuli for assessment of critical listening abilities when selected carefully for length and content. Students should listen and then answer questions posed by the examiner about the detection of false reasoning and prejudice, propaganda, or bias. Questions should also be posed that require the student to draw inferences, judge statements, and apply inductive and deductive reasoning. Multiple questions for each critical listening ability should be asked. Questions should be phrased at appropriate syntactic and semantic levels so as not to interfere with the student's comprehension. In addition to answering questions, students can express what they heard in the advertisement or speech.

An alternative procedure would involve presenting oral information and then having students detect whether they were hearing fact or opinion, for example, or having them infer what might happen in a given situation. This approach is different from the critical listening tasks that students must engage in during their daily living. However, the approach provides some information about their critical listening skills.

Analysis

Systematic recording of the student's responses to the various questions presented is necessary. The examiner should note whether the responses appear to follow a consistent pattern (e.g., correct responses to natural situations and incorrect responses to contrived situations, or correct responses to factual questions but incorrect responses to opinion questions).

Interpretation

A student who consistently answers questions incorrectly is likely to have difficulty with critical listening in a classroom setting and in other daily living situations. Professionals should consider providing intervention for the student's deficient critical listening, either through direct intervention or indirect consultative services.

Question Asking and Answering

Areas Assessed

The informal assessment task for question asking and answering provides information primarily on comprehension and production of linguistic features. Within a conversation, this task can also provide data on discourse. The student's ability to ask and to answer questions appropriately also has strong implications for survival language skills.

Administration

The student should be engaged in both asking and answering questions if an insufficient number of questions have been generated during other directed tasks. Specific tasks for asking questions might include the following:

1. Establish a quiz game format in which the response is supplied and the student must generate the question, like "Jeopardy."

2. Direct the student to ask a question, given an imaginary situation (e.g., "How would you ask a stranger sitting next to you on the bus what time it is?"). Request the individual to generate two or more alternate ways to ask the same question.

3. Role play situations with the student that require question-asking behavior (e.g., you role play the math teacher and the student role plays someone who has been out of school for several days and is missing assignments).

Tasks for answering questions might include these:

1. Role play interviewing the student for a job.

2. Present questions that request action (e.g., "Would you mind moving over a seat?"), or state information (e.g., "Can you believe we're having another test in science?"), and determine if the student understands what the appropriate responses would be.

3. Ask questions with the same semantic intent with increasing syntactical complexity, and determine if the student comprehends the question (e.g., "Who is our president?" "What is the name of the person we call President?" "You know the name of our president, don't you?"). These questions should be interspersed throughout the assessment, not presented consecutively.

Analysis

The student's spoken questions should be transcribed and analyzed for their syntactic structure and semantic intent. A variety of question forms should be evident, and questions should be stated clearly enough to communicate their intended messages. The questions should also be analyzed for their adherence to pragmatic rules. Older students may know how to ask questions, but communication is impaired if they ask in a way that offends their listeners.

Responses to questions asked by the examiner should be recorded and analyzed to determine what question types were comprehended. Comprehension is demonstrated by answering with the appropriate category of response (e.g., answering a "who" question with a name), although the answer may not always be accurate or "correct."

Interpretation

Students who fail to comprehend all question types directed at them are at a severe disadvantage academically, socially, and vocationally, since this is an assumed ability by the middle grades. Interference with test taking in the classroom and with demonstration of informational listening skills are probable accompanying deficit areas.

Students who fail to produce a variety of question forms have restricted strategies for gaining new information about the world around them. Extreme concern should be expressed if students fail to ask adequate questions during the assessment process, even when they are directed to do so.

Word Retrieval

Areas Assessed

The informal assessment task for word retrieval provides information on comprehension and production of linguistic features and on discourse. While the administration suggestions below are contrived situations, word-retrieval problems noted during this task are also likely to be observed within natural discourse samples. This directed task does not need to be completed if word-retrieval skills are not suspect.

Administration

The examiner should determine the presence or absence of a semantic deficit by obtaining a baseline measure of receptive vocabulary. The student's ability to define words, to identify likenesses and differences, and to state synonyms and antonyms could be measured (Wiig and Becker-Caplan, 1984), or formal receptive vocabulary tests could be administered. The student's receptive vocabulary performance should be compared to either chronological or mental age to confirm or refute the presence of a semantic deficit.

Once the presence or absence of a semantic deficit has been documented, naming accuracy and rate should be measured by a variety of tasks such as sentence completion, naming an item upon description, rapid automatic naming, and word association (Wiig and Becker-Caplan, 1984). Snyder and Godley (1992) recommend that the examiner systematically assess those intrinsic and extrinsic variables that influence naming behavior. The following are intrinsic variables that affect naming:

1. the frequency with which words occur (i.e., the more frequently a word occurs, the easier it is to retrieve);

2. the age of acquisition (i.e., the earlier the word is acquired, the easier it is to retrieve);

3. the category type (i.e., prototypic categories such as fruits and vegetables are easier to retrieve than words from well-defined categories such as months of the year in which there is a small set of semantic features);

4. the degree of abstractness (i.e., the more concrete the word, the easier it is to retrieve); and

5. the word class (i.e., it is easier to name concrete nouns than to name verbs, adjectives, and abstract nouns).

According to Snyder and Godley (1992), the following extrinsic variables influence naming:

1. whether the naming is in context, such as that required in a sentence-completion task, which is easier than confrontational naming (i.e., naming a pictured object);

2. syntactic requirements (i.e., the more difficult the sentence construction, the more difficult the word-retrieval task);

3. whether the task requires discrete naming, which is easier than continuous instances of naming; and

4. priming, which is the influence of the preceding word or words on the individual's ability to retrieve or recall a target word.

Both the intrinsic and extrinsic variables need to be taken into account when assessing a student's word-retrieval abilities. The examiner should also assess the behaviors that are indicative of word-finding difficulty, such as the nature of word substitutions (e.g., semantically related errors, phonologically related errors, visual perceptual errors, same grammatical class errors) and performance characteristics such as accuracy (e.g., Is the target word retrieved on the first response? What is the speed of the response?).

If a semantic deficit is determined to be present, the examiner should attempt to restrict words to be retrieved to those known to be within the student's current vocabulary. If no semantic deficit is found, words commensurate with the documented receptive vocabulary level can be used.

Analysis

Data should be examined to determine the presence of a semantic deficit, a word-retrieval problem, or a combination of the two. If it is unclear which problem is more pervasive (i.e., low vocabulary or lack of word-retrieval skills), Wiig (1983) has suggested an analysis of the student's response to multiple choices. For example, if a student is pausing to find a word, supply a choice of three or four words; the individual with low vocabulary will not necessarily be assisted by multiple choice, whereas the individual with word-retrieval problems will appear to recognize instantly the desired word.

Interpretation

Everyone experiences word-retrieval problems some of the time. However, if word-retrieval problems are consistently present not only in naming confrontation situations but also during discourse, then a deficit area is in need of intervention. Students found to have deficient vocabulary, either with or without the presence of word-retrieval problems, should also be considered for intervention.

FORMAL ASSESSMENT INSTRUMENTS

To this point, this chapter has focused on informal assessment procedures for evaluating cognition, language, and communication behaviors of preadolescents and adolescents. Additionally, many formal tests have been published that assess a multitude of isolated variables. When selecting formal tests to use with the older school-age population, we encourage examiners to refer to pages 139–141 for a discussion on how to critique standardized assessment instruments. Examiners may also wish to refer to other resources that provide criteria for the evaluation of tests (American Speech-Language-Hearing Association Ad Hoc Committee on Instrument Evaluation, 1986). Having done this, examiners can cautiously proceed with selecting one or more standardized tests that are relevant to the student being assessed.

Historical Perspective on Standardized Tests

According to Madaus and Tan (1993),

The history of testing in Europe and the United States shows that changes or adaptations in testing technology were directed at making testing more efficient, manageable, standardized, objective, easier to administer, and less costly in the face of increasing numbers of examinees. (p. 55)

A post-World War II technological development, the high-speed optical scanner, "facilitated the deployment of large-scale, low-cost, multiple-choice testing programs of the 60s, 70s, and 80s" (Madaus and Tan, 1993, pp. 56–57). In the 1990s, there appears to be a negative reaction to these cheap, efficient, administratively convenient, multiple-choice tests.

Although testing has been used in American education as a policy tool since the 1840s, the nature and magnitude of testing changed dramatically after World War II (Madaus and Tan, 1993). In 1958, the passage of the National Defense Education Act marked the emergence of using testing as a tool in the national policy arena.

In the late 1960s, standardized tests were used to make decisions on whether to keep or kill programs. In the 1970s, standardized test performance was linked to graduation, promotion, and placement. In the 1980s, states expanded the use of test results to evaluate teacher and student effectiveness and to allocate resources to school districts. In the 1990s, we hear comments that encourage the creation of a national testing system for world-class standards that would allow America to compete more effectively in global affairs (Alexander, 1993; Costa, 1993; Madaus and Tan, 1993; O'Neil, 1993).

Madaus and Tan (1993) maintain that much of the mandated standardized testing that goes on today is bureaucratic rather than educational in its usefulness. They also state that testing is heavier in special education and bilingual programs. Thus, students with language disorders and differences may be particularly vulnerable to overtesting and the use and abuse of standardized tests.

PL 94-142, along with its accompanying regulations and amendments, is another federal windfall for the testing industry. PL 94-142 requires that tests and other evaluation materials be used to place students in programs, to assess areas of special need, and to evaluate the effectiveness of individualized educational programs (IEPs) of students with disabilities or other special needs (Madaus and Tan, 1993).

What does the future hold? According to Madaus and Tan (1993), the focus will revolve around "authentic" or "innovative" performance-based assessment. Such assessment has been, and will continue to be, touted as beneficial in that it drives instruction and learning in positive ways and focuses learning on higher-order thinking skills. At the same time, Madaus and Tan (1993) offer this caution:

Such claims about the efficacy of these assessments need to be carefully evaluated. It is not the form of the tests (e.g., multiple choice, performance task, portfolio, or product to be evaluated) that is important in determining the impact of a testing program on students, teachers, and schools. Instead it is the use to which the results are put. (p. 73)

Critique of Standardized Tests

A standardized test has four aspects that are standardized (American Speech-Language-

Hearing Association Ad Hoc Committee on Instrument Evaluation, 1986):

1. Test content is fixed.

2. Administrative procedures are prescribed.

3. Responses are scored using predetermined criteria.

4. Test scores are interpreted by reference to norms or performance criteria.

Examiners who use standardized tests need to find answers to the following questions for each test selected (American Educational Research Association, American Psychological Association, and National Council on Measurement in Education, 1985; American Speech-Language-Hearing Association Ad Hoc Committee on Instrument Evaluation, 1986; Boyce and Larson, 1983; Larson and McKinley, 1987):

1. Is there a clearly stated purpose and definition of the population(s) with whom the test is to be used?

2. Is the test content relevant to the purpose of the test?

3. What stimulus presentation is used to elicit a response?

4. What response mode is used to determine if a response is correct?

5. Is the test valid for the population to which it will be administered? Does it have content validity?

6. Is the test reliable for diagnosing a communication disorder? Does it have intrajudge and interjudge reliability?

7. What is the rationale on which the test is based? Is it based on empirical data, clinical experience, theoretical constructs, or a combination of these?

8. Does the test avoid cultural and sexual stereotyping and biases?

9. Does it assess communication behaviors in a natural context and in a dynamic, ongoing fashion?

10. Are procedures for recording and analyzing responses clearly specified?

11. Are normative data available on the preadolescent or adolescent population being assessed?

12. Is the sample size adequate? Has the representative sample from the population been adequately described?

13. Are the manual instructions to the examiner and to the student clear and concise?

14. Does the test documentation clearly list the qualifications needed (e.g., education, experience, certification) by the examiner to administer the test?

These questions must be answered to ensure that the test is appropriate for the preadolescent or adolescent and is a valid and reliable measure of performance.

Worthen and Spandel (1991) cite seven common criticisms of standardized tests:

1. Standardized tests do not promote learning.

2. Standardized achievement and aptitude tests are poor predictors of individual students' performance.

3. Test content and curriculum content frequently are mismatched.

4. Standardized tests too frequently dictate what is taught in the classroom.

5. Standardized tests too frequently mislabel students in ways that are harmful to the students.

6. Standardized tests are too frequently racially, culturally, and socially biased.

7. Standardized tests measure only limited student knowledge and behaviors.

According to Worthen and Spandel (1991), there are some pitfalls to be avoided when using standardized tests:

1. Do not use the wrong tests.

2. Do not assume test scores are infallible.

3. Do not use a single test score to make a decision.

4. Do not forget to supplement test scores with other information.

5. Do not set arbitrary minimums for performance tests.

6. Do not assume that tests measure all the content, skills, or behaviors of interest.

7. Do not accept uncritically all claims made by test authors and publishers.

8. Do not interpret test scores inappropriately.

9. Do not use test scores to draw inappropriate comparisons.

10. Do not allow tests to drive the curriculum.

11. Do not use poor tests.

12. Do not use tests unprofessionally.

Table 6.12 presents a variety of tests that the examiner might choose when assessing an older student's cognition, language, and communication behaviors. A number of variables have been summarized for each test, including age range, primary area(s) assessed, theoretical construct stated, content validity, interjudge reliability, normative data, stimulus presentation (modality and type of auditory input), and response mode. The information cited in the "Age Range" column matches what the author(s) of the test reported in the examiner's manual; however, at times the age range cited by the author(s) was discrepant from the age range sampled for the normative data. Likewise, information recorded in the columns labeled "Theoretical Construct Stated," "Content Validity," "Interjudge Reliability," and "Normative Data" was taken from the perspective of the author(s) of the test. We do not necessarily concur with the conclusions drawn by the writers of the tests. For example, Vallett (1981) stated that his test was based on Piagetian theory and explained no further. Although a "yes" was recorded in the "Theoretical Construct Stated" column, it is questionable whether this variable warranted credit.

The information in Table 6.12 recorded in the columns "Primary Areas Assessed," "Stimulus Presentation," and "Response Mode" was taken from our perspective. This information was gathered by carefully reviewing the test materials.

Related Assessment Instruments in Other Disciplines

In addition to using formal tests designed to measure cognition, language, and communication of preadolescents or adolescents,

TABLE 6.12	FORMAL TESTS OF COGNITION, LANGUAGE, AND COMMUNICATION											
TESTS	**AGE RANGE**	**PRIMARY AREAS ASSESSED**				**THEORETICAL CONSTRUCT STATED**	**CONTENT VALIDITY**	**INTERJUDGE RELIABILITY**	**NORMATIVE DATA**	**STIMULUS PRESENTATION**		**RESPONSE MODE**
		THINKING	**LISTENING**	**SPEAKING**	**WRITING**					**MODALITY**	**TYPE OF AUDITORY INPUT**	
Clinical Evaluation of Language Fundamentals–Revised (CELF–R) (1987) Semel, E., Wiig, E., Secord, W. The Psychological Corporation San Antonio, TX	5.0 – 16.11	—	X	X	—	Yes	Yes	Yes	Yes	A & V	W/S/Cs	O/Pt
Detroit Tests of Learning Aptitude (3rd ed.) (DTLA–3) (1991) Hammill, D. Pro-Ed Austin, TX	6.0 – 17.11	X	X	X	—	Yes	Yes	No	Yes	A & V	W/S/Cs	Pt/O/Wr
Diagnostic Achievement Battery–2 (DAB–2) (1990) Newcomer, P. Pro-Ed Austin, TX	6.0 – 14.11	—	X	X	X	No	Yes	No	Yes	A & V	W/S/Cs	O/Pt/Wr
Expressive One-Word Picture Vocabulary Test: Upper Extension (EOWPVT–UE) (1983) Gardner, M. Academic Therapy Publications Novato, CA	12.0 – 15.11	—	—	X	—	No	Yes	No	Yes	V	W	O

* Criterion-referenced	A — Auditory	Cs — Connected Speech	G — Gesture	O — Oral
** Rating Scales Only	Og — Other Gesture	P — Phrases	Pf — Performance	Pt — Pointing
	S — Sentences	V — Visual	W — Words	Wr — Written

(continued)

TESTS	AGE RANGE	PRIMARY AREAS ASSESSED				THEORETICAL CONSTRUCT STATED	CONTENT VALIDITY	INTERJUDGE RELIABILITY	NORMATIVE DATA	STIMULUS PRESENTATION		RESPONSE MODE
		THINKING	LISTENING	SPEAKING	WRITING					MODALITY	TYPE OF AUDITORY INPUT	
Expressive One-Word Picture Vocabulary Test–Revised Edition (EOWPVT–R) (1990) Gardner, M. Academic Therapy Publications Novato, CA	2.0 – 11.11	—	—	X	—	No	Yes	No	Yes	V	W	O
Fullerton Language Test for Adolescents (2nd ed.) (1986) Thorum, A. Consulting Psychologists Press Palo Alto, CA	11 – 18	—	X	X	—	No	Yes	Yes	Yes	A & V	W/P/S	O/PF
Inventory of Essential Skills (1981) Brigance, A. Curriculum Associates North Billerica, MA	Grade 6 – Adult	X	X	X	—	No	Yes**	No	No*	A & V	W/S/Cs	O/PF/ WR
Let's Talk Inventory for Adolescents (1982) Wiig, E. Charles E. Merrill Columbus, OH	9 – Young Adulthood	—	—	X	—	No	Yes	Yes	Yes	A & V	Cs	O
Peabody Individual Achievement Test–Revised (PIAT–R) (1989) Markwardt, F., Jr. American Guidance Service Circle Pines, MN	5.0 – 18.11	—	X	X	X	No	Yes	No	Yes	A & V	W/S	O/PT/ WR

* Criterion-referenced	A — Auditory	Cs — Connected Speech	G — Gesture	O — Oral
** Rating Scales Only	OG — Other Gesture	P — Phrases	PF — Performance	PT — Pointing
	S — Sentences	V — Visual	W — Words	WR — Written

(continued)

TABLE 6.12—(Continued)

Tests	Age Range	Primary Areas Assessed				Theoretical Construct Stated	Content Validity	Interjudge Reliability	Normative Data	Stimulus Presentation		Response Mode
		Thinking	Listening	Speaking	Writing					Modality	Type of Auditory Input	
Peabody Picture Vocabulary Test–Revised (PPVT–R) (1981) Dunn, L., Dunn, L. American Guidance Service Circle Pines, MN	2.5 – 40	—	X	—	—	No	Yes	Yes	Yes	A & V	W	Pt
Receptive One-Word Picture Vocabulary Test (ROWPVT) (1985) Gardner, M. Academic Therapy Publications Novato, CA	2.0 – 11.11	—	X	—	—	No	Yes	No	Yes	A & V	W	Pt
Receptive One-Word Picture Vocabulary Test: Upper Extension (ROWPVT–UE) (1987) Gardner, M. Academic Therapy Publications Novato, CA	12.0 – 15.11	—	X	—	—	No	Yes	No	Yes	A & V	W	Pt
Test of Adolescent/ Adult Word Finding (TAWF) (1990) German, D. Riverside Publishing Chicago, IL	12.0 – 80.0	—	X	X	—	Yes	Yes	No	Yes	A & V	W/S	O/Pt
Test of Adolescent and Adult Language 3 (TOAL 3) (1994) Hammill, D., Brown, V., Larsen, S., Wiederholt, J. Pro-Ed Austin, TX	12.0 – 24.11	—	X	X	X	No	Yes	Yes	Yes	A & V	W/S	O/Wr

* Criterion-referenced	A — Auditory	Cs — Connected Speech	G — Gesture	O — Oral
** Rating Scales Only	Og — Other Gesture	P — Phrases	Pf — Performance	Pt — Pointing
	S — Sentences	V — Visual	W — Words	Wr — Written

(continued)

TESTS	AGE RANGE	PRIMARY AREAS ASSESSED				THEORETICAL CONSTRUCT STATED	CONTENT VALIDITY	INTERJUDGE RELIABILITY	NORMATIVE DATA	STIMULUS PRESENTATION		RESPONSE MODE
		THINKING	LISTENING	SPEAKING	WRITING					MODALITY	TYPE OF AUDITORY INPUT	
Test of Concept Utilization (1972) Crager, R., Spriggs, A. Western Psychological Services Los Angeles, CA	5 – 18	X	—	—	—	No	Yes	Yes	Yes	A & V	S	O
Test of Language Competence– Expanded Edition (1989) Level 1 Level 2 Wiig, E., Secord, W. Psychological Corporation San Antonio, TX	5.0 – 9.11 9.0 – 18.11	X X	X X	X X	— —	Yes Yes	Yes Yes	Yes Yes	Yes Yes	A & V A & V	W/S W/S	O O
Test of Language Development– Intermediate (2nd ed.) (TOLD–I:2) (1988) Hammill, D., Newcomer, P. Pro-Ed Austin, TX	8.6 – 12.11	—	X	X	—	Yes	Yes	No	Yes	A	W/S	O
Test of Nonverbal Intelligence (2nd ed.) (TONI–2) (1990) Brown, L., Sherbenou, R., Johnsen, S. Pro-Ed Austin, TX	5.0 – 85.11	X	—	—	—	Yes	Yes	No	Yes	V	G	P/Og

TABLE 6.12—*(Continued)*

* Criterion-referenced	A — Auditory	Cs — Connected Speech	G — Gesture	O — Oral
** Rating Scales Only	Og — Other Gesture	P — Phrases	Pf — Performance	Pt — Pointing
	S — Sentences	V — Visual	W — Words	Wr — Written

(continued)

TABLE 6.12—(Continued)												
TESTS	**AGE RANGE**	**PRIMARY AREAS ASSESSED**				**THEORETICAL CONSTRUCT STATED**	**CONTENT VALIDITY**	**INTERJUDGE RELIABILITY**	**NORMATIVE DATA**	**STIMULUS PRESENTATION**		**RESPONSE MODE**
		THINKING	**LISTENING**	**SPEAKING**	**WRITING**					**MODALITY**	**TYPE OF AUDITORY INPUT**	
Test of Pragmatic Language (TOPL) (1992) Phelps-Terasaki, D., Phelps-Gunn, T. Pro-Ed Austin, TX	5.0 – 12.0	—	—	X	—	Yes	Yes	Yes	Yes	A & V	S/Cs	O
Test of Problem Solving– Elementary (TOPS) (1984) Zachman, L., Barrett, M., Huisingh, R., Jorgensen, C. LinguiSystems East Moline, IL	6.0 – 11.11	X	—	—	—	No	Yes	Yes	Yes	A & V	S	O
Test of Problem Solving– Adolescent (TOPS) (1991) Zachman, L., Barrett, M., Huisingh, R., Orman, J., Blagden, C. LinguiSystems East Moline, IL	12.0 – 17.11	X	—	—	—	Yes	Yes	Yes	Yes	A & V	Cs	O
Test of Word Finding (TWF) (1989) German, D. Riverside Publishing Chicago, IL	6.6 – 12.11	—	X	X	—	Yes	Yes	No	Yes	A & V	W/S	O/Pt
Test of Word Finding in Discourse (TWFD) (1991) German, D. Riverside Publishing Chicago, IL	6.6 – 12.11	—	—	X	—	Yes	Yes	Yes	Yes	A & V	S/Cs	O

* Criterion-referenced	A — Auditory	Cs — Connected Speech	G — Gesture	O — Oral
** Rating Scales Only	Og — Other Gesture	P — Phrases	Pf — Performance	Pt — Pointing
	S — Sentences	V — Visual	W — Words	Wr — Written

(continued)

TESTS	AGE RANGE	PRIMARY AREAS ASSESSED				THEORETICAL CONSTRUCT STATED	CONTENT VALIDITY	INTERJUDGE RELIABILITY	NORMATIVE DATA	STIMULUS PRESENTATION		RESPONSE MODE
		THINKING	LISTENING	SPEAKING	WRITING					MODALITY	TYPE OF AUDITORY INPUT	
TABLE 6.12—*(Continued)*												
Test of Word Knowledge (TOWK) (1992) Wiig, E., Secord, W. The Psychological Corporation San Antonio, TX	5.0 – 17.0	—	X	X	—	Yes	Yes	Yes	Yes	A & V	W/S	O/Pᴛ
Test of Written Language (2nd ed.) (TOWL–2) (1988) Hammill, D., Larsen, S. Pro-Ed Austin, TX	7.6 – 17.11	—	—	—	X	No	Yes	Yes	Yes	A & V	S/Cs	Wʀ
The Word Test–R (Elementary) (1990) Huisingh, R., Barrett, M., Zachman, L., Blagden, C., Orman, J. LinguiSystems East Moline, IL	7.0 – 11.11	—	—	X	—	No	Yes	No	Yes	A	W/S	O
The Word Test (Adolescent) (1989) Zachman, L., Barrett, M., Huisingh, R., Orman, J., Blagden, C. LinguiSystems East Moline, IL	12 – 17.11	—	—	X	—	No	Yes	No	Yes	A & V	W/S	O
Vallett Inventory of Critical Thinking Abilities (1981) Vallett, R. Academic Therapy Publications Novata, CA	4 – 15	X	—	—	—	Yes	Yes	No	No*	A & V	W/P/S/ Cs	O / Pꜰ

* Criterion-referenced	A — Auditory	Cs — Connected Speech	G — Gesture	O — Oral
** Rating Scales Only	Oɢ — Other Gesture	P — Phrases	Pꜰ — Performance	Pᴛ — Pointing
	S — Sentences	V — Visual	W — Words	Wʀ — Written

(continued)

TABLE 6.12—*(Continued)*		PRIMARY AREAS ASSESSED				THEORETICAL CONSTRUCT STATED	CONTENT VALIDITY	INTERJUDGE RELIABILITY	NORMATIVE DATA	STIMULUS PRESENTATION		RESPONSE MODE
TESTS	AGE RANGE	THINKING	LISTENING	SPEAKING	WRITING					MODALITY	TYPE OF AUDITORY INPUT	
Woodcock Language Proficiency Battery–Revised (WLP –R) (1991) Woodcock, R. Riverside Publishing Chicago, IL	2.0 – 90.0+	X	X	X	—	No	Yes	Yes	Yes	A & V	W/S/Cs	O/ Wʀ/Pꜰ
Woodcock-Johnson Psycho-Educational Battery–Revised (WJ–R) (1990) Woodcock, R., Johnson, M. Riverside Publishing Chicago, IL	2.0 – 90.0+	X	X	X	—	No	Yes	No	Yes	A & V	W/S/Cs	O/Pᴛ/ Wʀ
Writing Process Test (WPT) (1992) Warden, M., Hutchinson, T. Riverside Publishing Chicago, IL	Grades 2 – 12	X	—	—	X	Yes	Yes	Yes	Yes	A & V	Cs	Wʀ

* Criterion-referenced	A — Auditory	Cs — Connected Speech	G — Gesture	O — Oral
** Rating Scales Only	Oɢ — Other Gesture	P — Phrases	Pꜰ — Performance	Pᴛ — Pointing
	S — Sentences	V — Visual	W — Words	Wʀ — Written

speech-language pathologists should be aware of additional data that can be gleaned from tests administered by other professionals. For example, intelligence tests administered by psychologists can be a source of information.

To what extent the intelligence test may be used by the speech-language pathologist is contingent upon whether the speech-language pathologist adheres to the strong or weak cognitive hypothesis. According to Casby (1992), the strong cognitive hypothesis states that cognitive development accounts for and is a prerequisite to language development. The weak cognitive hypothesis states that cognitive abilities make certain meanings available for language (e.g., social and language-specific sources), and language has its own specific sources; more specifically, language can influence development in cognition.

Casby (1992) reviews literature demonstrating that individuals such as those with developmental delays or retardation may have language skills that surpass their cognitive or mental ages. Despite these findings, the strong cognitive hypothesis or cognitive referencing model continues to influence criteria of eligibility for who receives speech-language services in the schools (Casby, 1992; Cole, Mills, and Kelley, 1994). Casby found that 31 states use the strong cognitive hypothesis as the basis for their eligibility criteria for speech-language services. Casby (1992) stated,

> Certainly, cognitive and linguistic skills are highly correlated, yet it has not been established that cognition serves as a necessary or sufficient prerequisite to language development. There is now

incontrovertible evidence that the strong cognitive hypothesis does not accurately reflect the relationship between cognition and language. Eligibility decisions that rely on the strong cognitive hypothesis are thus no longer appropriate. (p. 201)

Cole, Mills, and Kelley (1994) conducted a study to examine the agreement of various cognitive-language profiles to confirm or refute the cognitive referencing model. Their study concluded that the use of the cognitive referencing model or strong cognitive hypothesis to establish eligibility criteria for speech-language services is questionable. We concur with these authors and do not recommend that speech-language services for preadolescents and adolescents be based upon mental age/cognitive ability being greater than language age. Many students whose language age is greater than or equivalent to their mental age do and can profit from speech-language services.

Tests of reading and writing abilities can provide additional insight into the adolescent's linguistic system, as can annual tests of academic achievement. It is our contention that speech-language pathologists should be knowledgeable about other tests being completed with the student, and that these results should be integrated, as appropriate, with data gathered on the parameters discussed in this chapter. Does testing completed by other professionals support or refute findings by the speech-language pathologist? The speech-language pathologist should request that other examiners record oral responses of students verbatim, thus allowing the opportunity for later analysis by the clinician.

An intelligence test like the *Wechsler Intelligence Scale for Children–Third Edition* (Wechsler, 1991) will provide both a verbal and a performance quotient. The verbal performance quotient of an individual relies heavily on oral communication skills. So, too, does the performance quotient rely on language when the stimulus presentation utilizes an auditory modality. The most commonly used intelligence tests should be familiar to speech-language pathologists, including the *Leiter International Performance Test–Revised* (Leiter, 1979), the *Slosson Intelligence Test–Revised* (Nicholson and Hibpshman, 1990), the *Stanford-Binet Intelligence Scale* (4th edition) (Thorndike, Hagen, and Sattler, 1986), the *Stanford-Binet Intelligence Scale* (Form L-M) (Terman and Merrill, 1973), the *Wechsler Intelligence Scale for Children–Third Edition* (Wechsler, 1991), and the *Wechsler Adult Intelligence Scale–Revised* (Wechsler, 1981).

Academic achievement tests with which speech-language pathologists may need to be familiar include the *Mini-Battery of Achievement* (Woodcock, McGrew, and Werder, 1993), *Diagnostic Achievement Test for Adolescents–Second Edition* (Newcomer and Bryant, 1993), the *Woodcock-Johnson Psycho-Educational Battery–Revised* (Woodcock and Johnson, 1990), *Diagnostic Achievement Battery–Second Edition* (Newcomer, 1990), and *Wide Range Achievement Test–Revised* (Jastak and Wilkinson, 1984).

Reading and writing tests with which speech-language pathologists may want to be familiar include the *Gray Oral Reading Tests–Third Edition* (Wiederholt and Bryant, 1992), *Gray Oral Reading Tests–Diagnostic* (Bryant and Wiederholt, 1991), *Test of Reading Comprehension–Revised Edition* (Brown, Hammill, and Wiederholt, 1986), *Writing Process Test* (Warden and Hutchinson, 1992), and *Test of Written Language–Second Edition* (Hammill and Larsen, 1988). Readers are encouraged to examine these assessment instruments for the cognitive, language, and communication behaviors they demand if the student is to respond accurately to test items.

SUMMARY

This chapter provided, by category, an extensive description of what behaviors to assess: cognition, comprehension and production of linguistic features, discourse (conversations and narrations), written communication, meta-abilities, nonverbal communication, and survival language skills. It placed an emphasis on an integrative assessment process (i.e., evaluating the ongoing, interactive dynamics of cognition, language, and communication behaviors).

The chapter proposed specific informal methods for assessing behaviors: case history forms, a learning style questionnaire, portfolios, analysis procedures for conversations and narrations, and directed tasks. It summarized formal tests that might be selected for older students according to a predetermined set of variables. In addition, it listed assessment instruments from related disciplines.

DISCUSSION QUESTIONS

1. Describe several specific informal assessment tasks that would permit the examiner to gather integrated information on cognition, comprehension and production of linguistic features, discourse, written communication, meta-abilities, nonverbal communication, and/or survival language skills.

2. Select two intelligence tests, two achievement tests, or two reading tests appropriate to administer to older students. Summarize and critique the tests for cognitive, language, and communication skills needed to complete items successfully.

SUGGESTED READINGS

Casby, M. (1992). The cognitive hypothesis and its influence on speech-language services in schools. *Language, Speech, and Hearing Services in Schools, 23,* 198–212.

Damico, J. (1991). Clinical discourse analysis: A functional approach to language assessment. In C. Simon (Ed.), *Communication skills and classroom success: Assessment and therapy methodologies for language and learning disabled students.* Eau Claire, WI: Thinking Publications.

LANGUAGE INTERVENTION WITH OLDER STUDENTS

7

GOALS:

To discuss how to structure intervention programs for older students

To present general intervention procedures

To illustrate selected specific intervention methods

To summarize commercial resources appropriate for preadolescents and adolescents

To explain how to implement educational and environmental system modifications that assist older students with language disabilities

Intervention with older students who have language disorders is paramount for their survival at school, at home, and in the community. Unfortunately, as involved professionals consider the myriad of challenges that at-risk youth face within their own families and communities, the provision of speech-language intervention may appear inconsequential. Intervention may be considered an extra, a "frill," and certainly an expense that can be crossed off the budget.

On the contrary, speech-language intervention for older students who have been diagnosed as having speech-language disabilities is one of the most crucial services to provide, since the crux of their problems often rests on their lack of adequate communication skills. Without intervention, the risk is great

that these youth will engage in antisocial behaviors and experience school performance failure leading to personal injury, incarceration, or a welfare-state adulthood.

Appropriate speech-language intervention that teaches the older student communication skills for academic, social, and vocational situations is the key to his or her ability to "fit" into society—to function as a family member, a lifelong learner, a citizen, a participant in leisure, and both a consumer and a producer of goods and services (Valletutti and Bender, 1982). This chapter addresses how speech-language pathologists can best intervene with older students to help them function as more effective communicators at school, at home, and in the community.

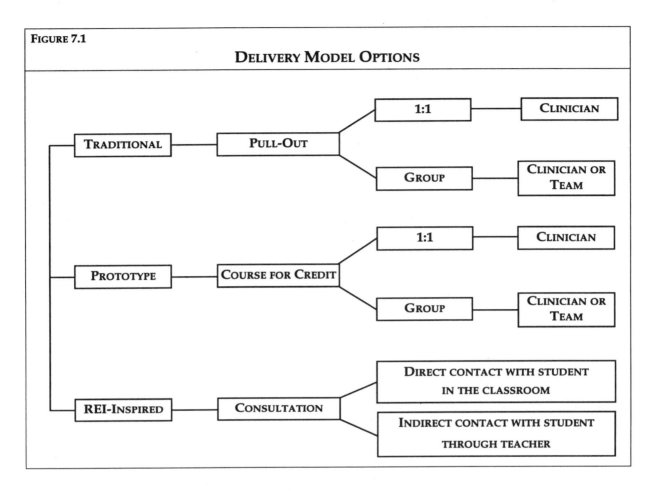

FIGURE 7.1

DELIVERY MODEL OPTIONS

SERVICE DELIVERY FOR INTERVENTION

Appropriate service models for older students must be selected or their cooperation with intervention will be minimized. Primary choices for service delivery are presented in Figure 7.1.

Traditionally, speech-language services have been delivered through pull-out models (i.e., removing a student from his or her classroom and providing speech-language services in an isolated therapy room). While younger children are excited to be singled out for such

attention, older children often react negatively. Perhaps they are being removed from a classroom where they are struggling to stay abreast. Others are removed from study periods. (This is equivalent to being removed from recess in earlier grades.)

Removal from a class or study period makes students with speech-language disabilities appear even more different than their peers. Yet they are at an age during which their desire to conform—not to appear different than their peers—is greatest. The undesired "visibility" of leaving an existing class or study period may sabotage speech-language intervention. The other disadvantage with the pull-out model across all age levels is the discontinuity of intervention and classroom instruction. Students are still expected to know the information presented while they are out of the class for intervention.

To coordinate speech-language goals and academic content, the model of choice has increasingly been collaborative consultation. This may take one of three basic forms (Simon and Myrold-Gunyuz, 1990):

1. *The formula model*—The speech-language pathologist and collaborative partner plan lessons weekly. Each then teaches a lesson to a different group of students in the classroom.

2. *The communication enhancement model*—The speech-language pathologist guest-teaches a demonstration lesson for all students while the classroom teacher assists.

3. *The curriculum-based model*—The speech-language pathologist notes the language of instruction in the classroom, then provides complementary lesson components and advises how language can be taught to students in an effective and efficient manner.

While classroom consultation is a viable, practical intervention model for preschool and elementary students, the educational system is structured counterproductively with respect to consultation at upper grade levels. With whom might a speech-language pathologist collaborate? Once students reach middle grades and beyond, classroom teachers focus on curricular content, almost to the exclusion of basic skills. Since oral language skills are

assumed to be intact by most classroom teachers, few will appreciate the benefit of taking class time to focus on language skills. And if a professional were to pull a small group aside within a classroom, that is frequently more embarrassing to a pre-teen or teen than resorting to the traditional pull-out model.

Consultation at the secondary level is probably most feasible when it occurs between the speech-language pathologist and another specialist (e.g., a guidance counselor, a learning disabilities specialist, a school-work transition liaison). These educators, like the speech-language pathologist, have a vested interest in the communication skills of students. Team-teaching situations involving the speech-language pathologist and another specialist can also be very powerful for effecting changes in preadolescents and adolescents.

The most effective intervention model, advocated by us since 1983, is the prototype service delivery model (Boyce and Larson, 1983; Larson and McKinley, 1987; Larson, McKinley, and Boley, 1993; McKinley and Larson, 1985). The essence of this model is that speech-language services are provided through a class that has the same requirements as any other course the student takes (i.e., it meets for so many minutes each week, a grade is given, credit is granted toward high school graduation). This model is midway between the traditional pull-out model and the much-advocated consultation model and is described further in Appendix J. Information on the program planning component of the prototype model is presented on page 296.

Choosing to implement a prototype delivery model does not negate other service delivery options. Many professionals organize their schedules so part of the day is spent delivering services through each of the major models. The main goal is to match the student's needs with the most appropriate delivery model. Failure to do so will sabotage even the most brilliant lesson plan. So too will failure to consider the paradigm shifts occurring, even as you read.

PARADIGM SHIFTS

The Van Riper Lecture Series (Kalamazoo, MI, May 1993) focused on new paradigm shifts that are radically changing how professionals view education in general and speech-language services in particular. Barbara Hoskins (1993) discussed four main principles of these new paradigms:

1. *Systems thinking*—Professionals are experiencing the leveling of hierarchies into networks, the collaboration with partners in the process, and the supporting of classrooms as systems. Relating this to delivery model options, speech-language services need to be integrated into the overall educational system. Once they are, gone will be the era when administrators and decision makers question why a student still needs speech-language services past the age of 10 years. They will understand that speech-language pathologists are part of the network that forms a successful support system for older students.

2. *Market driven*—Professionals are realizing an emphasis on choice and on flexible, accessible services. Focus is on the learner,

and the parents and the community are viewed as consumers. In our experience, once older students and parents understand the importance of speech-language services, they strongly advocate the continuity and expansion of these services. Speech-language pathologists seeking to create strong programs for older students would be well-advised to spend considerable effort on educating consumers about their services.

3. *Focus on diversity*—Professionals are placing renewed emphasis on integrating students with special needs into the mainstream and into heterogeneous groups. Schools are no longer expected to be a "melting pot" for cultural diversity, but rather they are to be a "salad bowl"—institutions that allow, even encourage, individual identities of all students. By the year 2000, as many as one-third of the children receiving speech-language-hearing services will be from Black, Hispanic, Asian, and Native North American cultures (American Speech-Language-Hearing Association, 1988). They will be served by predominantly white, middle-class professionals (Crago, 1990). As Crago and Cole (1991) pointed out, "A culturally sensitive refocusing of our assessment and intervention practices is long overdue" (p. 100).

4. *Practical results*—Professionals are developing an orientation toward demanding results, especially given the economic crunch of the late 1980s and early 1990s. Attention is directed toward

relevant goals, performance-based assessment, classroom-based intervention, and asking the question, "What does this student really have to learn to function?" Practical results will be a primary measurement to evaluate the effectiveness of intervention, regardless of the service delivery model chosen.

THE ROLE OF ETHNOGRAPHY IN INTERVENTION

In 1974, Hymes described a new area of study called "the ethnography of speaking," which examines the role of speaking in the socialization of children. Anthropology and linguistics were brought together not in an attempt to establish communication universals, but to preserve the complexity of language use. Duranti (1988) explained,

> Ethnographers . . . like the people they study . . . struggle both to capture and maintain the whole of the interaction at hand. The elements of one level (e.g., phonological register, lexical choice, discourse strategies) must be related to elements at another level (e.g., social identities, values). . . . Ethnographers act as linking elements between different levels and systems of communication. (p. 220)

An ethnographic approach is different from a pragmatic analysis approach because there is stronger concern for the sociocultural context of language use.

Ethnography is critical when intervening with minority students. Speech-language pathologists from the majority culture will not typically share assumptions, values, or communication patterns with children from minority cultures. Thus, formulation of appropriate intervention strategies is prevented when professionals lack awareness of the importance of the cultural-socialization relationships within a given minority population.

Crago and Cole (1991) described nine basic assumptions that characterize the ethnographic approach. These nine assumptions should become part of the foundation upon which solid, practical intervention goals and activities are created:

1. "The everyday details of life can be made comprehensible" (p. 107). Study the details of people's everyday life experiences and build knowledge of what people say, what they do, and what people say they ought to say or do. Incorporate these details into intervention.

2. "Accurate description requires extensive contact" (p. 108). Learn extensively about the minority cultural groups treated. Only then are appropriate speech-language services delivered.

3. "Interpretation is an inherent part of observation" (p. 108). Seek and capture accurate interpretations of people's beliefs and actions to select appropriate times, forms, places, and people for intervention.

4. "Analysis is an iterative spiral and not predetermined" (p. 108). Start with an initial set of questions during intervention and collect the response data. This should lead to more questions. Analysis during intervention is ongoing.

5. "All descriptions are partial and subjective" (p. 109). Understand your influence on any findings and results. Describe and account for your own life situations that might contribute to partiality. Open, honest reckoning may lead to more productive clinical outcomes.

6. "Descriptions have emic and etic dimensions" (p. 109). (*Emic* refers to the people being investigated [e.g., the minority students]; *etic* refers to the outsider studying the people [e.g., a speech-language pathologist].) Shape etic frameworks to suit the client at hand, who may or may not fit into such a mold. Recognize how your perspectives, actions, and interpretations are seen by clients.

7. "More than one perspective is needed" (p. 110). Gain multiple perspectives on a student's functioning. Avoid misinterpretations such as deficiency interpretations of cultural differences by tapping into culturally informed points of view.

8. "Both macro and micro levels of analysis are needed" (p. 110). Use language samples to pinpoint important gaps that are not culturally related (micro level). Document how language is integrated with cultural and socioeconomic dimensions (macro level).

9. "Themes are generalizable from the careful study of a small number of people" (p. 111). Gather information on the communicative interactions of a few families within a particular cultural group, as it can be relevant to several children on your caseload.

Damico and Damico (1993) echoed the need to respect the complexity of the relationships between language and social skills when considered from a diversity perspective. As speech-language pathologists are called upon more and more to recommend interventions for students from culturally and linguistically diverse backgrounds, it is critical that the students' home languages are not seen as detriments and that their home cultures are not devalued in any way (Damico and Damico, 1993). Rather, professionals should assist students from diverse backgrounds to become more empowered in the educational system (Damico and Armstrong, 1991).

DIRECT SERVICES

Assessment includes an appraisal of the student and his or her educational and environmental systems. Similarly, intervention focuses on direct services to students and on indirect services to the systems in which they function.

UNIQUE ASPECTS OF SERVING OLDER SCHOOL-AGE CHILDREN

Direct services to older school-age children have unique aspects compared to serving younger children. While not an exhaustive list, the more crucial aspects include mutual planning, motivational issues, a learning strategies approach, and available counseling.

Mutual Planning

A profile of relative strengths and weaknesses should have emerged from the assessment results. Moreover, this information should have been explained to the student in such a way that awareness of the language disorder was established. Mutual planning of goals and objectives by the student and the involved professionals should occur at the outset of intervention and periodically throughout the process. This mutual planning is essential to the student's assuming responsibility for the modification of the language disorder.

The planning process should have no "hidden agenda." Professionals should communicate openly and honestly about what needs to be accomplished and why it is to be done. After goals and objectives are identified, the student should assist in ranking them by importance. Certainly, professionals can provide guidance by pointing out when prerequisite objectives are necessary to reach top-ranked goals. However, unlike younger children who have no investment in the goal-setting process, older children must fully participate if they are to be active and cooperative learners during intervention. Otherwise, goals may be self-defeating.

The age of the child also affects the selection of goals and objectives to be emphasized. In general, goals for pre-teens and youth in early adolescence should focus on developing the language necessary for academic progress and personal-social growth (i.e., peer group acceptance). Goals for students in late adolescence should focus on developing the language necessary for enhancing voca-

tional potential and personal-social growth (i.e., one-to-one long-term relationships). In middle adolescence, any or all of the three areas (i.e., academic progress, personal-social growth, and vocational potential) might be emphasized.

Motivational Issues

Motivation can sometimes be enhanced by using contracts, offering speech-language intervention as a course for credit, providing grades for speech-language intervention, scheduling speech-language services within existing time modules, developing and using supportive titles for speech-language services, considering carefully the area of the school where services are provided, and encouraging an intrinsic desire to improve communication. Each of these motivational issues is described below.

Contracting

Some students seem to be motivated to learn when they sign a contract that specifies goals for communication performance and the time frame within which the goals are to be accomplished. When using contingency contracts with preadolescents and adolescents, the professional should make the contracts appear adultlike and official (Larson and McKinley, 1985b). The contract should be developed jointly with the student and should specify the consequences for positive performance or lack of performance. The professional should be flexible when developing the contract and should allow sufficient time for the student to help shape its content.

Course for Credit

Another motivational consideration is recognition of the student's efforts by offering speech-language intervention as a course at the middle-school or junior-high level and as a course for credit (e.g., one-half credit per semester) at the senior-high level. Students invest at least as much time and energy working on their communication skills as they do on other skills taught in courses for credit. If a decision is made to offer speech-language intervention as a course for credit, then it should be determined whether this is to be an elective course or whether a required course can be waived for speech-language intervention (i.e., credit for speech-language intervention substitutes for the required course credit).

Assume for a minute that speech-language courses have been established and that they may be taken either as electives or as waivers for required classes. The speech-language pathologist and the student need to determine which option is most suitable (i.e., elective or substitute). Major considerations when making this decision include these:

1. Is the student attempting to function in required mainstream courses but failing, or nearly failing, one or more? If so, is the failure resulting from poor comprehension of vocabulary and concepts, or from the high cognitive demands of the curriculum? When one or both factors are contributing significantly to failure in a required course, a rationale can be built for the student to receive a waiver from that course on the grounds that insufficient language and cognitive skills inevitably prevent success in the course. When the speech-language course replaces the class being failed, prerequisite language and cognitive abilities become goals and objectives in the student's individualized plan.

2. What other electives are in competition with the speech-language course? Students with language disorders, especially those who need intervention at the secondary level, frequently wish to take vocationally oriented classes which usually are offered as electives. These students need flexibility to take these electives because the courses are important for their future vocational success. Also, these students are often more motivated to participate in elective courses than in required courses. Since these same students may be at risk for dropping out of school, they must be kept in courses that spark their interest. If there are many electives in which the student is interested, it might be best to build a rationale for substitute credit. However, if a rationale for substitute credit is not appropriate, then the student should be counseled to take speech-language intervention as an elective course. Other elective vocational courses might then be taken outside the regular school day.

Grading

Offering speech-language courses entails giving grades for student performance. There are several options for grading. Giving a letter grade or using a satisfactory/fail system, as other courses would, is appropriate. If the speech-language course is substituting for a required course, a letter grade may be mandatory when this is the grading policy for other required courses. Another option is to grade by progress, resulting in a description of performance and not a letter grade. Grading by progress most accurately reflects performance on individual goals and objectives, and could possibly be combined with other mandatory grades.

Even when speech-language intervention is not organized as a course for credit, grading should be explored as an option. As much as grades appear to be aversive to students, they are inherent in the student's educational experience. Grades are a way to give credibility to speech-language intervention. Several options exist regarding their use:

1. Have the student's performance in speech-language intervention contribute to a percentage of the student's grade in another course. For example, if the student is being removed from part of English class for speech-language services, propose to the English teacher that a portion of the student's grade be determined by speech-language performance.

2. Request a space on the student's regular report card for speech-language performance and record a letter grade or satisfactory/fail.

3. Include a progress report card with the student's regular report card.

The option(s) chosen for grading should be clarified with the preadolescent or adolescent. The student needs to understand that grading will occur and realize when and how grades will be reported. Deriving a grade to evaluate the student's performance may be accom-

plished in several ways. One alternative is to assign a percentage to each course requirement (e.g., 25 percent for class discussion, 25 percent for projects, 25 percent for examinations, and 25 percent for daily assignments).

Another way to derive a letter grade is to assign points for participation and work completed and to remove points for inappropriate behaviors. At the end of a grading period, a minimum number of points is needed for each letter grade.

A word of warning about grading should be given here. In school districts honoring speech-language intervention as a course for credit and permitting letter grades, other teachers and parents may raise validity questions: "Is an A or B given for speech-language of less value than an A or B earned for algebra?" "Should an A or B in speech-language contribute the same to class rank as an A or B in English?" Since class rank affects scholarship and college admission decisions—to name just a few issues—the impact of grading for speech-language intervention may have broad implications. At least one school district resolved the dilemma by disallowing speech-language grades in class-rank calculations. This was not a supportive decision for the adolescents with language disorders in that school system, but it was the best compromise that could be struck among the speech-language pathologist, parents, and teachers.

Scheduling

Another motivational issue to consider is scheduling the speech-language course so that the student receives appropriate intervention rather than token services. Meeting twice a week for 20 or 30 minutes using a pull-out model may not be sufficient to help the preadolescent or adolescent make significant progress in communication behaviors. What may happen during these short time blocks is that the student may experience success but become frustrated further when the intervention time cannot be extended.

A more viable means to schedule intervention is to use existing time modules and to have the administrator incorporate the course into the class schedule like all other subject areas. Meeting for full time modules will allow more time for intervention and will eliminate the problems in middle, junior, and senior high schools caused by students entering a class after 20 minutes of speech-language intervention, or leaving a class midway to go to intervention. This obvious entering and leaving causes disruptions and is one more way youth with communication disorders look different from their peers.

While an obvious solution to scheduling might appear to be removing students from study halls, we would urge caution. Some students offer such extreme resistance to intervention during study time that they refuse to participate. Others disrupt sessions so severely that they need to be removed. From the perspective of the professional, these youth may be using study hall time inefficiently for academic activities, but students may insist on study hall for social reasons or for relaxation. Still, other students, particularly those in early adolescence, often willingly accept being removed from study time for speech-language intervention. They would rather work on structured objectives and activities with the

speech-language pathologist than work on homework assignments for which they lack basic skills. (Sometimes homework assignments can be used as the medium for achieving speech-language goals.) Also, students may have few friends with whom to relate socially during study hall, and they may possess few acceptable relaxation outlets (e.g., reading a book, writing a letter).

When scheduling options during the regular school day fail, the speech-language pathologist might consider requesting an extended contract day. Some students would prefer not to use school time for speech-language intervention, or they may have no flexibility in their schedules to do so. However, they would agree to intervention before or after regular school hours. Secondary-level speech-language pathologists might consider working an extended schedule four days a week, rather than a regular five-day week, to accommodate the needs of these students.

Supportive Titles

The speech-language pathologist must consider and select supportive titles for courses. "Speech therapy" and "language therapy" may be unsupportive titles for students with communication disorders trying to appear similar to their peers. Better titles might be "individualized language skills" or "oral communication strategies." Speech-language pathologists should determine optimal titles for their courses, since preferences will vary according to geographical location.

The title selected is also important because it will appear on the student's report card and transcript. If speech-language intervention is offered as a substitute course, then professionals may have fewer options for course titles; the substitution may need to be reflected in the title (e.g., "alternative English," "functional science"). If intervention is structured as an elective course, usually more flexibility in titles exists.

Areas of the School

Providing speech-language services out of the mainstream areas of the school is frequently viewed negatively by older students. A room located in a part of the school that is perceived as part of the mainstream is less likely to carry a negative image.

Many times, because of overcrowded conditions, the speech-language pathologist cannot have a private classroom throughout the day that is large enough for groups of students to meet. However, a classroom somewhere in the building is generally open because secondary-level teachers have staggered preparation periods.

Given a willingness to be flexible and to tote their materials from classroom to classroom, speech-language pathologists can meet in areas of the school viewed positively by older students. As a toehold is gained for the profession of communication sciences and disorders at the middle and secondary levels, buildings being constructed or remodeled should take the speech-language pathologist's space needs into account.

Intrinsic Motivation

Note that motivational procedures mentioned thus far are appropriate extrinsic forms of reinforcement for youth. Students should

be assisted to realize that increasingly successful communicative acts are their own rewards. When extrinsic motivational systems such as points for appropriate communication behaviors have been established, students should eventually be weaned from such a system. Often this weaning process occurs naturally over a long break time from programming (e.g., summer vacation). Students arrive after the break and no longer ask for points (D. Boley, personal communication, 1986). They seem to be more willing to participate in speech-language intervention because they realize they are becoming more successful in communicating. We have noted that this change from extrinsic to intrinsic motivational forces often occurs between the eighth and ninth grades.

A Learning Strategies Approach

When choosing the overall approach to intervention with older students, speech-language pathologists may choose from among these:

1. the learning strategies approach;

2. the basic skills approach;

3. the functional curriculum approach; and

4. the tutorial approach.

For most preadolescents and adolescents, the learning strategies approach is the most appropriate. "*Learning strategies* are defined as techniques, principles, or rules that will facilitate the acquisition, manipulation, integration, storage, and retrieval of information across situations and settings" (Alley and Deshler, 1979, p. 13). Furthermore, the use of learning strategies assumes that youth with language disorders "despite limited academic skills . . . possess sufficient intellectual strengths to think abstractly and process information critically" (Weller et al., 1992, p. 96).

Emphasis in a learning strategies program is on *how* to learn (i.e., process) rather than *what* to learn (i.e., product). In a summary report on the 1993 Conference for School Supervisors and Administrators, Peters-Johnson (1994) quoted Lauren Hoffman, assistant director of program planning and development at the South Metropolitan Association, Flossmore, Illinois: "This new paradigm [in education] . . . will focus not only on content, but on learning how to learn" (p. 121). The latter focus infers strategies—an approach to intervention as viable now as when it was conceived in the 70s.

Advantages of this program type are numerous. Learning strategies allow students to make changes in response to immediate concerns, but also to generalize to other situations. The emphasis on how to continue learning is better suited than other program types to the ongoing adaptation that students will be facing in their lifetimes, living in a technologically oriented culture. According to de Bettencourt (1987), youth who attain competence in learning strategies maximize their learning efficiency and apply their metacognitive abilities successfully in both academic and nonacademic settings. Strategies that allow students to continue learning may be imposed by the adult providing intervention, but they are often most effective if they are generated by the students themselves (Levin, 1976).

In contrast, in a basic skills approach, skills are taught that approximate the student's achievement level. For example, if an adolescent has third-grade comprehension skills, then intervention tasks are designed to teach the next comprehension skills at that grade level. This approach makes the assumption that identifying and sequencing of prerequisite skills are possible; that past instruction has been inappropriately or incompletely delivered; and that students will benefit, in spite of a history of not benefiting, from similar intervention in the elementary grades. While the proposition of increased competence in basic skills is attractive, the reality is that limited time is available to older students, thus making it unlikely that enough progress can be made to reduce the gap between grade level and functioning level when using a basic skills approach.

In a functional curriculum approach, the focus is on equipping students to function in society (i.e., to teach them survival skills). This approach has merit in that, at least over the short term, students are equipped to function independently in society. A better approach would be to combine a functional curriculum approach with learning strategies. With the combined approach, intervention could focus on survival language for a specific situation (e.g., for using a microwave oven) and at the same time teach strategies for learning the language to use the next kitchen appliance still being invented (e.g., to ask questions for clarification, to highlight key ideas in the instruction manual).

The tutorial approach concerns itself with providing instruction in academic content areas. We would urge speech-language pathologists to resist the temptation to respond to classroom assignments as a primary goal of intervention. While providing tutorial assistance meets the immediate needs of preadolescents and adolescents, it is a short-term solution. Little time is left to intervene with the actual, underlying problems when every minute is spent on assisting students with academic assignments. At the same time, speech-language pathologists need to be very aware of academic assignments and use them as a medium during intervention. However, the focus should be on teaching strategies for learning the academic content, not merely tutoring that content. Using classroom assignments as the vehicle for teaching learning strategies helps students gain independence, whereas a simple tutoring approach keeps students dependent on adults for academic success.

Available Counseling

The focus of counseling during speech-language intervention is to give information to students about the impact of their language disorders on academic progress, personal-social growth, and vocational potential. Also critical is to obtain information from students about their perceptions of the disorders and to provide release and support for feelings associated with the disorders. The counseling is specific to problems associated with the communication disorders; it does not address topics in which speech-language pathologists are unqualified to intervene (e.g., domestic violence, suicide proneness). Preadolescents and adolescents with problems that extend beyond their communication disorders need

more help than empathic responses from speech-language pathologists; they need emphatic referrals to trained counselors. It is unethical and impossible to try to handle all of the problems associated with preadolescence and adolescence within the confines of the speech-language program.

Counseling about the communication disorder should not be a segregated part of intervention, but an integral part of the process. Opening each session with a "class meeting" is a recommended way to integrate counseling. The class meeting contains three parts:

1. self-reports on how successfully students have transferred two or three communication behaviors outside of the intervention setting;

2. issues or problems that are of primary concern to the students, particularly as they relate to communication disorders; and

3. opportunities for participants to reinforce themselves or to compliment one another.

Self-Reports

The self-report part of the class meeting targets two or three behaviors that the youth is trying to incorporate into daily living situations (e.g., accepting compliments appropriately, using mnemonic strategies to remember information). These are selected mutually by the speech-language pathologist and the student. Once appropriate use of the behavior is reported for 10 consecutive sessions (the number is arbitrarily selected), it is replaced with a different behavior. The reporting relies on the honesty of the student. While teens and preteens might occasionally misrepresent the truth, their peers in the intervention session tend to challenge these misrepresentations. Honesty is certainly desirable, but dishonesty does not destroy the value of self-reporting on communication behaviors outside the intervention setting. Whether honesty or dishonesty prevails, the value of students' thinking about their communication (i.e., metacommunication) is retained.

Issues

The issues part of the class meeting affords a routine mechanism for uncovering significant problems in the lives of youth. Some days there are no issues, and the class meeting proceeds quickly to the third part (compliments). Other days, problems surface that require referral to other professionals. If the speech-language pathologist happens to be team teaching with other specialists (e.g., guidance counselor, learning disabilities specialist), then a wider range of problems can be addressed as they surface.

When professionals are open recipients to the students' feelings and attitudes, they often absorb the brunt of listening to significant problems and determining the necessary referral course. On other days, problems surface that are appropriate to discuss within the speech-language program. These problems tend to be paramount to the students at that moment in time. Failure to address the problems would be detrimental to the remainder of the session. The best-planned lesson is doomed if students arrive at a session preoccupied with a burning issue or problem and it is dismissed as irrelevant. The best lessons

with preadolescents and adolescents use topics of deep interest to them, such as those that surface during the issues section of the class meeting, and weave these topics into existing goals for thinking, speaking, and listening.

When problems are addressed during issues time, it is often helpful to have students refer to a problem-solving model chart. Figure 7.2 is an example of such a chart. Whether this particular chart or an adaptation is used, the logical flow of the steps within the model tends to guide the discussion of the problem effectively. The professional monitoring the discussion should also mediate how a problem-solving model can assist in analyzing and resolving other difficult issues throughout the student's daily life.

Compliments

The third part of the class meeting is a time for students to reinforce themselves and to compliment one another. Professionals should be prepared to model compliments, since the individuals receiving intervention often have received few of them. Compliments should focus on actions (e.g., "I like the way you said 'Good morning' to me") rather than on physical attributes (e.g., "I like your shirt"). Initially, compliments may feel uncomfortable to students. However, even this discomfort has an advantage, because compliments can be used very successfully to eliminate insults among students grouped together. For every insult from one adolescent or preadolescent to another, have that person follow it with a compliment. In our clinical experiences, giving compliments is so aversive, initially, for youth that it extinguishes the "put-down" behaviors. Once students have seen professionals model

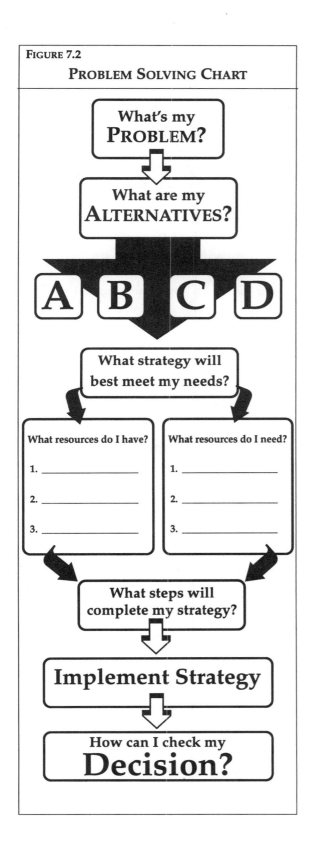

FIGURE 7.2

PROBLEM SOLVING CHART

What's my **PROBLEM?**

What are my **ALTERNATIVES?**

A **B** **C** **D**

What strategy will best meet my needs?

What resources do I have?

1. _____

2. _____

3. _____

What resources do I need?

1. _____

2. _____

3. _____

What steps will complete my strategy?

Implement Strategy

How can I check my **Decision?**

compliments (including self-compliments), have received a number of compliments during intervention, and have been "forced" to give compliments following insults, they gradually begin voluntarily to make positive comments about themselves and fellow peers. Once that begins, group cohesiveness often becomes stronger, students seem more willing to take risks to change communication behaviors, and their emotional support of each other may become evident inside and outside of the intervention sessions.

The class meeting takes approximately the first 5 to 10 minutes of the session if there are no issues and the meeting consists only of a review of objectives and compliments. The meeting may last the entire session if the issues or problems are weighty, are appropriate for group discussion, and are intertwined with intervention goals and objectives.

WHAT TO TEACH

Given the mutual planning of goals and objectives discussed in the previous section, it is important to use terms familiar to preadolescents and adolescents. We recommend the terms *thinking, listening,* and *speaking skills,* since those are common words and ones that likely surfaced during the assessment process. Important thinking, listening, and speaking skills to consider during intervention, including meta-abilities in these areas, are listed in Tables 7.1, 7.2, and 7.3, respectively. Behaviors cited in Table 7.1 have been summarized from Feuerstein (1979).

In addition, nonverbal communication behaviors and survival language skills may need to be taught. These skills, which are

TABLE 7.1 THINKING SKILLS		
INPUT PHASE	**ELABORATION PHASE**	**OUTPUT PHASE**
• Using senses to gather clear and complete information • Exploring a situation systematically • Naming objects and events consistently • Describing when and where events and objects occur • Recognizing events and objects as the same even when changes occur • Organizing information by several characteristics simultaneously • Knowing when and how to be precise and accurate	• Defining problems and determining what needs to be done • Using relevant information to a problem and ignoring irrelevant information • Forming a "good picture in the mind" about what must be done to solve a problem • Making a plan with needed steps to reach a goal • Remembering the pieces of information needed to solve a problem • Looking for relationships among separate objects, events, and experiences • Comparing experiences, objects, and events, for similarities and differences • Finding the category to which new objects, events, and experiences belong • Considering several different alternatives • Using logic to prove answers and to defend opinions	• Being clear and precise in language so the listener understands • Taking sufficient time to think through a response • Restraining from saying or doing something that will be regretted later • Using a strategy to help find answers • Talking about when and where input, elaboration, and output phases of thinking skills are used

TABLE 7.2	LISTENING SKILLS

COMPREHENSION OF LINGUISTIC FEATURES

Identifying morphological structures

Differentiating syntactical structures as incorrect

Comprehending sentence transformations

Comprehending sentences of various length and complexity

Comprehending semantic features

Applying informational listening skills

- Comprehending factual information and following directions
- Concentrating attention on the speaker
- Utilizing the time differential between thinking and speaking speeds
- Understanding main ideas and supportive details
- Formulating questions for clarification

Comprehending adolescent slang

Monitoring comprehension skills to identify when something was not understood

DISCOURSE

Applying critical listening skills

- Identifying the credibility of the source and/or speaker
- Recognizing inductive and deductive reasoning of the speaker
- Detecting false reasoning
- Recognizing propaganda devices
- Drawing inferences
- Judging statements

Listening to retell a story

Utilizing appropriate informational and critical listening skills during conversations

Recognizing when the application of listening skills failed and repair strategies need to be used (e.g., to ask for a repetition of the information, to acknowledge lack of comprehension)

TABLE 7.3	
	SPEAKING SKILLS

PRODUCTION OF LINGUISTIC FEATURES
Using simple and complex sentences to express ideas clearly and concisely
Using sentence fragments appropriately
Using figurative language
Using specific language and applying strategies when struggling to retrieve a word
Monitoring whether the sentence structure used conveyed the message appropriately and accurately

DISCOURSE
Using cohesion devices appropriately while telling or retelling a story, making a report, explaining a process, or conversing
Producing language that fulfills eight functions of communication: to give information, to get information, to describe, to persuade, to self-disclose, to indicate a readiness for further communication, to solve problems, to entertain
Applying rules of conversation appropriately across and within various social contexts
• Initiating and closing conversations appropriately • Selecting appropriate topics • Maintaining topics • Switching topics in an orderly fashion • Making contributions to the conversation informative • Making contributions to the conversation truthful • Making contributions to the conversation relevant • Making contributions to the conversation clear, brief, and orderly • Switching to formal registers as appropriate
Engaging in narrative and metanarrative skills during storytelling and retelling
• Summarizing/categorizing stories subjectively and objectively • Analyzing and critiquing the story • Generalizing the story's meaning
Recognizing when the application of speaking skills failed and repair strategies need to be used (e.g., to repeat the story, to rephrase instructions)
Using the language of language to analyze and discuss various communication situations

summarized in Tables 7.4 and 7.5, must be intact for the student to function adequately in academic, social, and vocational situations. Chronological-age expectations should be set for these skill areas (i.e., nonverbal communication and survival language), even for individuals who have mental ages much younger than their peers. Why? Because nonverbal communication behaviors and survival language skills are so basic to independent daily living.

Students deficient in these areas stand out as "odd" or "different" both to adults and to other youth. They may even be viewed as "dangerous." For example, it may be considered "cute" for a young child with Down's

syndrome to hug a complete stranger, but this behavior is viewed as inappropriate by middle grades, even if the student is functioning mentally at a much lower level. By late adolescence, the hugging behavior could even be viewed as an assault, especially if the perpetrator is much larger physically than the recipient. Thus, the mental- versus chronological-age expectations become blurred by the middle grades. Clearly, teaching the student to have nonverbal communication behaviors and survival language skills more like those of their age-matched peers is the safer and more desirable course of intervention.

Finally, written language skills are summarized in Table 7.6. The intent of Table 7.6 is not to include all potential reading and writing skills, but rather to provide a selective list that relies heavily on language and cognitive skills. The content for Table 7.6 has been extrapolated from Creaghead and Tattershall (1991) and Isaacson (1991).

Reading and writing goals are included along with the other five areas (i.e., thinking,

---

TABLE 7.4
NONVERBAL COMMUNICATION BEHAVIORS

- Matching oral and nonverbal messages
- Determining whether oral and nonverbal messages of others match or mismatch
- Detecting emotion through facial expression
- Displaying emotion through facial expression
- Recognizing the impact of distance (i.e., proxemic behavior) on the message
- Maintaining socially acceptable distance
- Maintaining appropriate eye contact

TABLE 7.5
SURVIVAL LANGUAGE

- Comprehending language for specific situations (e.g., school classroom, restaurant, grocery store)
- Comprehending language for multisituational settings (e.g., money, signs)
- Producing language for specific situations
- Producing language for multi-situational settings

TABLE 7.6				
WRITTEN LANGUAGE				
GENERAL SKILLS				
READING	• Identifying types of written material to read (e.g., textbook, storybook, newspaper) • Identifying major discourse genres (e.g., narrations, personal journals, instructions) • Predicting directions and content on the basis of page format		WRITING	• Creating single-proposition sentences • Composing compound and complex sentences • Combining sentences into cohesive paragraphs • Using an appropriately diverse vocabulary while avoiding the repetition of favorite words • Applying writing conventions (e.g., punctuation, spelling, penmanship) to compositions so they are presentable to others
EXPOSITORY TEXT				
READING	• Deriving main ideas from headings, subheadings, visual aids (e.g., pictures, charts, graphs), and typography (e.g., bold, italics, underscore) • Following multistep directions		WRITING	• Stating the overall objectives in a topic sentence and establishing a clear direction and purpose • Sequencing directions and actions appropriately • Transitioning cohesively from one idea to the next • Using variety, originality, imagination, and logic, as needed, to develop the overall objective
NARRATIVE TEXT				
READING	• Visualizing the action sequence of a story to retell or to answer comprehension questions • Determining the characters' feelings and plans so that understanding is gained to know why characters do what they do		WRITING	• Providing a well-detailed background • Developing a "real" central figure • Selecting and maintaining the appropriate voice for telling the story

listening, speaking, nonverbal communication, and survival language) when they are essential to reaching objectives set for academic performance, personal-social interactions, and vocational achievement. Reading and writing become part of the speech-language intervention process when they support, rather than hinder, the acquisition of oral communication skills.

At about the third-grade level (i.e., 8–9 years of age), children increasingly use their sentence-level knowledge and narrative discourse processing skills in reading (Snyder and Downey, 1991). Before that age, children appear to focus much of their processing efforts on reading at the word level (Chall, 1983). Between 8 and 9 years, the decoding process is sufficiently mastered to the point where it can be automatically applied to print (Chall, 1983).

> At this point, children expend less effort on the phonological and lexical processing required for decoding and word recognition and begin to allocate more attention and processing resources to the syntactic and discourse operations required for the higher order processing of text (connected discourse). Thus it is at this stage that children are thought to move into fluent reading. (Synder and Downey, 1991, p. 130)

Youth with language disorders do not attain decoding automaticity and are thought to become "stuck" at the early stages of reading, thus preventing progress to the more advanced stages of reading for meaning (Chall, 1983). The different dimensions of language processing appear to have an impact on reading at the word and text levels (Kamhi and Catts, 1989).

Some researchers (Kamhi and Catts, 1986, 1989; Wallach and Miller, 1988) suggest that reading-related oral language skills develop as school-age children interact with formal instruction and written texts. Fawcett (1994) cited the intricate interconnections among language processes and noted "that growth in oral language supports growth in written language and vice versa" (p. 39). Thus, there appears to be reciprocity in the oral-written

language relationship (Snyder and Downey, 1991), and intervention may justifiably include speaking, listening, reading, and writing goals and activities.

HOW TO INTERVENE

From the earlier description in this chapter of the class meeting, it is perhaps apparent that intervention with older school-age children should be student centered. Objectives and activities need to be authentic, meaningful, and relevant from the student's perspective, not just the professional's viewpoint.

Not only are the students guided toward goals for what to learn, but a major part of intervention is helping them understand why to learn. Anyone who has worked with older school-age children knows that special programming is not as readily embraced by them as by younger children. The power of the sticker to reinforce desirable behaviors during intervention has typically faded. The most powerful replacement is a strong intrinsic motivation to learn better communication skills for improved functioning in academic, personal-social, and/or vocational settings. And the best way to trigger intrinsic motivation is for students to understand their own strengths and deficits, to accept responsibility for improving their skills, and to realize the benefits of adequate thinking, listening, speaking, reading, and writing skills.

For professionals to assist youth in developing these skills, and their intrinsic motivation in the process, they need to play the role of a mediator. A mediator constantly adapts his or her input to the special needs of the students so the input is within the student's level of proficiency (Damico, 1992). The professional may also act as a mediator between the student and his or her language output. Thus, mediation is a primary aspect of intervention.

Mediation

How students learn new behaviors is the topic of an ongoing theoretical debate. Traditional behaviorists would have us believe that learning involves a stimulus-response (S-R) situation (Skinner, 1957). Piaget (1959) revolutionized how we think about learning by interspersing an "O" between the "S-R"—in effect, reminding us that the stimulus-response is affected by the organism ("O") receiving the stimulus and generating the response.

Learning of the S-R or S-O-R type is direct exposure learning. The organism (student) interacts with the stimulus, derives meaning, and formulates a response. Direct exposure learning does not explain, however, the vast amount of learning that takes place, according to Feuerstein (1979). He posits that mediated learning experiences account for much of our learning, especially by children who cannot have direct exposure experiences. For example, most of what we know about history is acquired through mediation, not through direct exposure. Mediation is different from direct exposure in that some human (H)—a teacher, a parent, a sibling, a friend—comes between the stimulus and the organism and/or between the organism and the response. Figure 7.3 illustrates how mediation compares to other theoretical explanations for learning.

FIGURE 7.3

THEORETICAL EXPLANATIONS FOR LEARNING

S-R

Stimulus-Response Learning

S-O-R

Direct Exposure Learning

$S \twoheadrightarrow H \twoheadleftarrow O \twoheadrightarrow H \twoheadleftarrow R$

Mediated Learning Experience

The "human" involved in mediation frames, filters, and schedules the stimuli. He or she may cause certain aspects of the stimuli to be salient and other aspects to be suppressed. For example, in teaching the social significance of World War II, the mediator might focus on the shifts in attitude that occurred and deliberately not focus on the details of the war itself. When teaching writing, the mediator might provide a critique of the content and deliberately ignore spelling and punctuation errors.

Feuerstein (1980) contends that there is an intention to transcend the immediate teaching situation during mediation. Even something as simple as asking a student to close the door can be mediated. Simply saying, "Close the door" does not mediate. But if you say, "Please close the door because there's a strong draft in the hallway and I'm afraid the wind might ruin our art projects," then you have established a reason for closing the door that goes beyond the immediate situation. You have established a relationship between closing the door and preventing a problem (destruction of art projects) and have modeled how to anticipate predictable mistakes.

Mediation certainly occurs from birth onward. "Good" parents mediate without having the label for it. They are constantly scheduling stimuli for their children such as when and where to eat, and how much. "Do's" and "don'ts" are followed by explanations that go beyond the immediate need. "Don't touch the stove. You'll get burned." "Pet the doggie. He likes you." "Put your shoes on. We're going to Grandma's." The immediate needs are to avoid touching the stove or to pet the doggie or to put on shoes, but the "good" parent adds information that goes beyond the immediate need and draws connections between actions and results. "Good" teachers do the same.

The more mediation a child has, the more capable he or she becomes to learn independently through direct exposure to stimuli. So states Feuerstein's (1980) theory of *cognitive modifiability*. When a young child arrives at school with a history of appropriate mediated learning experiences, his or her cognitive

functioning is adequate. When mediated learning experiences have been lacking, deficient cognitive functioning is the result.

When children past the age of 10 experience concomitant cognitive deficiencies and language disorders, a lack of mediated learning experiences can almost always be traced in their development (Feuerstein, 1980). In some youth, cognitive ability is greater than their language age; in others the pattern is reversed. In either case, intervention can be very effective, for as language skills increase, the student's cognitive functioning often improves. And as students think better, they communicate better.

One of the greatest travesties in the provision of speech-language services is denying students intervention simply on the basis that they are currently communicating better than their cognitive levels would indicate. When both language and cognition are lagging years behind chronological-age expectations, intervention is warranted regardless of any discrepancy that might exist between the two measures (Casby, 1992). Provision of the mediated learning experience that has been lacking is a prime focus of intervention whether language exceeds cognition, whether cognition exceeds language, or whether both are equally impaired.

Granted, some individuals are so neurologically impaired that mediation is generally unsuccessful. Mediation is not a panacea. There are individuals who require such an investment of the professional's time to make minor cognitive and language gains that one questions the efficacy of such intervention. This is not the population being addressed in this text. Rather, the older school-age child with inclusion into regular education all or part of the day is modifiable, and mediation is paramount for the development of adequate cognitive functioning.

Bridging

Bridging is another essential aspect of intervention that should occur concurrently with mediation. While the professional mediates, the student bridges. *Bridging* involves the application of a new idea, concept, or skill to a different situation. For example, if the student has just learned how to interrupt politely, he or she describes a situation when this skill might need to be used in a community setting. Or the student is given an assignment to interrupt someone politely the next day and then to report back on the experience.

Bridging might also be thought of as "transferring" or "generalizing." We prefer the term *bridging* because it sounds more concrete to students. You cannot bridge for your students. Rather, you guide students to do the bridging through the questions asked and the time allowed. Without the consistent inclusion of bridging in intervention, students will make minimal gains in using their new communication behaviors in other settings.

During bridging, students apply new behaviors and strategies learned within intervention sessions to novel academic, personal-social, or vocational situations. Professionals structure intervention so students engage in bridging, but only the students themselves can make a meaningful application. The application should be specific enough to demonstrate the understanding of how to apply the new behavior or strategy in other relevant situations. Table 7.7 provides examples of strong bridges, in contrast with weak bridges, for a variety of behaviors and strategies.

Within Table 7.7, only one guide question for each new behavior or strategy is indicated. This is not to imply that only one probing question would be used. Rather, the professional should generate many ongoing questions about each behavior or strategy that will trigger bridging responses from students throughout the intervention process. When weak bridges are given (e.g., the first response in Table 7.7, "In math class"), professionals should ask follow-up questions that encourage expansion (e.g., "When, in math class, might you switch topics of conversation with the teacher?").

A common pattern is for older students to generate no bridges, or weak bridges, initially. The realization of an application for what is being learned in an educational situation appears foreign to many students. However, with guidance from the adult mediator(s), preadolescents and adolescents gradually improve the quantity and quality of their bridges. The improvement is facilitated by the provision of a partial bridge by the speech-language pathologist and the encouragement of its completion by the student. The following transcript, taken from a group session, illustrates this facilitation of bridging that may occur when students are reluctant or unable to bridge:

	STRONG AND WEAK BRIDGING BY STUDENTS		
TABLE 7.7			
NEW BEHAVIOR OR STRATEGY	**PROFESSIONAL'S GUIDE QUESTION**	**STRONG BRIDGE**	**WEAK BRIDGE**
Switching topics (of conversation) appropriately	When might you have to switch topics when talking with a teacher at school? (academic bridge)	When I have two things to ask, like what assignments I'm missing and what's on the test.	In math class
Formulating questions for clarification	Are there times when you want to ask questions for clarification, but it's not appropriate? (personal-social bridge)	I want to ask my mom something but she's on the telephone; I want to ask my friend something, but he's taking a make-up exam.	At school; at home
Making a plan to reach a goal	Who earns a living by making plans? (vocational bridge)	City planners; architects; air traffic controllers	Adults; everybody

Professional: We have been practicing giving clear messages. We made it a rule to use the fewest words possible, but still to communicate the message. Think for a minute. Where else is it important to give clear messages using the fewest words possible?

Young Adolescents: (No response after waiting five to ten seconds)

Professional: Suppose you are at a pay phone. You need a ride home. You put your money in the phone and discover it is a long-distance call to your home. The voice message tells you to deposit another coin. You now have no more money. When you call from a pay phone, you can only talk for three minutes long distance before depositing more money. How would giving a clear message be important in this situation?

Young Adolescent 1: Better tell Mom to pick you up. Tell her to get there fast.

Professional: Good idea! You'd really want to get right to the point of your message when you're stranded at a pay phone. Now think for a minute about telegrams, like a Western Union message. You've been studying about telegrams and the Morse code in history. Why is it important to send short messages when wiring a telegram?

Young Adolescents: (No response after waiting five to ten seconds)

Professional: Does anyone know . . . is it free to send a telegram or does it cost money?

Young Adolescent 2: Don't know.

Professional: Let's think about sending messages to other people when we can't see them. It costs to mail a letter. It costs to make a phone call. Do you think a telegram will be free?

Young Adolescent 2: No, people gotta pay.

Professional: All right. When people send a telegram, they have to pay so much for each word. So why would it be important to send a telegram using the fewest words possible?

Young Adolescent 2: So it don't cost much.

Professional: Good thinking! So it doesn't cost as much. Sometimes sending a clear message may save us money. Let's think of another situation. You are in the middle of study hall and you need to tell your friend something. How will clear messages help now?

Young Adolescent 3: You better tell your friend fast. O' else the teacher may catch you and put your name on the board.

Professional: In our school, that's true. In this case, sending a clear message could help you to avoid trouble. You've done a good job of bridging some examples of when and why it is important to give clear messages using the fewest words possible.

From the transcript, notice how the professional assisted the young adolescents to think about a particular communication behavior as it affected their lives. Sometimes this process is facilitated by the use of a hands-on activity, rather than relying on students answering questions (e.g., bring in a telegraph key and practice formulating actual telegrams). With frequent exposure to the general procedure of bridging, students gradually begin to generate spontaneous responses that result in positive transfers in daily communication.

Application of Mediation and Bridging

No matter what the focus of intervention or the objectives, mediation and bridging become general principles that guide the process. Common questions and statements that emerge time and time again are these:

When using a written task to facilitate an oral communication activity:

What do you see that looks familiar on this page? Where have you seen that before? What looks different?

What do you think we are to do on this page? What were the cues you used to figure that out? Where else have you seen those cues?

What strategies could you use to do this task? (Or, What do you have to think about to do this task?)

Where else have you used those strategies? (Or, Where else have you had to use that kind of thinking?)

What mistakes might you make while doing this task?

When is another time you have made that mistake?

How could you prevent the mistake from happening?

When engaging in an oral communication activity without the benefit of a written task:

Today we're going to [describe task]. When/where have you ever had to do [task]?

If I didn't know how to do [task], here's one consequence: [describe]. What could happen to you if you don't know how to [task]?

Here's what I need to think about while I do [task]. Tell me what you'll think about. Where else do you do that kind of thinking?

At this point, you might be making several observations. First, the level of questioning may strike you as "high." Observe the comparable questions that appear in textbooks and in teacher-student exchanges in the middle grades and beyond. Students are expected to handle thought-provoking questions. Your mediation will help them handle higher-level questions across a variety of settings.

Second, the prevalence of metacognition and metalinguistics is apparent. Students are repeatedly being asked to think about their thinking and to communicate about their communication. This is intentional and sets intervention for older students apart from that which professionals do with younger children.

Children younger than age 10 are not usually expected to engage in metacognitive discussions about the skills being taught and why they need to be learned. To do so could be developmentally inappropriate. Bliss (1993) stresses the importance of not explaining the communication act or commenting on its importance to children or adolescents. However, we believe that as children mature, especially those who lack mediated learning experiences, explaining the significance of learning various communication skills (and equally important, having them bridge the significance of the skills to meaningful academic, personal-social, and vocational settings) are essential components of intervention. These components also promote the intrinsic motivation of the student to improve communication skills.

A difference between intervening with children past age 10 and with those younger than age 10 is that older students are capable of "meta" activities like

- thinking about their thinking;

- thinking about their talking;

- talking about their thinking; and

- talking about their talking.

Extending this to written communication, they can also

- think about their writing;

- write about their thinking; and

- write about their writing.

Likewise, "meta" activities can encompass thinking, talking, or writing about their listening and/or reading. This ability to engage in higher-level cognitive discussions and tasks should be routinely incorporated into intervention as students learn how to learn. The

"good" mediator helps students select meaningful skills to learn, structures questions and activities so students understand why the skills are important, and provides opportunities to bridge the skills to relevant academic, personal-social, and/or vocational situations.

Enhancing Oral Communication

Traditional intervention procedures have systematically taught phonology (articulation), syntax (grammar), semantics (concepts), and pragmatics (social communication, functional language) as isolated skill areas. Of these, until recently, pragmatics was often ignored in deference to the other three areas. In contrast, current philosophy is to teach the natural interactions among the skill areas and to make pragmatics the "umbrella" that encompasses the other skills. Figure 7.4 compares the two approaches.

Most older students have some type of oral language system, albeit an ineffective or inefficient one. The challenge during intervention is to help students use the system they do have in the most appropriate way possible. How can they use their current language to communicate better in daily living situations?

This is not to imply professionals will avoid working on articulation problems or grammatical errors of older students. However, when phonology or syntax or semantics are addressed in intervention, the mediation will relate to a pragmatic base. In other words, the student will be assisted to see that his or her articulation errors are causing intelligibility problems in academic situations and rejection or ridicule in personal situations and, therefore, there are strong pragmatic and social

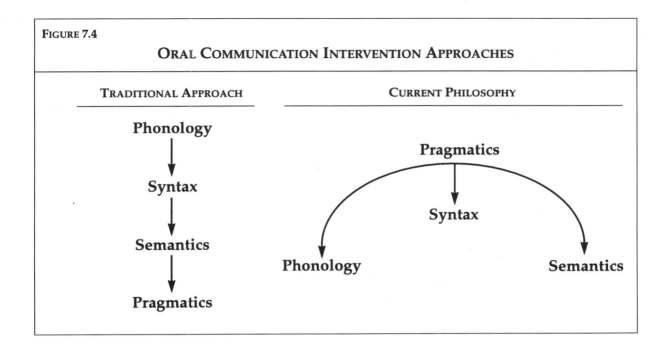

FIGURE 7.4

ORAL COMMUNICATION INTERVENTION APPROACHES

TRADITIONAL APPROACH | CURRENT PHILOSOPHY

Phonology
↓
Syntax
↓
Semantics
↓
Pragmatics

Pragmatics
↓
Syntax

Phonology   **Semantics**

communication reasons for taking responsibility for correcting the articulation errors.

When pragmatic and social communication skills are the primary deficit area, there is a growing call for speech-language intervention (Walker, Schwarz, Nippold, Irvin, and Noell, 1994). Children who have weak social skills and problematic peer relations in the early years of their school careers risk a host of negative outcomes (e.g., low self-esteem, under-achievement, juvenile delinquency, dropping out of school) (Strain, Guralnick, and Walker, 1986). Preventing these negative developmental outcomes hinges on proactive, systematic social skills training (Walker et al., 1994).

Mediation and bridging are an integral part of an oral communication intervention program. Students should be guided to understand what they are being taught and why, and they should be given opportunities

to bridge the new skill or concepts to novel situations.

Intervention activities should be relevant and contextually based with a focus on the communication process, not the end product. Activities that produce communication breakdowns (e.g., referential communication tasks or barrier games that are slightly higher than the student's skill level) can produce great learning moments when a "safe" environment —one allowing youth to experiment and make mistakes—is set. (Referential communication activities are further explained in the section beginning on page 184.) Discussion should center on why the speaking or listening task succeeded or failed. Was the success or failure due to actions of the speaker or the listener or both? The purpose of this discussion is not to focus blame but to determine how to send and/or receive successful oral messages.

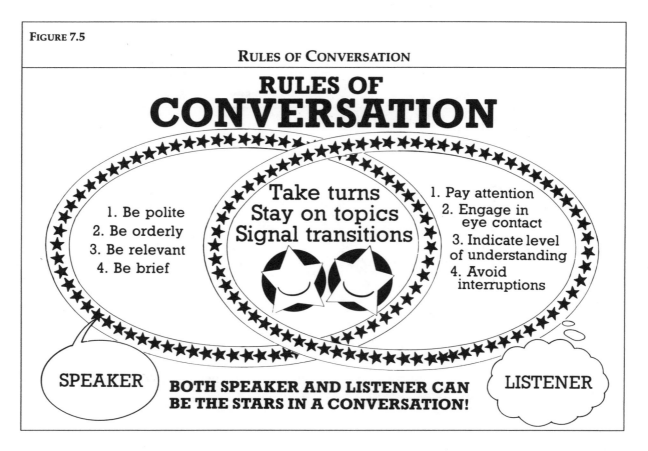

FIGURE 7.5

RULES OF CONVERSATION

This type of discussion assumes basic conversational rules are intact or can be taught to the students in the group. Basic rules of conversation based on Grice's (1975) fundamentals are summarized in Figure 7.5 and should be provided graphically for students as in the poster shown. Ideas for teaching these rules have been provided in detail by Schwartz and McKinley (1984).

Enhancing Written Communication

Traditionally, teachers have asked students to complete assignments that include a page or less of writing and that stress subject-area concepts (Applebee, Auten, and Lehr, 1981). These same teachers have emphasized mechanical aspects of writing (spelling, punctuation) over text-forming aspects and have usually asked students to write about information already known to them so they are not looking for novel ideas. Increasingly, teachers in individual schools across the country are now stressing process over product and are using writing as means for learning (e.g., "journaling").

For students to become better writers, they need to write more and to do so by completing meaningful, authentic activities. Writing needs to serve as a tool for learning rather than as a means to display acquired knowledge (Applebee et al., 1981). Like oral communication, written language needs to be seen as a process with a number of distinct aspects.

One simple formulation is to use an instruction sequence of prewriting, writing, and editing (Applebee, 1981; Perl, 1979), which is equivalent to Stewart's (1991) planning, translating, and reviewing stages cited in Chapter 6.

Prewriting

Prewriting involves thinking about a topic, gathering information, talking, and reading. In authentic writing situations, this period may extend for weeks or even months. In classroom situations, some teachers allow students just over three minutes (Applebee et al., 1981)! Most writing assignments in school begin with the expectation that the student already knows what to write and can rapidly start.

Discussion of a topic is an excellent technique that can be used to enhance both written and oral communication. One way to collaborate within the school setting is for the classroom teacher or learning disabilities specialist to formulate a writing assignment and then allow time for the speech-language pathologist to have students discuss the topic, formulate strategies for gathering and organizing the information to complete the assignment, and outline or map the amassed data. The outline or map might be accomplished through word-processing software or with traditional recording methods.

Writing

Writing involves the composing process. The topic is developed on paper (or computer screen). Concern should be on expressing ideas, not on formulating sentences. Multiple drafts will be needed before the various sections of writing support each other. In contrast, some teachers require only one draft and do little to mediate the notion that cohesive writing almost always requires a successive refinement process. Unless the written piece is very short, students should anticipate and be required to produce more than one draft. Using a word-processing package and saving the document on disk for use in sequel drafts is strongly recommended. Mediation should be used to help students focus on sections needing greater clarity or stronger arguments. Students should also bridge to situations when various writing expectations will be demanded of them (e.g., writing a letter or paper to persuade versus writing to tell a story).

Editing

Editing involves "polishing"—attending to spelling, punctuation, usage, and other mechanics. When teachers have a "first-and-final draft" mentality (and some do), that copy is also surrounded by demands for accuracy and neatness—a rather unrealistic expectation even for the best writers among us. While word processing helps greatly to omit the "messiness" factor, the writing and the editing phases should still be approached as separate, albeit related, factors.

When teachers comment on student papers, they function in much the same way as an editor's evaluation. In authentic writing situations, the editing would be acted upon and students would write another draft, using the editorial suggestions and revisions to produce a better manuscript. Unfortunately, in many school situations, the editorial comments simply become private criticism for the author that may or may not prove beneficial. After all, educators cannot assume that students' reading of their critiques (if indeed they're read at all) results in learning how to correct their errors.

Writing should be motivated by a need to communicate to a reader who does not already know what is going to be said (Applebee et al., 1981). The best lessons for older students view writing as a vehicle for learning, which emerges naturally from other activities. When oral and written communication skills are interwoven in clinical activities, the power of language to create meaning is maximized, and "meaning-making is the general purpose of all forms of language text or all skills" (Damico, 1992, p. 10).

Specific Intervention Methods

Many volumes would be needed to delineate the many specific methods (i.e., procedures and materials) that could be used for teaching thinking, listening, speaking, nonverbal communication, survival language, and written language skills. Methods abound and vary with the theoretical underpinnings selected for intervention. Instead of attempting to present many methods superficially, a few representative methods will be presented here with some depth. These methods have been selected because they are ones we advocate for older students with language disorders. They are consonant with our theoretical constructs presented in Chapter 2, and with the recommended general program approach of learning strategies.

Within the discussion of each specific method, we describe procedures, discuss materials, highlight areas of emphasis, list sample bridging questions that could be asked by the adult providing intervention, and summarize potential strategies that could be mediated for the student. The selected specific methods are these:

1. referential communication activities;

2. narrative storytelling activities;

3. expository discourse activities; and

4. word-finding activities.

Referential Communication Activities

Referential communication activities, also known as "barrier activities," emphasize the communication functions of giving and getting information. To perform these functions, adequate speaking and listening are required. This ability to express and to comprehend informative messages is a function repeated many times by competent communicators throughout a typical day. However, students with language disorders often have difficulty engaging in precise message formulation and reception. Referential communication activities increase this precision.

Referential communication activities are appropriate for preadolescents and youth in all stages of adolescence. By altering the content and the level of difficulty, the activities become adaptable to any age and ability level.

Procedure

Referential communication activities require a minimum of one speaker and one listener. They are seated near each other with a physical barrier (i.e., a screen) between them. The speaker and the listener have identical sets of materials that are concealed from each other by the screen. The speaker explains to the listener how to construct or reconstruct an identical two- or three-dimensional model that the listener cannot see.

Barrier activities may involve more than one speaker and one listener simultaneously. One speaker may give directions to many listeners. Numerous speakers could collaborate on sending a clear message to one or many listeners; this is a common communication experience (e.g., a committee deciding how to word a statement; two parents agreeing on what to say after their child has misbehaved).

Another option for including more than one speaker and one listener during referential communication activities is to appoint one or more observers. The observer is free to study the model the speaker is describing and to observe the responses of the listener. The observer can often see firsthand when and why any communication breakdowns are occurring. The format of assigning "speaker-listener-observer" roles is based upon the idea that people can more easily focus on the relation between speaker (message) and listener (response) when not enmeshed in one of those roles (Shantz, 1981). It may be that "vicarious" role reversal occurs by the observer, thus making it an effective experience.

Whatever combination of participants is used during barrier activities, the outcome is natural communication. There is a reason for the speaker to formulate a message and a reason for the listener to attempt to understand it. All participants, including any observers, are afforded the opportunity to observe the effects of adequate and inadequate communication.

The adult providing intervention may use a number of variations during referential communication activities:

1. *Questions for clarification versus no questions.* Questions for clarification should be allowed initially between the listener and the speaker. They should not only be encouraged, but modeled by the adult providing intervention. If the student's message has been too general, saying, "I've got n [4, 2, or however many] like that. I'm not sure which one you mean. Can you help me?" is more effective than either saying, "Which one?" or guessing which referent the speaker intends (e.g., "Is it this one?") (Robinson, 1981).

   As participants become more proficient in producing and comprehending messages, occasional sessions might be held during which questions for clarification are not allowed. During and after these sessions, students should discuss and bridge their experiences (e.g., How did the rule of "no questions" affect your understanding of the message? Was the activity more or less difficult when questions were not allowed? What question(s) would you have asked if you could have? In what other situations have you been where you were not allowed to ask questions for clarification?).

2. *State versus state-restate.* The usual sequence of events during barrier activities is for the speaker and the listener to compare models after the message has been given and questions for clarification, if allowed, have been asked.

Another option is for the listener to restate the entire message to the speaker before the comparison of models is shared. The restatement may also be accomplished sequentially (i.e., as the speaker gives one part of a step-by-step message, the listener restates the information). Restatement may allow for identification of the source of any communication breakdowns and permit repair.

3. *Gestures versus no gestures.* Initially, gestures that help to clarify the spoken message may be allowed, especially for students who need the activity to be as concrete as possible. Gestures might be particularly tempting to use when spatial orientation is an important attribute to describe. Disallowance of gestures that substitute for description (e.g., pointing to a piece of the model rather than describing it) should be enforced most of the time. However, occasional use of gestures will allow the opportunity for discussion concerning how the oral message becomes modified with and without accompanying gestures.

4. *Partial message versus complete message.* When students begin referential communication activities, they are more likely to be successful if partial messages are sent and received in sequential order. Later on, speakers should be required to send the entire message at once, and listeners should be required to receive the whole message prior to beginning the response. This requires memory strategies, thus making the level of the task more difficult.

5. *Questions for information versus clarification.* This variation of referential communication activities requires the listener to ask questions for information rather than questions for clarification. The speaker in turn supplies responses to these questions rather than initiating the content of the message. For example, if wh-questions are allowed, then the questions might include: "What shapes are used?" "What size is the triangle?" and "Where is it placed?" The activities could also be structured to require the listener to ask yes-no questions. The speaker remains in control of the model to be duplicated. However, the listener must employ careful questioning strategies to obtain all the necessary information to complete the activity successfully.

6. *Time limit versus unlimited time.* This variation introduces the impact of time pressure on the fluency and efficiency of the message. When students are given a structured time limit (e.g., one minute) to send a message, more planning must occur than when messages have no restrictions. Discussion should focus on how speakers and listeners alter their behaviors when time is of the essence.

Materials

Materials for referential communication activities may be either two- or three-dimensional. In both cases, the materials should be sophisticated enough so they do not cause embarrassment to the older student. Regardless of the material selected, two or more identical sets will be needed.

The adult providing intervention should mediate for the student that the model constructed or reconstructed with the materials is secondary to the communication process occurring. Referential communication has not been successful until the speaker and the listener share a common meaning for the message. When communication breakdowns occur, they should be analyzed and repaired. Depending upon the focus of the barrier activity, the materials may be natural or contrived. For example, actual objects may be used (i.e., natural materials), and the speaker must describe to the listener how to orient them to one another. On the other end of the spectrum, materials may be contrived, such as drawing two-dimensional representations of objects.

An additional material that is sometimes desirable during referential communication activities is a tape recorder. With a tape recorder, the speaker's message can be recorded and replayed to prevent discrepancies between what was perceived to have been communicated versus what actually was communicated.

Areas of Emphasis

The most common areas of emphasis during referential communication activities are speaking and listening. The role of the student engaged in the activities may alternate between speaker and listener, or one role may be assigned throughout. Regardless of the specific content of an activity, ongoing opportunities are available for producing and comprehending clear messages. The roles of speaker-listener are easily replaced by writer-reader when a focus on written language is desired.

If the content of the referential communication activities is carefully planned, then areas of emphasis may also include thinking behaviors, nonverbal communication, and survival language. For example, thinking may be emphasized more specifically if the materials selected require application of spatial, quantitative, and qualitative concepts. Nonverbal communication may be emphasized if messages that could be more easily communicated with gestures, or a combination of gestures and oral language, are utilized. For example, give each student a group of pictures illustrating such actions as someone waving a flag, starting a lawn mower with a pull rope, and bouncing a ball. Through gestures, the student can communicate to the receivers what picture is to be matched. Also, using the technique of gestures versus no gestures (discussed in the "Procedure" section on pages 184–186) provides a means for focusing upon nonverbal communication.

An emphasis on survival language behaviors during referential communication activities is best accomplished when tasks from the student's natural environment are planned. Activities chosen should relate as closely as possible to situations in which the student would actually be placed. For example, have the student give a message about how to find several items in a storage closet or drawer.

Bridging Questions

Speech-language pathologists using referential communication activities might consider asking these bridging questions during or after the activities:

1. In what other situations has it been important to communicate a message clearly?

2. Tell me about a time when you were talking and a breakdown in communication occurred (i.e., you were the cause of the breakdown). What were the consequences?

3. Tell me about a time when you were listening and a breakdown in communication occurred (i.e., you were the cause of the breakdown). What were the consequences?

4. Give an example of when you asked a question for clarification. Did it prevent a communication breakdown?

5. You have just been prevented from using gestures and eye contact when saying your message. When else are you prevented from using nonverbal communication?

Strategies to Mediate

A partial list of strategies that the professional could mediate for youth during referential communication activities includes these:

1. visualizing the information being spoken or listened to (i.e., seeing the model "in your mind");

2. using a plan to organize the information (i.e., what is most important to say first, next, last?);

3. concentrating attention on the speaker when in the role of a listener (i.e., blocking out distractions);

4. knowing how and when to ask a question for clarification;

5. using appropriate concepts (e.g., spatial, quantity, quality) to make messages concise; and

6. taking the listener's perspective when producing a message.

Narrative Storytelling Activities

A wide array of discourse-level skills are needed for successful participation in social and academic pursuits. One essential narrative skill is storytelling. As children reach adolescence, the ability to comprehend and to produce larger units of language becomes increasingly important for peer acceptance and academic survival. Whereas younger children often receive help from teachers and parents to fill in narrations, adolescents are often not helped.

Narration activities can be used during preadolescence and during early, middle, and late stages of adolescence. They should be chosen with the student's social-emotional level and interests in mind.

Procedure

Westby (1991a) has suggested three levels of activities for enhancing narrative skills. Goals for each level have been summarized as follows (Westby, 1991a):

Early Stage—Provide exposure to literate language. Structure interactions to facilitate reporting.

Middle Stage—Facilitate understanding of relationships among character traits, emotions, and events. Require the child to structure the narrative.

Advanced Stage—Facilitate comprehension of more complex embedded narratives. Facilitate metanarrative skills. (p. 351)

Although it is desirable for older students to be performing at the highest level of activity, they may need to acquire more concrete behaviors before abstract abilities such as metanarrative skills develop. Obviously, activities recommended at the early, more concrete, level (Westby, 1985) to provide exposure to literate language for young children (e.g., "show and tell" time, dramatization of nursery rhymes) are not appropriate at the preadolescent and adolescent levels. However, exposure can be promoted through activities such as listening to "Books on Tape" that are of interest to older students; watching movies, home videos, or Public Broadcasting System literary presentations based upon any of the "Books on Tape" (e.g., *The Other Side of the Mountain*, Valens, 1975); and listening to old-time radio dramatizations such as Orson Wells's *War of the Worlds.*

Hoggan and Strong (1994) summarized 20 strategies that might be used to teach narrative skills and thus achieve the goals cited by Westby. The strategies are organized into the categories of "pre-story presentation," "during-story presentation," and "post-story presentation." All 20 strategies are appropriate to use at the preadolescent level, and all but "dramatic play" are appropriate during adolescence.

Pre-story presentation strategies include establishing a preparatory set, summarizing the story before it is presented, engaging in semantic word mapping (to help students understand word relationships and concepts), and using think-alouds (e.g., asking students to make predictions about a story's topic).

A few of the during-story presentation strategies are questioning (e.g., to extend thinking, to obtain information, to engage in problem solving) and episode mapping. Post-story presentation strategies include such items as clarifying internal states of characters, story retelling, and story-grammar cuing. *Scaffolding* is the term often used for this cuing. "Scaffolding is the use of leading questions that help the speaker organize [the] story" (Page and Stewart, 1985, p. 25).

Garnett (1986) has suggested that a chart listing major elements of a story can be used as a guide for narrators and for discussion after the story. Table 7.8 suggests the content of this chart. Preadolescents, or those less skilled in narration, should be guided to use the concrete scaffolding items first (e.g., setting, events), both when listening to stories and when telling them. As narrative skills emerge, abstract elements of a story (e.g., theme, moral) should receive focus. When these more skilled adolescents hear stories that they retell, they should be able to answer all of the questions listed in Table 7.8. When they tell stories, the beginning is marked by a description of setting and the ending is marked by a conclusion, but the elements listed in between vary in sequence and as to whether they need to be included.

As students become familiar with various elements of narration and practice logical sequencing of the elements, they should be encouraged to remind themselves of the questions to be answered during the narration. Long-term reliance on a visible chart or on someone to ask the questions of them should be discouraged.

TABLE 7.8

A SUGGESTED CHART OF STORY ELEMENTS TO BE USED AS A GUIDE FOR NARRATORS

BEGINNING	SETTING OF STORY	Who are the main characters? Where does the story take place? When does the story take place?
	THEME OF THE STORY	What is the main idea (theme) of the story?
	EVENTS OF THE STORY	What happens to the characters?
	GOAL(S) OF THE CHARACTERS	What are the characters trying to do?
	MOTIVE(S) OF THE CHARACTERS	Why are the characters trying to reach the goal(s)?
	ATTEMPTS	What happens when the characters try to reach the goal?
	REACTIONS OF THE CHARACTERS	What are their feelings? What are their plans?
ENDING	CONCLUSION	How does everything turn out? What lesson (moral) did you learn from the story?

Page and Stewart (1985) and Westby (1991a) emphasize the importance of direct instruction in improving cause-and-effect relationships as a general means to developing narration skills. Emphasis should be on relationships that are most essential to stories, including the effects of the environment on people, animals, and events; the effects of various types of people (e.g., the "do-gooder," the "villain") and animals on events; the effects of events on feelings and, conversely, the effects of feelings on events; and the knowledge that much behavior is intentionally planned. Through mediation and discussion, students should be presented with questions such as these:

1. How do you identify emotions?

2. What causes feelings?

3. What do people do when they feel a certain way?

4. What would you predict [character name] will do in this situation? Why?

At the highest level of narration, late adolescents should discuss themes, plots, and/or morals of stories (Westby, 1991a). They should talk about the structure of narratives and how to vary structure intentionally for different purposes (i.e., metanarrative skills). Adolescents might tell stories from the perspectives of different characters, or tell a similar story with different endings. For example, *Choose Your Own Adventure* books, *Twist-A-Plot* books, and similar series allow each story to be completed in several dozen ways. A *Choose Your Own Adventure* book could be read to the student, followed by informational and critical listening questions concerning characters and events. At the frequent decision points within the story, the student can be asked which choice to select and why. Following completion of the story once, or in a number of different ways, the student can reformulate it using the assistance of self-imposed scaffolding questions.

Throughout narrative storytelling activities, professionals should be particularly aware of oral expression difficulties that interfere with clear formulation or reformulation (e.g., word-retrieval problems, verbal mazes, inappropriate use of sentence fragments, nonspecific language including lack of pronoun references). These problems must be addressed before adequate narrative skills can be expected.

Materials

The primary materials needed for narrative skill building activities are books, audiotapes, videotapes, and playback equipment. The books and tapes selected should provide models for well-structured narrations. Selection might be based on what is currently being studied in the student's classroom. Middle- and secondary-level English teachers are a good resource for selecting quality literature that is of interest to most preadolescents and adolescents. When the selected books are

not available on tape, service groups in high schools are often willing to assume responsibility to tape the necessary books.

When books not on tape are used for narrative storytelling activities by professionals, they should be read to the student, or paraphrased, so the primary task remains one of listening, not reading. In some cases, it might be desirable for the student to follow along in the book as it is being read, so that both auditory and visual modalities are used. Usually, it is not appropriate during oral language intervention that the primary task of adolescents should be that of reading stories.

Areas of Emphasis

Speaking and listening are the most often emphasized areas during narrative skill building activities. Listening is primary when reformulation tasks are presented; speaking is necessary during both formulation and reformulation tasks. Written language skills can be emphasized by requesting the student to formulate or reformulate a story in writing. By analyzing and discussing various aspects of stories, meta-ability skills are emphasized.

Thinking and nonverbal communication can be focused upon if the tasks are structured appropriately. For example, requesting the student's underlying reasoning for why a particular choice was made within a *Twist-a-Plot* story places emphasis on thinking during the activity. Asking the student to predict how the facial expression just described in the story will affect the feelings of another character places emphasis on nonverbal communication. Survival language skills are often not emphasized when the narrative activities focus on fiction.

Bridging Questions

Adults providing intervention might consider asking these bridging questions during or after storytelling tasks:

1. In the story, one of the main characters felt very [emotion]. When is a time you felt that way? What event led to your feeling that way?

2. What happens when the setting of a story is never explained? Think of a time someone tried to tell you something and you did not know the setting. Think of a time you tried to tell someone else a story and forgot to tell the setting.

3. In some stories, you can predict how the characters will feel or act next. When (besides in stories) do you predict something that will happen? How can predictions help you?

4. I prepared you for listening to the story by telling you the title and the topic of the story. How did that help you understand what the story was about? How could knowing the titles and topics of stories help you in social studies? In science?

5. The group has been talking about cause and effect. Tell me something funny that happened in the story. Together, let's figure out what caused it to be funny.

Strategies to Mediate

A partial list of strategies that the professional could mediate for youth during narrative storytelling activities includes these:

1. asking key questions of yourself to help organize the narrative (i.e., scaffolding);

2. listening for the major organizational structure of a narrative;

3. using cohesion devices to connect ideas in the narrative together (i.e., to make the narrative easier for listeners to understand);

4. predicting outcomes of events as a way to remember "what happens next";

5. describing the setting of a story first, before much action is begun; and

6. pretending you are a character in the story, and everything happens to you as you retell the story from that character's perspective.

Expository Discourse Activities

When someone explains the rules of a game, delineates how to make something, engages in "show-and-tell" communicative behavior, or describes the characteristics of an object or idea, expository discourse skills are being used. Nelson (1993) defines *expository discourse* as "discourse that conveys factual or technical information" (p. 358). Referential communication, which was summarized earlier, is one aspect of expository discourse.

Success in school relies on expository discourse competence because expository text structure is used in most content textbooks and teacher lectures (Nelson, 1993). Students are at risk when they do not understand the complex language of expository discourse (e.g., directions, predictions, facts, specifications, dates, conclusions).

Procedure

Expository text can be viewed from both comprehension and production perspectives. Older students are simultaneously expected to listen to lectures; to derive main ideas and relevant details from their textbooks while reading; to write expository texts of their own (e.g., book reports, answers to essay questions); and to engage in activities such as oral report giving, discussing, and defining.

Intervention might begin with teaching students to recognize different discourse structures, beginning with narrative structure (Nelson, 1988; Wallach, 1990; Westby, 1989). Students could then be taught to contrast narrative and expository texts (Nelson, 1993). Expository text structures to teach include these patterns of organization:

1. by comparing and contrasting;

2. by problem and solution;

3. by cause and effect;

4. by chronological sequence (i.e., episodic sequence);

5. by order of importance (i.e., hierarchical);

6. by category (i.e., topical cluster or list); and

7. by physical location.

Major patterns of organization could be visually displayed for students, like the poster shown in Figure 7.6.

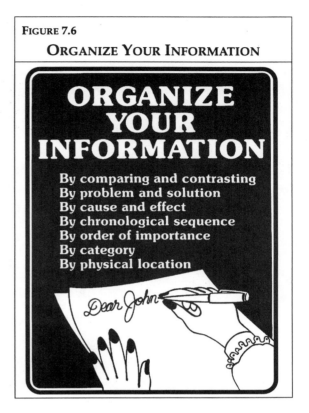

FIGURE 7.6

ORGANIZE YOUR INFORMATION

These additional expository text macro-structures have been cited (Nelson, 1993; Westby, 1991b):

- by description; and

- by matrix (i.e., the intersection of several categories).

When students understand expository text structures, they can follow the outline of a teacher's lecture, organize their notes, apply mnemonic strategies, and prepare their own papers more efficiently.

Initially, the adult providing intervention may set up the expository text structure, then coach the student to fit additional pieces of information into the organization. Mediation may be provided to explain the structure that is chosen and why it is an appropriate choice for the factual or technical information presented.

Students should receive practice in inferring structures, first with assistance, then without. Text excerpts from the student's curriculum and/or classroom lecture snippets could be used. While expository discourse skills are being acquired, the adult should frame the structural cues so the student recognizes them as independently as possible. Scaffolding support should be offered (e.g., Why did ___

happen?; List the features of ___ ; Give examples of ___ ; Give the steps in doing ___).

Westby (1991b) emphasized that the framing-of-cues process should help students recognize key words that may signal different kinds of expository text. Sample key words are listed in Table 7.9 for the different expository text structures cited earlier. These key words are often in the form of conjunctions and logical connectors and serve as text cohesion devices. Intervention should include focusing

TABLE 7.9

KEY WORDS FOR DIFFERENT EXPOSITORY TEXT STRUCTURES

TEXT STRUCTURE	KEY WORDS
COMPARING AND CONTRASTING	same, different, however, but, on the contrary, similar, dissimilar, yet, still, common, alike, rather than, instead of, compare, contrast
PROBLEM AND SOLUTION	one problem, the problem is, the issues are, a solution(s) is (are)
CAUSE AND EFFECT	if, then, because, reason, affected, influenced, resulted in, therefore, since, thus, hence, consequently, cause, caused, effect, net effect, result, consequence
CHRONOLOGICAL SEQUENCE (episodic sequence)	first, second, third, after that, antecedent, before that, preceding, next, last, in order, subsequent, proceeding, finally, eventually, gradually
ORDER OF IMPORTANCE (hierarchical)	first, second, third, most, least, all, none, some, always, never, more, less, _____+er, _____+est, frequent, infrequent
CATEGORY (topical cluster or list)	group, set, for instance, another, an illustration of, such as, an example of, like, category, class
PHYSICAL LOCATION	here, there, left, right, above, below, north, south, east, west, around, on top, under, bottom, front, back, forward, backward, side
DESCRIPTION	defined as, called, labeled, refers to, is someone who, is something that, means, can be interpreted as, describe, procedure, how to
MATRIX	interpret, intersection, come together, overlap, influenced by, simultaneously, at the same time, converge

on these key words and making certain that students comprehend their meaning. Key words might be stressed during oral exchanges, highlighted in discourse being read, and edited in when students are writing their own expository text.

Materials

The student's curricular materials should be used whenever possible when teaching expository discourse skills. Textbooks, supplemental reading, handouts, and tests can all be analyzed with the student for text structure and key words. Classroom lectures and teacher directions can also be used and are best captured on video- or audiotape for ongoing benefit. Simulated lecture and direction segments can be created in lieu of capturing "the real thing." Still, simulations should be as realistic as possible so that students are exposed to expository text structures as they will naturally occur in their environment.

Areas of Emphasis

The most common areas of emphasis during expository discourse skills intervention are speaking, listening, reading, and writing. Analysis of text structure also requires thinking and meta-ability skills. Intervention should incorporate both comprehension (listening, reading) and production (speaking, writing) aspects. As key words are identified while listening or reading, they should be noted, then used by the student when speaking and writing.

Nonverbal communication is not generally emphasized while working on expository discourse skills. However, students might be taught that cues can be obtained by watching a teacher's nonverbal communication. For example, it would not be unusual for teachers to list items on their fingers as they are announcing them or to emphasize "first, next, last" nonverbally when giving directions with a chronological sequence.

Survival language skills are emphasized in the sense that understanding expository text is crucial to a student's survival in school (Nelson, 1993). Expository discourse is also common in vocational settings, into which the student must ultimately fit.

Bridging Questions

Professionals using expository discourse activities might consider asking these bridging questions during or after the activities:

1. We just analyzed a section in your textbook and decided it fit the organizational structure called _____. When else have you heard or read information organized by that structure?

2. We've been reading information organized by category. Now you've been given some new information. How would you fit the new information into the existing categories?

3. Your teacher has given you an assignment to write about some aspect of World War II. What are some choices of text structure, and how would what you write change with the structure? (For example, a student could write about the major chronological events of World War II or focus instead on the causes of the war and the net effects.)

4. You need to organize a three-minute speech in which you introduce yourself to the class. You decide to organize your speech using a "comparing and contrasting" structure. What are some questions you could ask yourself to prepare for your speech?

5. Sometimes reports are organized by describing the problem and then giving solutions. What are some topics you could organize that way? Sometimes it is easier to organize reports by the order of events (i.e., first, next, last). What are some topics you could organize that way?

Strategies to Mediate

A partial list of strategies that the professional could mediate for youth during expository discourse activities includes these:

1. organizing information by several characteristics simultaneously (e.g., chronological and problem and solution) and seeing how text structure would alter accordingly;

2. using relevant information once a text structure is chosen and ignoring irrelevant information;

3. looking for relationships among separate objects, events, and experiences, then selecting the expository discourse macrostructure that can reflect these relationships;

4. using logic to defend the text structure chosen for spoken or written discourse assignments; and

5. taking sufficient time to think through the text structure that is to be comprehended or produced.

Word-Finding Activities

Word-finding difficulties are common in many children and adolescents with special needs. While the problem has been recognized for some time, word-finding intervention programs have not kept pace with diagnostic procedures (German, 1993). Word-finding problems affect all aspects of an individual's life in social, academic, and, ultimately, vocational settings. The problems reveal themselves in discourse (e.g., when relating experiences or events), which impacts negatively on conversations.

Adequate word-finding ability is essential to these communication functions: to give information, to get information, to describe an ongoing event, to persuade the listener, to self-disclose, to solve problems, and to entertain. In short, word finding is one of the most pervasive communication skills that can be taught to students experiencing deficits. During word-finding activities, strategies are taught that eliminate or minimize the interference of word-finding problems during communicative exchanges.

Procedure

German (1992, 1993) outlines a word-finding intervention model that focuses on three areas:

1. remediation;

2. self-advocacy instruction; and

3. compensatory modification.

During remediation, the student learns word-retrieval strategies such as these:

• attribute-cueing strategies;

- semantic alternatives;
- associate cueing; and
- reflective pausing.

When teaching attribute-cueing strategies, emphasis is placed on phonemic cueing (i.e., instructing how the initial sound[s] or syllables in a word can be used to cue the target word). Similarly, graphemic cueing takes advantage of the initial letter(s) or spelling to cue the target word. Another type of attribute cueing is imagery cueing, which uses visualization of the referent to cue the target word. Gesture cueing uses a mime of the action associated with the target word.

Semantic alternatives include synonym substituting and category name substituting. To use synonym substitution, the student must first understand the concept of synonym. Students are taught it is appropriate to substitute a synonym for a word that is difficult to retrieve (e.g., *cook* for *chef*). In contrast, students who understand vocabulary categorization concepts could be taught to substitute a category name for a difficult-to-retrieve word (e.g., *vegetable* for *celery*).

In associate cueing, the adult planning word-finding activities for the student would explain how thinking of a word highly associated with the target word can provide a reminder of the difficult-to-retrieve word. For example, the student could think of the associated word *cake* to retrieve *birthday*. Other people can also provide associated words to cue the student when word-finding blocks occur. Associate cueing is good for building the retrieval strength of technical academic terms and names of important people, places, and events.

Reflective pausing is a good strategy for students who are fast but inaccurate namers. Students are taught to use pausing appropriately with the goal of reducing the retrieval of inappropriate words. When using reflective pausing, the student stops when trying to retrieve a word, remains silent rather than blurting out a competing (inaccurate) response, and applies one of the attribute-cueing or semantic-alternatives strategies described. The student might also admit to the listener that he or she "can't remember the word right now" to minimize the effects of the pause.

Techniques that help to reinforce word-finding strategies include segmenting, rhythm, rehearsal, and rapid-naming exercises. For students who understand syllabication, the use of segmenting can assist in retrieving multisyllabic words. Students divide words into syllables, then rehearse saying them. Likewise, a rhythm technique can be used with students who have syllabication skills. Again, using multisyllabic words, students tap for each syllable as they are rehearsing aloud.

When students do not have syllabication skills, a straight rehearsal technique can still help them to improve word retrieval. Multisyllabic words are repeated five times, for example. For students with slow retrieval speed, rapid-naming exercises might be used (e.g., practice 10 target words written or pictured on cards and attempt to improve the overall time it takes to flip through the 10 cards and name them). Words used for practicing word-retrieval strategies and techniques should come from the student's world. Words should be relevant to school, home, work, and recreational settings.

In addition to the direct remediation activities with students just described, focus should also cross over to self-advocacy instruction (German, 1993). First, students should become knowledgeable about the retrieval strategies that are best for their particular word-finding deficits. Students are then taught self-monitoring techniques (e.g., tallying when and how many times they engage in a particular gesture) and self-instruction sequences (e.g., what self-talk message might be used to cue a semantic alternative word choice such as "Let me think. To what category does the word that I'm trying to find belong? Oh, yes, it's a country in South America").

Another aspect of self-advocacy is teaching students to identify the impact of language settings, contexts, times of day, and the vocabulary itself on word-retrieval skills (German, 1993). Some situations will trigger more word-finding problems than others, and students should become knowledgeable about the parameters of those situations. As students progress through intervention for word-retrieval deficits, they should gradually learn to self-apply retrieval strategies and techniques and establish knowledge of the compensatory modifications that can be made for them.

The compensatory modification focus within word-finding activities should be implemented concurrently with the self-advocacy component (German, 1993); in this way, the student takes ownership of the word-retrieval problem. Instructional modifications are made that facilitate a student's word-finding skills. Collaboration with teachers, parents, and work supervisors identifies modifications that can be made in the classroom, at home, and on a job site. Older students, particularly those in high school and in postsecondary educational settings, should participate in conversations with teachers about modifications. Some compensatory modifications that might be used include altering tests to put less demand on retrieval skills (e.g., having an open-book exam), allowing additional time to complete a task, and providing multiple-choice formats when a retrieval block occurs. Similarly, family members and employers might allow more time for responses and reduce the number of stressful speaking situations that precipitate more word-finding problems.

Materials

The primary materials needed for word-finding activities are relevant vocabulary lists derived from a student's school, home, work, and community settings. Using words that are immediately meaningful for the student motivates that individual to learn word-retrieval strategies and to engage in word-finding techniques that will generalize to new terms that constantly surface.

Maintaining a notebook of words being studied is critical. Many helpful recording forms are also available in German's (1993) *Word Finding Intervention Program*.

Reinforcement materials may be needed to motivate younger students. For example, while engaged in the rehearsal technique, students may say a word five times and then get to move ahead on a game board, or perhaps they toss a pair of dice and say a word the number of times specified on the dice.

Areas of Emphasis

Thinking and speaking are the most often emphasized areas during word-finding activities. Self-advocacy instruction, encompassing self-monitoring and self-instruction sequences, involves primarily thinking and meta-ability skills. Speaking skills are paramount to demonstrate word-finding ability.

Nonverbal communication is also focused on when gestures are taught as an attribute-cueing strategy. Also, students may be asked to self-monitor inappropriate gestures (i.e., secondary characteristics) that sometimes occur during word-finding blocks.

Survival language is an area of emphasis during word-finding activities to the extent that vocabulary is chosen from home- and community-based settings (e.g., terms are selected from the language of restaurants and banks).

Bridging Questions

Adults providing intervention might consider asking these bridging questions during or after word-finding activities:

1. If you develop word-finding skills, how can that help you in school?

2. Tell about a time when you didn't use your word-retrieval strategies. What were the consequences?

3. You've asked your teachers to make some compensatory modifications in their classrooms. When you get a job, could you ask your employer to modify anything? If so, what? How would you ask?

4. When else could you use self-monitoring skills besides while retrieving words?

5. You've identified situations when it's harder for you to retrieve words and why. Is it ever hard for you to do other communication tasks, like listening? If so, describe the situations. What are some strategies you could use to listen better?

Strategies to Mediate

A partial list of strategies that the professional could mediate for youth during word-finding activities includes these:

1. organizing information by several characteristics simultaneously (e.g., recognizing that numerous categories could be used when applying the semantic alternatives strategy, such as ice cream fitting into the categories of desserts, dairy, and frozen foods);

2. knowing when it is important to be precise and accurate (e.g., there are times when only the exact word will do, such as the password to certain computer files);

3. using relevant information and ignoring irrelevant information (e.g., picking out the key words to remember from a teacher's instructions);

4. considering different alternatives (e.g., if one strategy fails, can another one be substituted?); and

5. restraining from saying something that will be regretted later.

Commercial Resources for Older Students

Many commercial resources have been developed for preadolescents and adolescents in the last decade. Table 7.10 summarizes some of the resources that professionals might consider when intervening with youth. The table is not intended to be a critique of the commercial resources available, but rather a summary of key information. Each commercial resource has this summary information: resource name, author(s), publisher, copyright, area(s) of modification, age or grade level at which the resource is appropriate, documentation, natural versus contrived procedures, and natural versus contrived materials. Several of the columns in Table 7.10 are self-explanatory; however, the latter three may not be. A description of these three categories follows.

The column called "Documentation" refers to whether the commercial resource includes information concerning the philosophical tenets, theoretical premises, or literature support underlying the material. A cursory glance at Table 7.10 will reveal that numerous commercial resources fail to provide documentation for users. The lack of documentation is alarming, because a resource may conflict with theoretical constructs of other approaches and resources utilized during intervention. If a resource does not have documentation, then users should spend considerable time studying it before choosing it for a given student, to make certain that the resource is appropriate.

The column called "Natural/Contrived Materials" refers to how similar or dissimilar the materials are to everyday situations. Materials can be aligned on a continuum from natural to contrived. The most natural material for a student would be none, or materials identical to those located in actual communi-

cation situations (e.g., real money, real job application forms, real menus from restaurants). Absence of materials is also considered natural, because much of the time when normal adolescents are engaged in conversations, no materials are selected by them (i.e., a group of adolescents frequently carries on a conversation removed from the here and now). Contrived materials refer to those that are artificial to everyday contexts (e.g., flash cards used to learn new vocabulary).

While it might be tempting to think that naturalistic materials are always better than contrived, the effectiveness of the materials depends on the objectives and the student. Contrived materials are often good for teaching strategies. They can act as a catalyst for generating more naturalistic discussion among students. In our clinical experiences, we have found it disastrous to attempt a discussion with early adolescents without the assistance of some contrived material that triggers their interest in bridging questions. On the other hand, by the time they are dismissed from intervention, students should be able to communicate appropriately when naturalistic materials are used.

The column called "Natural/Contrived Procedures" refers to how similar or dissimilar the procedures are to everyday situations. Natural procedures for preadolescents and adolescents include those that replicate most closely daily communication situations (e.g., conversing with a friend, asking a teacher a question in the classroom). On the other end of the continuum are contrived procedures, which differ the most from daily communication situations. For example, a drill-and-practice

TABLE 7.10	COMMERCIAL RESOURCES FOR OLDER STUDENTS				
RESOURCE	**AREA OF MODIFICATION**	**SUGGESTED AGE OR GRADE**	**DOCUMENTATION**	**NATURAL/ CONTRIVED MATERIALS**	**NATURAL/ CONTRIVED PROCEDURES**
ALP: Active Listening Program (1986) van der Laan, C. Thinking Publications Eau Claire, WI	Listening	Grade 6–Adult	Yes	Contrived	Contrived
Communicate (1986) Mayo, P., and Waldo, P. Thinking Publications Eau Claire, WI	Listening Speaking	Grades 5–12	Yes	Contrived	Natural/ Contrived
Communication and Self-Esteem (CASE) Study (1992) Marquis, M.A., and Addy-Trout, E. Thinking Publications Eau Claire, WI	Thinking Social Comm-unication	Grades 6–12	Yes	Natural/ Contrived	Natural/ Contrived
CORT Thinking Lessons (1981) deBono, E. Pergamon Press New York, NY	Thinking	Grades 5–12	Yes	Contrived	Natural
Daily Communication: Strategies for the Language Disordered Adolescent (1984) Schwartz, L., and McKinley, N. Thinking Publications Eau Claire, WI	Thinking Listening Speaking Nonverbal Comm-unication Survival Language	Grades 6–12	Yes	Natural/ Contrived	Natural/ Contrived
Daily Problem Solving Activities: Transitioning to Independence (1993) Gruen, A., and Gruen, L. Thinking Publications Eau Claire, WI	Thinking Listening Survival Language Writing	Grade 10–Adult	Yes	Contrived	Natural/ Contrived

(continued)

TABLE 7.10—*Continued*

RESOURCE	AREA OF MODIFICATION	SUGGESTED AGE OR GRADE	DOCUMENTATION	NATURAL/ CONTRIVED MATERIALS	NATURAL/ CONTRIVED PROCEDURES
Face to Face: Facilitating Adolescent Communication Experiences (1993) Hess, L. Communication Skill Builders Tucson, AZ	Speaking Listening Social Communication	Ages 12–19	Yes	Natural/ Contrived	Natural/ Contrived
Figurative Language: A Comprehensive Program (1992) Gorman-Gard, K. Thinking Publications Eau Claire, WI	Thinking Metalinguistics Speaking	Grades 4–12	Yes	Contrived	Natural/ Contrived
HELP: Handbook of Exercises for Language Processing (Volumes I, II, III, IV) (1980) Lazzari, A., and Peters, P. LinguiSystems East Moline, IL	Listening Speaking	Grades 4–Adult	No	Contrived	Contrived
Job-Related Social Skills: A Curriculum for Adolescents with Special Needs (1991) Montague, M., and Lund, K. Exceptional Innovations Ann Arbor, MI	Social Communication	Ages 15–22	Yes	Natural/ Contrived	Natural/ Contrived
Just for Laughs (1993) Spector, C. Communication Skill Builders Tucson, AZ	Thinking Metalinguistics Listening	Age 10–Adult	Yes	Contrived	Contrived
Let's Talk: Intermediate Level (1984) Wigg, E., and Bray, C. Psychological Corporation Austin, TX	Speaking	Grades 5–10	Yes	Natural/ Contrived	Natural/ Contrived

(continued)

TABLE 7.10—*Continued*

RESOURCE	AREA OF MODIFICATION	SUGGESTED AGE OR GRADE	DOCUMENTATION	NATURAL/ CONTRIVED MATERIALS	NATURAL/ CONTRIVED PROCEDURES
Life Skills Workshop: An Active Program for Real-Life Problem Solving (1992) Hannon, K., and Thompson, M. LinguiSystems East Moline, IL	Survival Language Reading Writing	Age 12–Adult	No	Natural/ Contrived	Natural/ Contrived
Life Works: A Transition Program for High School Students (1994) Dalke, C., and Howard, D. LinguiSystems East Moline, IL	Survival Language	High School	No	Natural/ Contrived	Natural/ Contrived
Make-It-Yourself Barrier Activities: Barrier Activities for Speakers and Listeners (1987) Schwartz, L., and McKinley, N. Thinking Publications Eau Claire, WI	Thinking Listening Speaking Writing	Grade K–Adult	Yes	Contrived	Natural
Mind Benders (1978) Harnadek, A. Midwest Publications Pacific Grove, CA	Thinking	Grades 7–12	No	Contrived	Contrived
125 Ways to Be a Better Listener (1992) Graser, N. LinguiSystems East Moline, IL	Listening	Grade 7–Adult	Yes	Natural/ Contrived	Natural/ Contrived
125 Ways to Be a Better Thinker (1993) Zachman, L., Barrett, M., Huisingh, R., Blagden, C., and Orman, J. LinguiSystems East Moline, IL	Thinking	Grades 7–12	Yes	Natural/ Contrived	Natural/ Contrived

(continued)

TABLE 7.10—*Continued*

RESOURCE	AREA OF MODIFICATION	SUGGESTED AGE OR GRADE	DOCUMENTATION	NATURAL/ CONTRIVED MATERIALS	NATURAL/ CONTRIVED PROCEDURES
PALS: Pragmatic Activities in Language and Speech (1988) Davis, B. Pro-Ed Austin, TX	Speaking Listening Reading Writing	Secondary Level	No	Natural/ Contrived	Natural/ Contrived
POW! Personal Power! (1992) Gajewski, N., and Mayo, P. Thinking Publications Eau Claire, WI	Thinking Speaking Listening Social Comm- unication	Ages 11–18	Yes	Contrived	Natural/ Contrived
Pragmatic Language Trivia for Thinking Skills (1990) Marquis, M.A. Communication Skill Builders Tucson, AZ	Thinking Speaking Listening Social Comm- unication	Ages 11–18	Yes	Contrived	Natural/ Contrived
Problem Solver (1986) Waldo, P. Thinking Publications Eau Claire, WI	Thinking Speaking	Grades 5–12	Yes	Contrived	Natural/ Contrived
Problem Solving for Teens: An Interactive Approach to Real-Life Problem Solving (1990) Gray, B. LinguiSystems East Moline, IL	Thinking	Grades 7–12	No	Natural/ Contrived	Natural/ Contrived
Question the Information: Techniques for Classroom Listening (1992) Danielson, J., and Sampson, L. LinguiSystems East Moline, IL	Listening Study Skills	Grades 6–12	No	Natural/ Contrived	Natural/ Contrived

(continued)

TABLE 7.10—*Continued*

RESOURCE	AREA OF MODIFICATION	SUGGESTED AGE OR GRADE	DOCUMENTATION	NATURAL/ CONTRIVED MATERIALS	NATURAL/ CONTRIVED PROCEDURES
Referential Communication: Barrier Activities for Speakers and Listeners (Parts One and Two) (1985) McKinley, N., and Schwartz, L. Thinking Publications Eau Claire, WI	Thinking Listening Speaking Writing	Grades K–5 (Part One) and Grade 6–Adult (Part Two)	Yes	Contrived	Natural
Scripting: Social Communication for Adolescents (1994) Mayo, P., and Waldo, P. Thinking Publications Eau Claire, WI	Speaking Social Comm-unication	Grades 5–12	Yes	Contrived	Natural/ Contrived
Skillstreaming the Adolescent: A Structured Learning Approach to Teaching Prosocial Skills (1980) Goldstein, A., Sprafkin, R., Gershaw, N., and Klein, P. Research Press Champaign, IL	Thinking Social Comm-unication	Ages 12–18	Yes	Contrived	Natural/ Contrived
Social Language for Teens: Tackling Real-Life Situations (1993) Turnbow, G., and Proctor, D. LinguiSystems East Moline, IL	Listening Speaking Social Comm-unication Nonverbal Comm-unication	Grades 5–12	Yes	Natural/ Contrived	Natural/ Contrived
SSS: Social Skill Strategies (Books A and B) (1989) Gajewski, N., and Mayo, P. Thinking Publications Eau Claire, WI	Thinking Speaking Social Comm-unication Nonverbal Comm-unication	Grades 6–12	Yes	Contrived	Natural/ Contrived
A Sourcebook of Adolescent Pragmatic Activities (Revised) (1994) Weinrich, B., Glaser, A., and Johnston, E. Communication Skill Builders Tucson, AZ	Speaking Listening Nonverbal Comm-unication	Grades 7–12	Yes	Natural/ Contrived	Natural/ Contrived

(continued)

TABLE 7.10—*Continued*

RESOURCE	AREA OF MODIFICATION	SUGGESTED AGE OR GRADE	DOCUMENTATION	NATURAL/ CONTRIVED MATERIALS	NATURAL/ CONTRIVED PROCEDURES
Study Smart: An Educational Activity to Reinforce Study Skills (1990) Mayo, P., Gajewski, N., and Rajek, A. Thinking Publications Eau Claire, WI	Study Skills	Grades 5–12	Yes	Contrived	Contrived
Tackling Teen Topics: Problem Solving Activities for Adolescents (1992) Murray, D., Herron, N., and Housel, S. Communication Skill Builders Tucson, AZ	Thinking	Adolescents	No	Contrived	Natural
Teaching Functional Academics: A Curriculum Guide for Adolescents and Adults with Learning Problems (1982) Bender, M., and Valletutti, P. Pro-Ed Austin, TX	Survival Language	Grade 9–Adult	No	Natural	Natural/ Contrived
Thinking with Language, Grades 4-6 (1992) Krassowski, E. Burke Communication Skill Builders Tucson, AZ	Thinking Speaking	11–16 years	Yes	Contrived	Natural/ Contrived
TOPS Kit—Adolescent (1992) Zachman, L., Barrett, M., Huisingh, R., Orman, J., and Blagden, C. LinguiSystems East Moline, IL	Thinking Reading	Ages 12–18	Yes	Natural/ Contrived	Natural/ Contrived
Transfer Activities: Thinking Skill Vocabulary Development (1986) Mayo, P., and Gajewski, N. Thinking Publications Eau Claire, WI	Thinking Study Skills Writing	Grades 5–12	Yes	Contrived	Natural/ Contrived

(continued)

RESOURCE	AREA OF MODIFICATION	SUGGESTED AGE OR GRADE	DOCUMENTATION	NATURAL/ CONTRIVED MATERIALS	NATURAL/ CONTRIVED PROCEDURES
TABLE 7.10—*Continued*					
Vocabulary to Go (1987) Danielson, J. LinguiSystems East Moline, IL	Listening Speaking	Grades 3–8	No	Contrived	Contrived
Vocabulary Maps (1993) Hamersky, J. Thinking Publications Eau Claire, WI	Thinking Listening Speaking	Grades 5–12	Yes	Natural/ Contrived	Contrived
Vocabulary Victory! (Levels A–D) (1991). Brigance, A. LinguiSystems East Moline, IL	Thinking Reading	Grade 4–Adult	No	Contrived	Contrived
The Walker Social Skills Curriculum The ACCESS Program: Adolescent Curriculum for Communication and Effective Social Skills (1988) Walker, H., Todis, B., Holmes, D., and Horton, G. Pro-Ed Austin, TX	Social Communication Study Skills	"Middle and High School"	Yes	Natural	Natural
Word Finding Intervention Program (1993) German, D. Communication Skill Builders Tucson, AZ	Word Finding	Children– Adults	Yes	Natural/ Contrived	Natural/ Contrived
Warm-up Exercises: Calisthenics for the Brain (Books I, II, III) (1984, 1985, and 1992) Kisner, R., and Knowles, B. Thinking Publications Eau Claire, WI	Listening Speaking	Grade 5–Adult	No	Contrived	Contrived
The Word Kit—Adolescent (1991) Lanza, J., and Wilson, C. LinguiSystems East Moline, IL	Listening Speaking	Grades 6–12	No	Contrived	Contrived

exercise is one in which people do not typically engage in a daily situation.

The professional should select the procedure that is most appropriate for the given student and objective. Adolescents who are initially learning a new behavior may be greatly assisted by using a one-on-one, drill-and-practice procedure. However, as behaviors are acquired, it is important to move procedures toward normal communication. Failure to do this will lessen the degree to which behaviors are likely to be transferred. Before dismissal from intervention, students should be able to communicate successfully when natural procedures are used.

Some professionals consistently use contrived materials and contrived procedures with adolescents, and thus fail to move them along the continuum toward more natural contexts. Intervention using contrived materials and procedures uses a high amount of one-on-one work with structured intervention programs. To reiterate, this is appropriate for some students some of the time. However, in our clinical experiences, the benefits of intervention for the student in other situations will not be apparent until procedures and materials become more natural.

Many commercial resources that have contrived materials and procedures can be moved along the continuum toward "naturalistic" through the general procedures of mediation and bridging explained previously in this chapter. For example, it is not unusual for some commercial materials to list an objective at the beginning of the activity and a brief summary of the procedures to use. With older students, this objective needs to be mediated before and during the activity if generalization of communication behaviors is to occur. Students also need to bridge the content of the objective that is specified in the commercial resource to other situations.

Focusing the activity so that students grasp its meaning and recognize its application in their lives results in the materials and procedures being less contrived and more natural. If professionals using the commercial materials fail to see the relevance of the prescribed objectives, a general rule is not to use that commercial resource. If the adults providing intervention cannot verbalize a strong rationale for students as to why they should learn a particular behavior specified in the commercial resource, then it will not be taught successfully. The recurring questions from preadolescents and adolescents—"Why do I need to learn this?" "When will I ever use this?"—compel each of us to examine our rationale for using a given resource on an ongoing basis.

INDIRECT SERVICES

Indirect intervention involves people from the student's educational and environmental support systems in activities that assist the youth to communicate more effectively. We are concerned primarily with those students who have language disabilities accompanied by problems within their support systems at school, at home, or in the community (e.g., they are having difficulty understanding the language that teachers use in the classroom, that parents use at home, or that supervisors use at work).

During indirect intervention, the speech-language pathologist attempts to affect positive modifications for the student without face-to-face contact with that student. More often, direct and indirect intervention are occurring simultaneously, and three-way interchanges will occur (e.g., a work supervisor, the student, and the speech-language pathologist are concurrently involved).

When the student's deficits revolve around language, two main choices can be made: Either the educational and environmental systems need to be modified to meet the existing performance of the student, or the student's performance must be changed to cope with the systems. Again, in reality, both activities may occur simultaneously. The adolescent would receive direct intervention in terms of how to change to fit the existing systems and, during indirect intervention, modifications that teachers, families, and employers can make would be the focus. This section of the chapter will focus on the modifications that could be made for the older student with language disabilities.

MODIFICATIONS OF THE EDUCATIONAL SYSTEM

When the educational system is modified to meet the language needs of older students, changes might occur in these areas:

- the organization of curriculum materials;
- the oral language of the educator during classroom discourse; and
- the written language of textbooks and other printed materials.

When approaching modifications of the educational system, professionals need to remember that deficiencies could exist in the system itself, which compound the older student's language disability. For example, the curriculum materials may be sequenced inappropriately, demand cognitive abilities that exceed the student's present capacity, or require written responses that surpass the student's ability level. (See Appendix D for how to analyze the curriculum.) The oral language of the teacher may be too rapid, complex, or disorganized for the older student to comprehend. Perhaps the teacher is using too many unfamiliar vocabulary terms or lengthy sentences. (See Appendix B for how to analyze the teacher's language.) Likewise, the written language of the textbook and other materials may be too complex or may contain an abundance of novel terminology.

Organization of Curriculum Materials

The overall organization of curriculum is typically generated by a curriculum committee that formally reviews specific content areas every few years. Often this process is linked with new textbook selection.

Speech-language pathologists should make known to administrators, department heads of specific academic areas, and classroom teachers that they are uniquely qualified to appraise the language and cognitive demands of the curriculum as they affect students with language disorders and learning disabilities. We urge speech-language pathologists to volunteer for curriculum committees in their local communities.

In some schools, volunteering to serve on a curriculum committee meets with quick approval. In other places, the voluntary request will be suspect and the speech-language pathologist may have to launch a campaign to educate others as to how the discipline of communication sciences and disorders may contribute positively to the outcome of the curriculum committee.

Often, professionals can make inroads on elementary-level curriculum committees before they can at the middle and high school levels. A phone call from the elementary principal to the secondary principal may remove roadblocks more quickly than other approaches, assuming the elementary principal speaks positively about the benefit of input from speech-language pathologists.

Once appointed to serve on a curriculum committee, the speech-language pathologist should analyze the language and cognitive demands of the curriculum as well as its organization from a developmental language standpoint. A determination should be made whether the curriculum is sequential or spiral in nature. Recall that in a spiral curriculum, skills gradually build upon each other; in a sequential curriculum, content and skills are relatively independent and each new topic provides a "fresh start" for the student.

If the curriculum is to be implemented with both normal students and those with disabilities, a cross-section of performance may be needed from both groups. Through these types of efforts, some schools develop alternative curricula or "schools within schools" to serve at-risk students and those with marginal academic skills. The pendulum swings back and forth in education as to whether such

tracking of students is "good" policy or "bad." In the 1990s, one of the passwords is "inclusion," and a modified curriculum is to occur in response to every individual's unique needs. The reality of implementing this concept in a classroom with dozens of students remains challenging.

Speech-language pathologists should also be involved when committees are formed to review and modify curriculum in special education areas. Special education curriculum naturally includes language and communication as areas to teach. However, the scope and sequence of objectives may be organized inappropriately, or important objectives may be missing. Relevant objectives may not be considered, especially if special education aligns itself in a parallel fashion with general education and teaches the same curriculum, only at a slower rate. For example, social communication objectives might be totally overlooked because they are not part of the curriculum for general education students.

In some cases, language goals might be buried in other areas of the curriculum. For example, the concept of "left-right" might be a goal tucked in the "adaptive physical education" area of the curriculum. Teachers may fail to grasp the strong language component contained within such goals. Speech-language pathologists can assist other special educators in seeing the pervasiveness of language within their curricula.

Oral Language of the Educator During Classroom Discourse

Good teaching involves adjustment of the form and content of messages to reflect an awareness of the needs and feelings of students. When selecting discourse style for the classroom,

> teachers use a combination of prior knowledge about the expected linguistic and cognitive abilities of their students along with immediate verbal and nonverbal feedback. In this way, they adjust their speaking styles to fit the presumed capabilities of the children they teach. (Nelson, 1984, p. 175)

Students outside the educator's expected group norm for language facility will have difficulty succeeding in that teacher's classroom. Occasionally, educators will overshoot the majority of the group, as reflected by such student comments as, "Nobody understands what's going on! I think Mr. B. talks to himself most of the time." Teachers may also undershoot, as reflected by student comments such as, "This class is so easy, it's boring! She must think we are babies."

Once the speech-language pathologist has established a firm relationship with the classroom teacher, that teacher can be encouraged to use several speaking styles for his or her students. For example, the rate of delivery may need to be slowed down for some students to capture main ideas. Key phrases may need to be repeated and perhaps handed out in a study guide. When students look perplexed, a re-explanation, perhaps using more concrete language, should follow. If the teacher's spoken language is excessively cluttered by verbal mazes, false starts, and revisions, the use of clearer messages and questions should be encouraged. These teachers in particular might be encouraged to use listening guides that capture main ideas and relevant details

that students are expected to comprehend. If teachers are resistant to developing listening guides (and often those who are in need of the most change are the ones least likely to accept help and are the most defensive), then study guides can be developed independently by using notes from students who are performing well in the class. Politically, relationships remain more amiable in school settings when teachers are not forced to make modifications, even when those changes are desirable for students.

How the teacher responds to student requests for clarification, even those that seem unnecessary at the time, will set the learning tone in the classroom. Perhaps most of us can remember a teacher in our past who ridiculed or embarrassed students for asking a question or for confessing to a lack of understanding. Students attempting to survive in these classrooms quickly learned that it was safer to say nothing at all and to suffer the consequences (e.g., completing an assignment incorrectly) than to risk the ire of the teacher.

Speech-language pathologists should encourage teachers to remain receptive to student questions, to share that receptive attitude with students, and to resist making the assumption that the students' questions are irrelevant. For example, directions may appear clear to educators because of their familiarity with the material but be ambiguous to students. Rather than reacting negatively to a question, educators might pursue a student's perspective by countering with a question like, "What is confusing you about the directions?"

When student requests for clarification are global (e.g., "I don't get it! Say it again"), teachers should help these students to isolate the information that was not understood and then to restate the question more precisely. Often, students do understand some of the directions but they lack the necessary skill to ask a specific question about what was not understood.

Sometimes discourse rule differences between regular classrooms and resource programs may complicate school language for students with language disabilities. For example, if the resource room is informal and students can ask questions whenever they arise, students may have difficulty adjusting to teachers who expect questions for clarification only at particular times, such as before or after class. The student who blurts out questions informally may be judged by the classroom teacher as "bumbling" or rude (Donahue, 1985). A signal system might be devised between the teacher and the student so the student knows when the behavior is inappropriate. Also, during direct intervention, judging when to ask questions and when to hold them could be emphasized.

Teachers should also realize that indirect requests (e.g., saying, "Don't you know you're supposed to begin reading Chapter 6 as soon as the bell rings?" to stop a student from engaging in a conversation) are frequently misunderstood by students with language disabilities. Frequently, they miss the illocutionary force of indirect requests.

Rather than assuming that indirect requests for action are understood, the teacher could ask students to explain what is expected. Perhaps better yet for some students is for the teacher to make direct requests until compre-hension of indirect requests is taught as a specific communication skill.

Written Language of Textbooks and Other Printed Materials

For many older students with language disabilities, the reading level of classroom textbooks is too high for them to comprehend without modifications. One such modification is to color-code textbooks for students with some reading skills but for whom the amount of print is overwhelming. When color-coding textbooks, one color or several might be used. For example, a yellow highlight might be used for main ideas, a blue highlight for relevant details, and a green highlight for new vocabulary words. If multiple colors prove to be confusing to students, then the system should revert to a simple one-color approach. The challenge is to leave more words that are *not* highlighted than are highlighted. When multiple books from different subject areas are being coded, an identical system of colors should be used, which will require agreement among professionals.

Initially, classroom teachers should do the color-coding, since they are most familiar with the material and with their expectations for students' performance. However, during consultation, a plan should be devised whereby the students are gradually taught to color-code the textbooks themselves. The plan should also include who will be responsible for teaching the skill of color-coding to students.

Sometimes, the greatest resistance to color-coding comes from administrators who fear color-coding will damage textbooks. One solution is to start with older textbooks that will be phased out in the next few years and which may already be worn. Professionals should assure administrators that there will always be a group of older students who need the assistance of color-coded textbooks. Once books are coded, they will still be very useful to future students. Another solution is to obtain permission to photocopy chapters from the chosen textbooks and to teach color-coding skills through the use of those copies. Ideally, students should learn how to color-code for themselves, and they can practice only when they have their own copies. Color-coding may become increasingly more important as students enter postsecondary learning experiences and are expected to learn independently.

Another viable modification when it comes to the written language of textbooks is to make available audiotape recordings of the material. This permits students to listen and relisten to the printed information for specific content areas. A number of states, as well as the Library of Congress, have books on tape already recorded for visually handicapped students, and these tapes are often available to students with reading difficulties. A phone call to your state department of education can verify whether textbooks on tape are available and the procedures for obtaining them.

If textbooks on tape must be created, contact youth groups interested in service projects (e.g., the Honor Society, 4-H clubs, Boy Scouts and Girl Scouts, Thespians, etc.). At the same time, find someone in your agency familiar with audio equipment who can guide the volunteers to produce quality recordings. A local radio or television studio committed to youth might even let you use a professional recording studio free of charge during off hours.

Another modification that could be considered is to provide a summary of key ideas that students should glean from written material. As mentioned previously, teachers could also provide listening guides that summarize main ideas and relevant details of information delivered through lecture. Additional notes in class could be obtained through a "buddy" system. A "buddy" who takes concise, well-organized notes shares them with students struggling to grasp the information presented through lectures. The sharing may be accomplished through photocopies or hand copying of notes by students with language disabilities. With the burgeoning use of computers in schools, these data can also be transferred electronically from student to student.

While another option is tape recording teacher lecture information, it is a less desirable option because of the time it takes to relisten to the information. Frequently, the students who might need to tape record lectures are the same students who fall behind in their schoolwork. Often, time is not available to relisten to lectures. However, tape recording of instructions for completing an assignment might be very prudent and would require little time for relistening.

Some teachers might perceive infringement of academic freedom when tape recording is done. These teachers may refuse to allow taping in their classes, despite the best possible advocacy on the part of the speech-language pathologist. Professionals need to be aware that Section 504 of the Rehabilitation Act of 1973 and the Americans with Disabilities Act both state that reasonable accommodations must be made for individuals with disabilities. Reasonable accommodations might well include tape recording of information so it can be listened to again. Perhaps if other professionals are made aware of these legal requirements, they would be less likely to resist audiotaping (D. Vetter, personal communication, 1986).

MODIFICATIONS OF THE ENVIRONMENTAL SYSTEM

When the environmental system is modified to meet the language needs of older students, changes might occur in these areas:

- the oral language used within the environmental system;

- the structure of the learning environment away from the student's school program; and

- the attitudes and feelings toward the individual with the language disability.

Oral Language

Through information sharing, the speech-language pathologist can advise parents, siblings, employers, and others when their language is too rapid or too complex for the student with a language disability to comprehend. Through changing rate of speech, repeating information, and reducing the length of sentences, the level of frustration when communicating with preadolescents and adolescents with language disabilities can be greatly reduced. At the same time, during direct intervention, older students can be coached to request repetition of information and to ask others to slow down their rate of speech.

When students have reading skills, they could ask for written messages that summarize the oral language. This strategy would be particularly appropriate for employment settings (e.g., when a supervisor gives a string of oral directions, it could be reinforced with a printed list). Initially, the involved professionals could work with employers to implement this modification; ultimately, older students should self-advocate for the modification.

Learning Environment

The learning environment at home should match as closely as possible the variables involved in how the youth learns best. For example, if the student learns best when there are few distracting noises, the family should be encouraged to provide that environment at home. Realistically, not all households can accommodate the student's learning style, but other options exist, such as community libraries. Nonetheless, it is valuable information for many families to develop an appreciation for the learning style of the individual with the language disability and to recognize that a modified setting can frequently make learning a less frustrating experience.

Students pursuing postsecondary education would be particularly wise to know their learning style and to adapt their environment accordingly, whenever possible. So, too, could employers make reasonable environmental accommodations (and they are typically willing to do so), because increased productivity is likely to be the result. Employers also need to comply with the Americans with Disabilities Act, which states that reasonable accommodations must be made for people with disabilities.

Attitudes and Feelings

The most challenging modifications probably reside in the realm of attitudes and feelings. As children become older, there are more opportunities and years during which others can build up negative attitudes and feelings toward them and their language disabilities. Parents, siblings, peers, and employers are increasingly realizing that the language disability is not something that will be "outgrown." As language demands and expectations increase, many students with language disabilities do not keep pace. Their feelings of failure in school and their frequent lack of a strong support group of friends contribute to the likelihood of developing at-risk behaviors.

Even once armed with information about disabilities, parents and siblings cannot usually just "decide" to change attitudes and feelings about the family member with the language disability without the benefit of some type of counseling or support group. Sue (1981) cautions, however, that counseling is "a white, middle-class activity that holds many values and characteristics different from those of Third World groups" (p. 28). During counseling, there is typically an emphasis on verbal communication using standard English, an imposition of class-bound values (e.g., strict adherence to time schedules; an ambiguous or unstructured approach to problems; the seeking of long-range solutions and goals), and an assumption of culture-bound values by the counselor (e.g., using an analytic cause-effect approach; distinguishing between mental and physical well-being; encouraging verbal/emotional/behavioral expressions). These characteristics of counseling may be sources of conflict and misinterpretation by family members and peers who are not white middle class unless adjustments are made by the counselor to accommodate other language systems, different class-bound values, and alternative culture-bound values.

Employers may also be slow to change attitudes toward individuals with disabilities. Often a supported employment arrangement involving a job coach or a school-business partnership is the best way to begin changing attitudes and feelings. Speech-language pathologists should form alliances with school-work transition specialists, offer to analyze the language required in various employment settings, and then provide intervention ideas for students struggling with oral and written directions at work. Also, social communication skill resources (e.g., Gajewski and Mayo, 1989a, 1989b; Montague and Lund, 1991) should be shared with school-work transition staff members. The transition from school to work is discussed further in the next chapter.

SUMMARY

This chapter provided a broad overview of speech-language intervention programs for older students. It presented both direct and indirect intervention considerations. Direct intervention refers to activities involving individuals with language disabilities, while indirect activities refer to modifications that might be made in the educational and environmental systems of students to assist them in their functioning.

Numerous ideas were presented as to how to structure intervention programs for older students in a way that is acceptable to them. We advocate the prototype service delivery model, which includes such features as meeting for a predictable time each day or week, granting credit toward high school graduation for speech-language services, assigning a grade for performance, and carefully considering where service is delivered and what it is called. Unique aspects of serving older school-age children were discussed, including mutual planning, motivational issues, the use of a learning strategies approach, and the availability of counseling.

The chapter also explained general intervention procedures, particularly the concepts of mediation and bridging. The intent of mediation is to transcend the immediate teaching situation so that the concept or skill being taught has relevance to the student beyond the immediate need. During bridging, the student expresses a connection between what is being learned and a meaningful situation at school, at home, or in the community.

Specific intervention methods were explained for several critical areas often addressed in older school-age children with language disabilities: referential communication, narrative storytelling, expository discourse, and word-finding skills. The discussion described procedures for each of these areas and provided mediation and bridging ideas.

Commercial resources appropriate for older school-age children were presented. These resources are representative of those that professionals can select when focusing on oral communication goals. Many resources have been developed in the last decade, and the astute professional will use them to design individual educational programs for each student.

The last part of the chapter delineated some ideas for modifications in educational and environmental systems to assist older students with language disabilities. We advocate that students change to meet the existing expectations of these systems as much as possible and, at the same time, recognize that certain modifications within these systems could greatly reduce the frustration of older students with language disabilities, as well as that of their teachers, their employers, their families, and their peer groups. The best intervention programs work simultaneously to develop the language skills of the students to their highest potential and also to support reasonable accommodations that assist the learning process at school, at home, and in the community.

DISCUSSION QUESTIONS

1. Describe additional specific intervention methods that would modify the older student's oral, written, and/or nonverbal language behaviors.

2. Select several commercial resources designed for older students. Summarize and critique these resources for language intervention.

SUGGESTED READINGS

Larson, V. Lord, McKinley, N., and Boley, D. (1993). Service delivery models for adolescents with language disorders. *Language, Speech, and Hearing Services in Schools, 24,* 36–42.

Nelson, N. (1993). *Childhood language disorders in context: Infancy through adolescence.* New York: Macmillan.

YOUTH: 8
THEIR TRANSITION
TO THE FUTURE

GOALS:

To present the evolving roles of speech-language pathologists

To discuss the major transition points from preadolescence to adulthood

To encourage more efficacy research related to preadolescents and adolescents

To sound a call to action on behalf of our youth

An array of trends and developments will affect how educational professionals perform their jobs in the coming decade and how older students make the transition from the world of school to the world of work. For example, more than half of all jobs will require post-secondary education and training, but only 15 percent will require a college degree (Cetron and Gayle, 1990). Technical institutes will supply the remainder of the necessary education and training.

A future perspective is needed to understand how current trends will affect and shape the roles of speech-language pathologists and the transitions that older students face (Montgomery and Herer, 1994). Within this era of change, we must continue to examine

efficacy of service and maintain a commitment to action on behalf of older students. This chapter focuses on precisely these issues by addressing the evolving roles of professionals, major transition points for older students, efficacy of speech-language services, and a call to action.

EVOLVING ROLES

In response to paradigm shifts, the roles of speech-language pathologists have shifted and will continue to adjust in response to trends. Recall that these major paradigm shifts were noted in Chapter 5 in relation to assessment (Westby and Erickson, 1992):

- a shift away from discrete point, standardized tests to authentic, descriptive assessment;

- a shift away from client-centered assessment to taking into account the student's social systems;

- a shift away from assessing only spoken communication to also including written communication and problem solving;

- a shift away from focusing on student similarities to an awareness of diversity among students; and

- a shift away from using exclusively quantitative data to including qualitative data and procedures.

These paradigm shifts were cited and discussed in Chapter 7 in relation to intervention (Hoskins, 1993):

- a shift toward systems thinking (i.e., supporting classrooms as systems);

- a shift toward being market driven (i.e., providing choice and flexible, accessible services);

- a shift toward diversity (i.e., encouraging individual identities of all students); and

- a shift toward practical results (i.e., targeting relevant goals and demanding results).

In response to the paradigm shifts, these professional roles have already emerged, or probably will emerge, in the coming decade as we serve older students:

1. Speech-language pathologists as *consultants* in addition to or instead of direct service providers. According to Nelson (1993), the consultant role is receiving a great deal of attention, but little research supports its efficacy.

2. Speech-language pathologists as *teachers* (i.e., "they assume responsibility for conveying the curriculum to children whose language problems make it largely inaccessible to them under ordinary circumstances" [Nelson, 1993, p. 174]). The professional's attention extends beyond the student's ability to use language for social and academic purposes to include the learning of information and skills targeted in the regular curriculum. (This casts the speech-language pathologist into the role of assuming responsibility for academic development and behavior management.)

3. Speech-language pathologists as *co-teachers*. "They co-teach with other professionals, who assume a major responsibility for teaching the regular curriculum" (Nelson, 1993, p. 174).

4. Speech-language pathologists as *community educators*, helping administrators, parents, school boards, employers, and the students themselves understand the evolving roles that clinicians play, the importance of speech-language services, and their commitment to youth with language disorders.

5. Speech-language pathologists as *diversity experts* and professionals with expertise interacting with students who speak

English as a second language. Authentic, descriptive assessment and practical results will be in demand for students from diverse backgrounds.

6. Speech-language pathologists as *literacy advocates.* In addition to focusing on oral language ability, professionals will assist with written language goals (Casby, 1988; Nelson, 1993).

7. Speech-language pathologists as *researchers.* As the demand for documentation of results grows, professionals must find creative ways to use computer technology, portfolios, and other data-gathering methods to substantiate that relevant goals are being achieved. There will be increasing demands to be accountable and to demonstrate the efficacy of services.

8. Speech-language pathologists as *transition monitors.* As students move from the demands of elementary to middle school or junior high school, then to high school, and then to employment or postsecondary education, different language expectations surface. Speech-language pathologists can be key players in assisting the student to make the adjustments necessary to survive the transitions.

TRANSITIONS

Preadolescence and adolescence are developmental periods in which numerous transitions occur. Transitions can be trying, challenging, and exciting as they mark points of risk and opportunity within the students' development. Major transition points are noted in Figure 8.1.

There is some discrepancy in the literature as to whether students make these transitions with ease or difficulty. Researchers such as Simmons et al. (1979) suggest that students have serious problems making multiple simultaneous transitions. Other researchers find that most students make most changes in their lives successfully (Offer, Ostrov, Howard, and Atkinsen, 1988). Because students vary as to how or if they make these transitions, it is important that we analyze and discuss ways to assist students in making these changes. Epstein and MacIver (1990) state that the purpose for articulation activities (i.e., activities that occur at the time of transition) are to inform and prepare students, families, and educators about current educational practices and future educational expectations.

TRANSITION POINT ONE

The first transition point marks the change from elementary to middle grades or junior high school. Schools that encompass grades 5–8 or 6–8 are considered middle schools in contrast to junior high schools, which encompass grades 7–8 or 7–9 (Alexander and McEwin, 1989). Alexander and McEwin (1989) summarized these differences between middle schools and junior high schools:

- An interdisciplinary plan of instruction is used more in the middle school; a

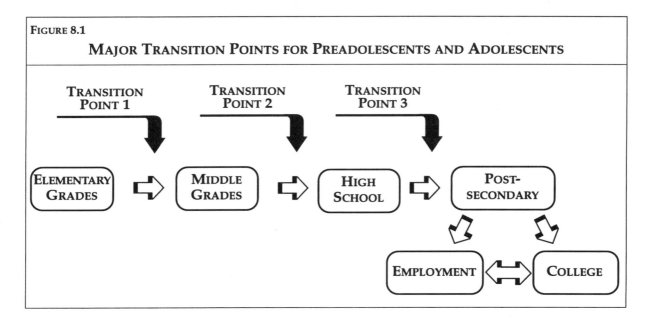

FIGURE 8.1

MAJOR TRANSITION POINTS FOR PREADOLESCENTS AND ADOLESCENTS

departmentalized plan of instruction is used more in the junior high school.

- Flexible scheduling is used more in the middle school; uniform daily periods are used more in the junior high school.

- Reasons for establishing middle schools are program and student related; reasons for establishing junior high schools are administratively related.

- Traditional exploratory subjects are required more in middle schools than in junior high schools.

- Random assignment for grouping in basic subjects and advisory programs is more common in middle schools than in junior high schools.

- Foreign languages are offered less frequently in middle schools than in junior high schools.

- A higher percentage of teachers and principals are involved in the decision to

organize middle schools than junior high schools.

As youth make the transition from elementary grades to the next level, informed professionals should instruct students about their upcoming school program and its requirements, procedures, and opportunities. The nature of this information changes depending on whether the transition is into a middle school or a junior high school. The list of differences between the two systems just presented might be helpful in planning for the students' transition.

The most common articulation activities used in the transition from elementary to middle or junior high grades are these (Epstein and MacIver, 1990):

- Elementary school students visit their next school for an information session or assembly.

- Elementary administrators and the middle or junior high school administrators meet together on articulation and programs.

- Middle-grade counselors meet with elementary counselors or staff.

Less frequent articulation practices include parents visiting their children's next school for orientation, teachers meeting together about courses and requirements, "big brother/big sister" programs (where a new student is guided by an older student at the new school), and elementary students attending regular (sample) classes at the middle or junior high school.

What difference does any of this information make for older students with language disorders? Virtually nothing has been written about the transition period for these youth. From our own experiences in consulting with school districts, we know that students are "at risk" for being dismissed from speech-language caseloads after the elementary school years. The reasons for this are varied:

- Language development charts have "run out" and many speech-language pathologists are not quite certain what to do once a child is past age 10.

- Speech-language services at middle and junior high schools are often limited and there is pressure to "clean up" the caseload before sending students off to a new school.

- Written language problems appear to be more problematic by middle grades than oral language disorders; thus, learning disabilities specialists assume a more major role as students age, while

many speech-language pathologists fade to the background, aware that communication problems still exist but not convinced that their continued involvement is as important as increased services to younger children.

- The students themselves may appear temporarily "caught up." By approximately fourth or fifth grade, many "delayed" youth are finally functioning at a concrete operational level of reasoning, even though their peers have been at that level for several years. (The problem is that students with language disorders often fail to make the transition into formal operational thinking, which many middle grade and especially junior high school teachers expect.)

- The students may appear to be making no progress and, therefore, continued intervention cannot be justified. (Recall the data cited in Chapter 3, where development is described as spurts followed by plateaus. Chances are that a student showing "no progress" is at a plateau.)

We have found that the best strategy is to retain older students on speech-language caseloads during the transition process into middle grades or junior high school before a dismissal decision is made. This ensures that students have successfully made the transition to the next level, understand the new rules and procedures, and are capable of adjusting to the higher language demands that are undoubtedly present.

With each new transition in the educational sequence, the assumption is made that students can handle higher-level concepts, more vocabulary, and greater independence as learners. Students with language disorders have a greater probability of succeeding after a transition if their speech-language clinicians remain involved through the process.

When students fail to adjust to the transition, and dismissal has already occurred, the process of referral, reassessment, and placement in intervention takes precious time. Clearly, this time lag is not desirable and is totally preventable if dismissal decisions are postponed until after major transition points in students' educational careers.

TRANSITION POINT TWO

The second transition point marks the change from middle grades or junior high school to senior high school. According to Epstein and MacIver (1990), the same primary articulation activities occur during this transition as they did from elementary to middle grades or junior high school: students visit the high school for an information session or assembly, administrators meet together on programs, and counselors meet together or with staff.

In many parts of the United States, particularly in urban areas, a very noticeable difference between middle schools and high schools is sheer size. "Experts repeatedly reaffirm the merits of smallness, and yet urban high schools remain Goliaths, as though there was virtue in bigness" (Maeroff, 1988, p. 638). George, Stevenson, Thomason, and Beane (1992) argue that the best high schools apply middle-school philosophy and

cite exemplary programs around the country. Unfortunately, these high schools remain in the minority to date.

A more realistic picture of today's high school has been painted by Sizer (1991), who describes it as a place where teachers need to interact with a hundred or more students each day, where teachers present material and expect students to display the information back to them, and where the school schedule is marked by rapid changes of subjects each period (each subject is planned by its teacher without any relation to any other subject). Add to this the growing concern in our high schools over violence and safety issues (Furlong and Morrison, 1994).

Precisely because high school campuses are so large, and the changes to be made are so consuming, the transition of students receiving speech-language services from middle school to high school is typically not a topic of concern to administrators. If anything, pressure may be exerted on professionals to dismiss as many students as possible from caseloads before their entrance into high school.

Again, we urge clinicians to assist students through the transition and then make dismissal decisions rather than engage in the more traditional, familiar, opposite scenario. For students with language disorders, high school brings a new set of demands and expectations: the acquisition of credits for high school graduation, the passing of minimal competency testing (in many states), and the planning of future years beyond high school (or at least the expectation that such planning should occur). Students with language disorders may need a modified graduation plan, direct assistance to meet minimum competency requirements, and counseling to make appropriate vocational choices based on their strengths and weaknesses. A knowledgeable speech-language pathologist can greatly assist with these issues.

Students with language disorders are also at great risk for dropping out of high school. They need the intervention, advocacy, and support that speech-language pathologists can provide. A significant reduction in the dropout rate is not only important to the students involved but should help solidify with administrators the importance of speech-language services at the high school level.

TRANSITION POINT THREE

The transition from high school to post-school life is the last major change made by adolescents. In the mid-1980s, the term *transition* became popular among educators working to prepare students for life after high school. According to the *Transition Resource Guide* (Heath Resource Guide, 1992), "The objective of transition is to prepare students to go directly into the job market, or to enter into higher education or training, to assist them in living independently, and to enable them to become contributing members of the community" (p. 1). This publication goes on to report that the Individuals with Disabilities Act (IDEA) of 1990, PL 101-476, which amends the Education for All Handicapped Children Act of 1975, PL 94-142, places a special emphasis on transition services. The IDEA legislation defines *transition services* as

a coordinated set of activities for a student, designed within an outcome-oriented process, which promotes movement from school to post-school activities, including postsecondary education, vocational training, integrated employment (including supported employment), continuing and adult education, adult services, independent living, or community instruction. (Heath Resource Center, 1992, p.1)

The IDEA mandates that students with disabilities begin preparing for transition by age 16. Transition services are to be written into each student's individualized education program or a separate individualized transition plan (ITP) must be developed. The speech-language pathologist should be a member of the team writing these plans, since speech, language, and hearing problems may be one of the disabilities that will need to be worked with or accommodated for in the student's post-school life.

Successful transition planning, according to Everson and Goodall (1991), is a visionary, individualized, and longitudinal process involving interagency and transdisciplinary processes. The remainder of this section will discuss two general types of post-school life transitions: (1) school to employment (work) and (2) school to postsecondary educational opportunities.

School-to-Employment (Work) Transition

The Forgotten Half

O'Neil (1992) refers to students not going on to postsecondary school as "the forgotten half" (i.e., 50 percent of our students are not bound for postsecondary education). These students are not prepared for postsecondary education nor are they prepared by the schools to enter the workforce.

A report by the Commission on the Skills of the American Workforce bluntly stated, "America may have the worst school-to-work transition of any advanced industrial country" (O'Neil, 1992, p. 7). Since no one has taken the initiative to link school-to-work transitions for young people, the young people themselves are left largely to their own devices.

The economic picture for the forgotten half is often one of periods of unemployment or underemployment (dead-end jobs). The absence of an effective system to assist these students in making a smooth transition from high school to the job market costs the United States dearly, both socially and economically. To ignore this problem places the United States at a disadvantage in participating in the global economy.

Although the gap between school and the workplace is wide, there are some positive signs (O'Neil, 1992):

- erosion of the wall separating academic and vocational programs;

- better information flowing to the schools about the skills, knowledge, and work habits that students need to be prepared for the workforce; and

- development of the interdisciplinary plans for transition from high school to life beyond resulting from the IDEA legislation.

It should be noted that several transition programs have been designed specifically to prepare high school students to enter the world of work. One such program is called Tech Prep, available in some schools throughout the United States, which prepares students for careers that require some education beyond the secondary level. The program allows students to take technically oriented courses at a community college or vocational technical college while they are still in high school. Some innovative high schools offer these courses right on their campuses too.

Types of Employment Options

Students with language disabilities who decide to work immediately after school may need support in seeking jobs, résumé writing, interviewing techniques, and following instructions for the job itself. The student with a disability might want to be aware of the types of employment options available, such as competitive employment, supported employment, and sheltered employment (Heath Resource Center, 1992). "Regular" employment (i.e., no support from outside the hiring agency) is certainly an option too.

Competitive employment provides the person with a mild or moderate communication disorder with regular supervision but not extensive follow-up because it is expected that the person will become capable of working alone. Students can be educated for competitive employment opportunities through various means:

- apprenticeships (i.e., students learn skills for specific occupations);

- internships (i.e., students are in a time-limited, paid or unpaid position in which they can sample a wide variety of jobs);

- on-the-job training (i.e., students work on the job while learning job duties); and

- transitional employment (i.e., students engage in a three-phase program: in phase one, participants receive total support services in a low-stress work environment; in phase two, they receive on-the-job training in local firms and agencies; and in phase three, they receive six months of follow-up services).

Each of these competitive employment options carries with it the expectation that ultimately the person is capable of functioning independently.

Supported employment provides integrated work in competitive environments and it uses a place-train approach as opposed to a train-place approach (Heath Resource Center, 1992). The individual is placed on the job and then provided intense training. There are four popular models of supported employment:

- *individual placement*, in which the person receives intensive on-the-job coaching from a job coach until he or she is proficient at the job;

- the *enclave model*, in which people are trained in small groups and supervised together in an ordinary work setting;

- the *benchwork model*, in which 8 to 15 people with disabilities perform contract work procured from a business; and

- the *mobile crew model*, in which individuals who need more support than others perform services as a team, moving from one job site to another (e.g., janitorial work or groundskeeping).

Sheltered employment occurs in settings in which people with disabilities (usually more severe disabilities) work in a self-contained unit, such as adult day programs, work activity centers, and sheltered workshops. According to the Heath Resource Center (1992),

> In an adult day program, individuals receive training in daily living skills, social skills, recreational skills, and prevocational skills. In work activity centers, workers receive similar training, but also learn basic vocational skills. In sheltered workshops, individuals do tasks such as sewing, packaging, collating, or machine assembly, and are paid on a piece-work basis. (p. 2)

Vocational Transition Team Process

Given these various types of employment options, it is important that the transdisciplinary team members follow a vocational transition process. Everson and Goodall (1991) recommend a five-step process as follows:

1. Convene the individualized transition planning team members. If the adolescent has a language disability, then the speech-language pathologist should be a member of this team. (This must begin no later than age 16 for youth with disabilities, whether or not they will seek employment after school.)

2. Develop personal profiles that list the types of future employment options available that are realistic for this youth (e.g., regular employment, competitive employment, sheltered workshop, supported employment). In addition, the file should address other adult lifestyle areas such as postsecondary education, community living arrangements, recreation/leisure activities, medical services, advocacy/legal needs.

3. Specify desired employment objectives and activities for this adolescent. As part of this process, the speech-language pathologist should conduct an assessment of the communication behaviors needed on the job and design a communication support system for the adolescent.

4. Implement transition objectives and activities which are critical to the adolescent's success (e.g., the speech-language pathologist might develop alternative communication systems, adapt materials, develop alternative performance strategies, facilitate functional communication, increase opportunities for communication interactions with peers and workers, and show how the adolescent might infuse communication behaviors in a variety of living, work, and leisure time activities).

5. Monitor, evaluate, and revise objectives and activities as they are needed as part of the transdisciplinary process for assisting adolescents with disabilities to enter the workplace.

Economic Trends and Policy Issues

Given the economic trends and policy issues facing the United States in the year 2000 and beyond, it is imperative that we prepare adolescents with language disorders to participate in the workplace. We need to examine the impact of these trends and issues on how speech-language pathologists might assist preadolescents and adolescents to become better prepared to enter the workplace and to become self-advocates within the workplace under such laws as the Americans with Disabilities Act (ADA). As we approach the year 2000, four key economic trends will shape the last years of the 20th century (Johnston and Packer, 1987):

The **American economy should grow** at relatively healthy pace . . . boosted by a rebound in the U.S. exports, renewed productivity growth, and a strong world economy. (p. xiii)

U.S. manufacturing will be a much smaller share of the economy in the year 2000. . . . Service industries will create all the new jobs, and most of the new wealth. (p. xiii)

The **workforce will grow slowly, becoming older, more female, and more disadvantaged**. Only 15 percent of the new entrants to the labor force over the years 1987 to 2000 were and will be native white males, compared to 47 percent in that category in the [early] 1980s. (p. xiii)

The **new jobs in service industries will demand much higher skill levels** than the jobs of today. Very few new jobs will be created for those who cannot read, follow directions, and use mathematics. Ironically, the demographic trends in the workforce, coupled with the higher skill requirements of the economy, will lead to both higher and lower unemployment: more joblessness among the least-skilled and less among the most educationally advantaged. (p. xiii)

This last trend has direct implications for adolescents with language disorders. It has been reported that 80 percent of the jobs in the year 2000 will require more than a high school education but less than a four-year college degree (Byrne, Constant, and Moore, 1992). Note that these statistics are even more dramatic than those cited by Cetron and Gayle (1990) in the opening paragraph of this chapter.

These four trends raise a number of important policy issues. Of the six policy issues raised by Johnston and Packer (1987) in the report entitled *Workforce 2000*, three have an impact on adolescents with language disorders:

- **We must accelerate our productivity in the service industries**. The prosperity of the U.S. will depend on each worker increasing his or her productivity in service areas such as health care, education, retailing, government, and other services.

- **We must integrate minority workers fully into the economy**.

  The shrinking of young people, the rapid pace of industrial change, and the ever-rising skill requirements of the emerging economy make the task of fully utilizing minority workers particularly

urgent between now and 2000. Both cultural changes and education and training investments will be needed to create real equal employment opportunity. (p. xvi)

- **We must improve the educational preparation of all workers**. "As the economy grows more complex and more dependent on human capital, the standards set by the American education system must be raised" (p. xiv).

As we raise our educational standards, it is important that every adolescent be encouraged to achieve his or her human potential. Failure to develop human potential is very costly, as Governor Arne Carlson of Minnesota noted in his state of the state address on January 26, 1993:

If a young person drops out of high school, goes on the welfare rolls for five years, then commits a violent crime and is committed to a prison for twenty years, it costs the state of Minnesota $500,000. If the same young person graduates from high school, completes technical school training, and works for twenty years at approximately a $24,000 level average over those 20 years, that individual contributes approximately $500,000 to Minnesota. The difference monetarily is approximately one million dollars per child.

Dropouts are financially expensive to society and often emotionally expensive to themselves. The dropout statistics are appalling (see Figure 8.2). The range varies from 4.6 percent in North Dakota to 15.2

Figure 8.2

HIGH-SCHOOL DROPOUT RATES, 1990

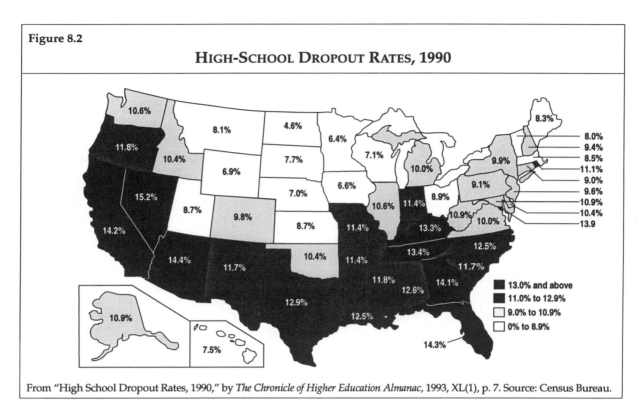

8.3%

8.0%
9.4%
8.5%
11.1%
9.0%
9.6%
10.9%
10.4%
13.9

■ 13.0% and above
■ 11.0% to 12.9%
□ 9.0% to 10.9%
□ 0% to 8.9%

From "High School Dropout Rates, 1990," by *The Chronicle of Higher Education Almanac*, 1993, XL(1), p. 7. Source: Census Bureau.

percent in Nevada, with states like Florida and California also showing high dropout statistics. If Governor Carlson's statistics are at all generalizable to states outside of Minnesota, then billions of dollars will be spent in the years ahead and a less productive workforce will be available for competing in the global economy.

The cost of America's failure to educate its people is staggering (Boyett and Conn, 1992):

- $219 billion annually for formal and informal training;

- $41 billion annually for welfare programs dominated by school dropouts;

- $16 billion each year in additional welfare costs because of teenage pregnancies (again dominated by school dropouts);

- $25 billion each year in lost productivity; and

- $240 billion each year in lost earnings and taxes over the lifetime of each year's dropouts because they couldn't get jobs at all or those they did get were marginal at best. (p. 271)

Given these four trends, the coinciding policy issues, and the cost projections, it is obvious that adolescents with language disorders will be placed at a disadvantage in entering the workforce and that the United States could be placed at a disadvantage in the global economy. Concerted effort must be made to educate adolescents in the necessary language skills (speaking, listening, reading, and writing) needed to be successful in the workplace.

In an Associated Press release (September 21, 1992) titled "Communication Skills Said Lacking: Businesses Say Workers Need Help," it was stated that most American businesses say workers need to improve their writing and talking. The business firms listed writing as one of the most valued skills but said that 80 percent of their employees at all levels needed to improve. Of particular importance to speech-language pathologists is the comment that 75 percent of the companies identified as a key problem interpersonal skills such as speaking with and listening to customers and other workers.

O'Neil (1992) stated that in one poll, only one-third of employers believe that recent high school graduates show the ability to read and understand oral instructions. It is becoming increasingly more difficult for employers to find entry-level workers (high school graduates) who can think on their feet, solve problems of several steps, and apply knowledge and skills to new situations. And yet, business management models (e.g., total quality management or continuous quality improvement) require workers to think and solve problems on the job, not with the aid of a distant manager.

Given the trends and policy issues facing us as part of the *Workforce 2000* (Johnston and Packer, 1987) initiative, the role of the speech-language pathologist with older students who need to prepare to enter the workforce is threefold: (1) to assess the communication pragmatic skills needed to be successful in a given workplace (see Chapter 6 for details);

(2) to teach thinking, listening, and speaking strategies for workplace success by developing working partnerships with the business community (see Chapter 7 for details); and (3) to assist adolescents in becoming self-advocates under such laws as the Americans with Disabilities Act (ADA) or Section 504 of the Rehabilitation Act of 1973.

Speech-language pathologists should teach adolescents with language disorders about their rights under the ADA (American Speech-Language-Hearing Association, 1992a, 1992b; Carey, 1992b; Williams, 1992) and how they can best be self-advocates under the law. Older students need to be prepared to function in a more open environment. We need to teach preadolescents and adolescents to take advantage of technology, which is increasingly being used as a way to overcome communication barriers. They need to know that they have the right to ask for workplace modifications that accommodate their handicapping conditions. At the same time, speech-language pathologists might also serve as resource people to businesses needing to comply with the ADA (American Speech-Language-Hearing Association, 1992a, 1992b).

For adolescents to be self-advocates (i.e., expressing their needs in a reasonable and informed manner) under the ADA, they must first know about the ADA and what the term *disability* means. Understanding the ADA's language is crucial to obtaining a clear grasp of the purpose, provisions, and objectives of this landmark federal civil rights legislation. In the ADA, *disability* is defined as a physical or mental impairment that substantially limits one or more of the major life activities. More specifically, a person with a disability is an individual who meets one or more of the following descriptions:

- The person has a physical or mental impairment that substantially limits one or more of the major life activities.

- The person has a record of such an impairment.

- The person is regarded as having such an impairment.

Major life activities include such behaviors as walking, speaking, seeing, hearing, breathing, learning, working, and caring for oneself.

Key regulations for nondiscrimination on the basis of disability are provided under the four ADA titles: Title I—Employment; Title II—Public Services; Title III—Public Accommodations; and Title IV—Telecommunications. Basic requirements of the ADA titles are summarized in Table 8.1.

Examples of accommodations under Title I for employees with hearing and/or speech impairment include the following:

- providing assistive listening and signaling devices, generic-type augmentative and alternative communication devices, and interpreter services;

- altering communication styles (e.g., ensuring speechreading cues, increasing patience, and using written communication if oral communication fails);

- modifying the work environment (e.g., reducing background noise, redesigning work space to accommodate an augmentative communication system); and

- modifying policies (e.g., permitting hearing-assistance dogs).

Under the ADA, the employer is to determine reasonable accommodations. A four-step process is to be used by the employer as follows:

1. Analyze the job function to determine its purpose and essential duties.

2. Consult with individuals regarding their limitations and need for accommodations.

3. Identify possible accommodations and assess their effectiveness in helping individuals perform essential job functions.

4. Consider the preferences of the person who is disabled and select an appropriate accommodation based on options available.

Each of the other ADA titles should be discussed in a similar way as it relates to the adolescent with a communication disorder. The article in the *American Speech-Language-Hearing Association* (*Asha*) journal by Williams (1992) titled, "What Do You Know? What Do You Need to Know?" should be read carefully. Another excellent book is Fersh and Thomas's (1993) *Complying with the Americans with Disabilities Act: A Guidebook for Management and People with Disabilities.* The speech-language pathologist, as a member of a team, can provide assessment and intervention procedures to assist the individual in developing communication behaviors needed to succeed in the workplace. Informing the person of his or her rights under the law is also critical.

School-to-Postsecondary-Education Transition

According to the most recent statistics available from the Department of Education at the time this text was printed, which are from 1989–90, 44.8 percent of students with

TABLE 8.1	
AMERICANS WITH DISABILITIES ACT REQUIREMENTS	
EMPLOYMENT	**PUBLIC ACCOMMODATIONS**
Employers may not discriminate against an individual with a disability in hiring or promotion if the person is otherwise qualified for the job. Employers can ask about one's ability to perform a job, but cannot inquire if someone has a disability or subject a person to tests that tend to screen out people with disabilities. Employers will need to provide "reasonable accommodation" to individuals with disabilities. This includes steps such as job restructuring and modification of equipment. Employers do not need to provide accommodations that impose an "undue hardship" on business operations. *Who needs to comply:* All employers with 25 or more employees must comply, effective July 26, 1992. All employers with 15–24 employees must comply, effective July 26, 1994. *For more information about employment issues, call the Equal Employment Opportunity Commission at 1-800-669-4000.*	Private entities such as restaurants, hotels, and retail stores may not discriminate against individuals with disabilities, effective January 26, 1993. Auxiliary aids and services must be provided to individuals with vision or hearing impairments or other individuals with disabilities, unless an undue burden would result. Physical barriers in existing facilities must be removed, if removal is readily achievable. If not, alternative methods of providing the services must be offered, if they are readily achievable. All new construction and alterations of facilities must be accessible. *For more information on accessibility issues, call the Access Board at 1-800-872-2253 (voice) or 1-800-993-2822 (TDD).*
	STATE AND LOCAL GOVERNMENT
	State and local governments may not discriminate against qualified individuals with disabilities. All government facilities, services, and communication must be accessible consistent with the requirements of Section 504 of the Rehabilitation Act of 1973.
TRANSPORTATION	**TELECOMMUNICATIONS**
New public transit buses ordered after August 26, 1990, must be accessible to individuals with disabilities. Transit authorities must provide comparable paratransit or other special transportation services to individuals with disabilities who cannot use fixed route bus services, unless an undue burden would result. Existing rail systems must have one accessible car per train by July 26, 1995. New rail cars ordered after August 26, 1990, must be accessible. New bus and train stations must be accessible. Key stations in rapid, light, and commuter rail systems must be made accessible by July 26, 1993, with extensions up to 20 years for commuter rail (30 years for rapid and light rail). All existing Amtrak stations must be accessible by July 26, 2010. *For more information on transportation issues, call the U.S. Department of Transportation at (202) 366-1656 (voice) or (202) 366-4567 (TDD).*	Companies offering telephone service to the general public must offer telephone relay services to individuals who use telecommunication devices for the deaf (TDDs) or similar devices. For more information about the ADA or to receive this information in alternative formats (e.g., Braille, large print, audiotape), contact: U.S. Department of Justice Civil Rights Division Coordination and Review Section PO Box 66118 Washington, DC 20035-6118 1-800-514-0301 1-800-514-0383 (TDD) (202) 514-0383 (TDD)

FIGURE 8.3

PERCENTAGE OF STUDENTS GRADUATING WITH HIGH SCHOOL DIPLOMA, BY DISABILITY CATEGORY

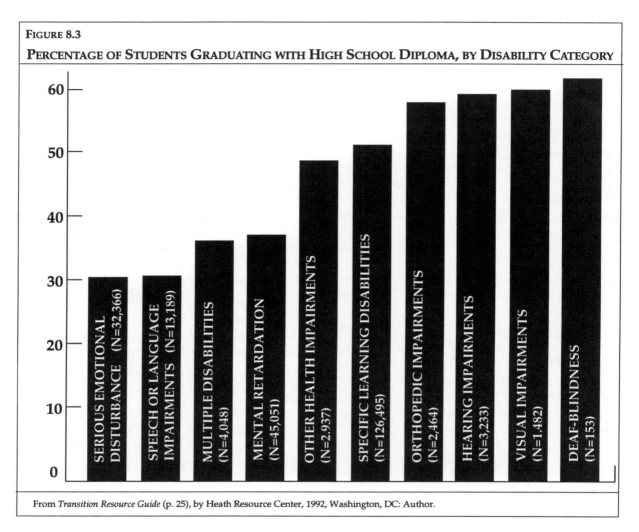

From *Transition Resource Guide* (p. 25), by Heath Resource Center, 1992, Washington, DC: Author.

disabilities graduated with diplomas, 27 percent dropped out of school, 13.3 percent had unknown status, 12.4 percent graduated with certificates, and 2.5 percent reached maximum age for school attendance. Figure 8.3 shows the percentage of students graduating with high school diplomas by disability category.

Students with specific learning disabilities represent the largest number of persons in a disability category, and slightly more than half (52 percent) earned high school diplomas. Other disability categories showing better statistics and the percentages of departing students who earned high school diplomas were as follows: visual impairments (61 percent); deaf-blindness (61 percent); hearing impairments (59 percent); and orthopedic impairments (58 percent) (Heath Resource Center, 1992). It should be noted that only 32 percent of those listed with speech or language impairments graduated with a high school diploma. In addition, Nelson (1994) cited a 32.5 percent dropout figure for students with "speech impairments" as reported in *Teaching Exceptional Children* published by the Council for Exceptional Children (1994).

Thus, approximately a third of the students with speech-language disabilities appear to graduate with a diploma, a third drop out, and a third are somewhere in between (i.e., they remain in school but fail to matriculate, they receive a certificate of attendance, or their status is unknown).

These figures should certainly alert speech-language pathologists to the role they need to play in junior and senior high school as well as on the transition planning team. To take advantage of many of the postsecondary educational opportunities, the student should have a high school diploma. Speech-language pathologists should be very concerned that only one in three students, who have a documented speech or language impairment as the primary disorder, is graduating from high school. Much potential is being wasted.

Transition Planning

Postsecondary education is any education beyond high school (i.e., trade or business schools, vocational technical schools, colleges, universities, and adult and continuing education programs [Heath Resource Center, 1994a]). "Education is not just about making a living; it is also about making a life" (Byrne, et al., 1992, p. 26). Regardless of the type of postsecondary education experiences that adolescents or young adults are seeking, early individualized transitional planning is imperative. Career awareness built in across all grade levels (K–12) can greatly assist this planning.

Getzel (1990) noted that without a coordinated transition plan, few students with disabilities will be able to take advantage of postsecondary educational opportunities. A good transition plan begins when students make the transition from elementary school to middle school or junior high school, and it continues beyond the senior year in high school. Table 8.2 provides a checklist of some variables that parents, students, and educators should consider starting at the junior high school level (Heath Resource Center, 1992).

Those students with language disorders who are going on to college should consider the following recommendations (adapted from the Heath Resource Center publication, *Getting Ready for College: Advising High School Students with Learning Disabilities* [1994b]):

1. **The basics need to be in place.** Speech-language pathologists can assist older students in

   - developing disability awareness (by encouraging self-advocacy);

   - understanding their language and learning disabilities;

   - understanding how their communication disorders affect social interactions with a wide array of individuals;

   - comprehending Section 504 of the Rehabilitation Act of 1973 and how it compares to PL 94-142 and IDEA (e.g., the student seeks and requests appropriate services under Section 504, whereas it is the responsibility of the schools [working with parents] to provide services under PL 94-142 and IDEA);

   - developing personal and skill development (by encouraging students to develop work-related skills and

TABLE 8.2

TRANSITIONAL PLANNING

IN JUNIOR HIGH SCHOOL: START TRANSITION PLANNING

- Become involved in career exploration activities.

- Participate in vocational assessment activities.

- Use information about interests and capabilities to make preliminary decisions about possible careers: academic vs. vocational, or a combination.

- Visit with a school counselor to talk about interests and capabilities.

- Make use of books, career fairs, and people in the community to find out more about careers of interest.

IN HIGH SCHOOL: DEFINE CAREER/VOCATIONAL GOALS

- Work with school staff, family, and people and agencies in the community to define and refine transition plan. Make sure that the IEP includes transition plans.

- Identify and take high school courses that are required for entry into college, trade schools, or careers of interest.

- Identify and take vocational programs offered in high school, if a vocational career is of interest.

- Become involved in early work experiences, such as job try-outs, summer jobs, volunteering, or part-time work.

- Re-assess interests and capabilities, based on real world or school experiences. Is the career field still of interest? If not, re-define goals.

- Participate in on-going vocational assessment and identify gaps of knowledge or skills that need to be addressed. Address these gaps.

Students who have decided to pursue postsecondary education and training prior to employment, may wish to consider these suggestions:

- Identify postsecondary institutions (i.e., colleges, vocational programs in the community, trade schools, etc.) that offer training in careers of interest. Write or call for catalogs, financial aid information, or applications. Visit the institution.

- Identify what accommodations would be helpful to address disability-specific needs. Find out if the educational institution makes, or can make, these accommodations.

- Identify and take any standardized tests (e.g., *PSAT, SAT, ACT*) necessary for entry in postsecondary institutions of interest.

- In senior year, contact Vocational Rehabilitation (VR) and/or Social Security Administration (SSA) to determine eligibility for services or benefits.

AFTER HIGH SCHOOL: PURSUE GOALS

- If eligible for VR services, work with a VR counselor to identify and pursue additional training or to secure employment (including supported employment) in your field of interest.

- If not eligible for VR services, contact other agencies that can be of help: state employment offices, social services offices, mental health departments, disability-specific organizations. What services can these agencies offer?

- If eligible for SSA, find out how work incentives apply.

- Find out about special projects in your vicinity (e.g., Projects with Industry, Project READY, supported employment models, etc.). Determine eligibility to participate in these training or employment programs.

- Follow through on decisions to attend postsecondary institutions or obtain employment.

From *Transition Resource Guide* (p. 24), by Heath Resource Center, 1992, Washington, DC: Author.

interests if college is delayed for some reason; making sure students' knowledge of study skills is adequate);

- increasing independent living skills;

- seeking part-time jobs or volunteer positions;

- requesting assessments, records, and course options in high school (requesting the high school to provide vocational assessment starting in the seventh grade);

- planning a four-year selection of college prep courses sufficient to allow the option of entering college;

- contacting the local vocational rehabilitation agency before graduating from high school; and

- taking advantage of testing provided under PL 94-142 and IDEA and in obtaining all special testing records before graduation.

2. **The college applications process needs to be completed** (i.e., getting ready to apply and deciding where to apply). First, in getting ready to apply to a college, the student with the help of professionals, should:

- consult with advisors to understand how much support was needed in high school and, therefore, how much help will be needed in college;

- consider how highly motivated he or she is to accomplish college work;

- decide whether arrangements for special testing conditions for the *PSAT, SAT,* and/or *ACT* are needed; and

- consider a wide array of postsecondary options, including community colleges, technical colleges, and universities.

Second, in deciding where to apply, the student should:

- visit colleges while in session;

- enroll in summer orientation sessions;

- take summer study skill courses; and

- search out personal contacts or follow other leads to find an appropriate advisor, friend, mentor, or teacher on campus.

The Guidelines for Success in Postsecondary Education

These major ideas will help adolescents or young adults to make the most of their postsecondary opportunities (Heath Resource Center, 1994a):

1. **Be capable of expressing needs to others and be open to change.** Students should consider new and different ways to do things and be involved.

2. **Plan ahead:**

- If in high school, adolescents should take time to think about their academic and career goals, main interests, and favorite subjects in school; to talk with appropriate educational personnel about their plans; and to take vocational tests that explore and identify their career interests, strengths, and weaknesses.

- If out of high school, adolescents should speak with a person at a local vocational rehabilitation office, community college, vocational technical college, or university.

- If in or out of high school, adolescents or parents should write to the Heath Resource Center for the booklet, *Transition Resource Guide* (Heath Resource Center, 1992), which will assist them in exploring a variety of postsecondary possibilities.

3. **Look for the best schools:**

   - Gather information about schools that offer education in the students' areas of interest.

   - Beware of the accommodations needed, given the students' language disorders.

   - Beware of the accommodations and services available at the schools that adolescents are most interested in attending. Can they accommodate students' needs?

   - Visit, if possible, the school(s) that students are most interested in attending and get a preadmission interview with an appropriate faculty member or administrator.

4. **Inquire about the admissions process:**

   - Do students need to take standardized admission tests?

- Are there special test-taking accommodations available that fit students' needs?

- Are preparatory courses required before students qualify for admission?

5. **Learn the services available.** The school should provide auxiliary aids, accommodations, and services that enhance access to persons with disabilities. A number of federal laws require that access be available, such as the Vocational Rehabilitation Act of 1973 (Section 504), the Vocational Education Act, and the Americans with Disabilities Act. It should be noted that the ADA does not replace Section 504 but reaffirms the Section 504 regulations for colleges and universities. Some of the types of adjustments and accommodations many postsecondary schools will make for persons with disabilities are:

   - pre-registration well in advance of classes so that the classes can be scheduled in such a way as to give students sufficient time to get from class to class;

   - flexibility in class scheduling so that if a class has been scheduled in a location that is not accessible, students may request that it be moved or, if not, a way is found for them to attend the class;

   - flexibility in course requirements so students may ask that one course be substituted for another (e.g., a deaf student might take an art course rather than a music course to fulfill the fine arts requirements);

- extended time for coursework or to complete a degree;

- test modifications such as extended time, oral versus written examinations, and use of tape recorders;

- notetakers for students having difficulty writing or listening to lectures and taking notes at the same time;

- special help for students with learning disabilities;

- interpreter services for deaf or hard-of-hearing students (it should be noted that interpreters are scarce, so determine ahead of time if the school can accommodate such a request); and

- special orientation programs for new students who have disabilities.

In addition, physical access should be carefully considered (e.g., classrooms, library, student union, dormitories, and recreational facilities).

It is the responsibility of students with disabilities to request the auxiliary aids, accommodations, and services just listed. Likewise, these requests should come well before the semester begins.

Publications that are excellent and most helpful for students considering postsecondary education are *Unlocking Potential: College and Other Choices for Learning Disabled People—A Step-by-Step Guide* (Scheiber and Talpers, 1987), and *Postsecondary Education and Career Development: A Guide for the Blind, Visually Impaired, and Physically Handicapped* from the National Federation of the Blind. In addition, the Heath Resource Center, One Dupont Circle NW, Suite 800, Washington, DC, has excellent resources and single copies free of charge. The Heath Resource Center is the national clearinghouse on postsecondary education for individuals with disabilities and is funded by the U.S. Department of Education. The following is a sampling of its publications: *How to Choose a College: Guide for the Student with a Disability; Education for Employment; Head Injury Survivor on Campus: Issues and Resources; Students Who Are Deaf or Hard of Hearing in Postsecondary Education; Learning Disabled Adults in Postsecondary Education; Strategies for Advising Students with Disabilities; Section 504, The Law and Its Impact on Postsecondary Education;* and *Resource Directory.*

EFFICACY OF SERVICES

Students, parents, related professionals, employers, and third-party providers will question the efficacy of service to students with language disorders until speech-language pathologists make the investigation of the effectiveness of their clinical services a high research priority (Damico, 1988; Larson and McKinley, 1987; Logemann, 1994; McKinley and Larson, 1990; Vetter, 1985, 1991). Clinical efficacy is "the ability to produce desired clinical results" (Damico, 1988, p. 51). It is the obligation of speech-language pathologists to provide services for preadolescents and adolescents with language disorders that are based on valid and reliable assessment data, that are humane, and that are offered in a cost-effective manner. Ultimately, these services should contribute to the quality of the student's life and to society as a whole (Vetter, 1991).

Given that the efficacy of our services should be conveyed to the consumer, it is interesting to note that there has been a lack of research on and demonstration of efficacy of services to preadolescents and adolescents with language disorders (Damico, 1988; Larson and McKinley, 1987; McKinley and Larson, 1990; Vetter, 1985, 1991). This situation may change in the future; the American Speech-Language-Hearing Association has several efficacy projects in progress (Logemann, 1994).

Damico (1988), using a case study format of a 12-year-old girl with a language disorder, discusses five factors that contribute to the lack of efficacy in the management of services. These five factors are fragmentation of language into discrete points during testing and intervention, therapist bias, acquiescence, lack of follow-up, and bureaucratic policies and procedures. Each of these factors is discussed briefly in the next sections.

FRAGMENTATION OF LANGUAGE

The fragmentation of language during the assessment process is problematic. Discrete point testing results in sets of language sub-components or splinter skills being assessed that are only tangentially related, if at all, to the ability to communicate in a wide variety of communication situations. Discrete point testing often results in reducing complex human communication behavior to a single score. This quantification of language into a single score often is a disservice to the student.

If discrete point tests are used to qualify a student for language intervention, plan remediation goals and objectives, and justify the dismissal of the student from the caseload, then failure to determine if the student can communicate in real situations may be the end result (Damico, 1988). When a complex behavior such as communication is fragmented, then the communication act is "stripped of its essential qualities of intentionality and synergy" (Damico, 1988, p. 57).

THERAPIST BIAS

Therapist bias can also affect the efficacy of services to students with language disorders. As Damico (1988) indicated, "Therapist bias is the phenomenon of an opinion or feeling influencing one's objectivity in the therapeutic situation" (p. 58). He stated that if there is a difference between the clinician's expectations and the client's behaviors, clinicians unconsciously modify what they perceive to be the communication performance outcomes of the student so that the clinicians' expectations are maintained.

ACQUIESCENCE

The speech-language pathologist's willingness to acquiesce (i.e., to agree to the impressions of others without dispute) is another factor that affects efficacy. Damico (1988) notes that this frequently happens with clinicians who are insecure in their judgment of their clinical competency.

LACK OF FOLLOW-UP

A lack of follow-up by the speech-language pathologist has been cited (Damico, 1988; Larson and McKinley, 1987) and contributes to the lack of efficacy. Follow-up should take the form of re-evaluation if a student is dismissed from the caseload, re-evaluation during the intervention process, and research to determine the long-term benefits of speech-language intervention on the student's quality of life.

BUREAUCRATIC POLICIES AND PROCEDURES

Despite the passage of PL 94-142 in the 1970s and the more recent PL 101-476, the educational system does not legally seek the *optimal* opportunity or service delivery for each student, but rather the *adequate* service for each student. There is a big difference between optimal services and adequate services. As Damico (1988) states so cogently, the system constrains our best efforts on behalf of the student:

> We determine how the individual child can fit into a service plan which emphasizes minimal compliance with federal regulations, generation of numbers sufficient to meet funding formulae, and procedures and data collection that give the illusion of efficacy and accountability. (p. 61)

Damico states that the factors most easily modifiable are those of discontinuing discrete point assessment and engaging in follow-up activities. If speech-language pathologists are

to demonstrate the efficacy of their services, then these modifications must be adopted. In Chapter 5, we discuss a model of assessment that examines language from a holistic perspective (i.e., functional, descriptive, authentic, dynamic, student centered, and multidimensional). Implementing the principles set forth in these components, in the lists of what communication behaviors to assess, and in the procedures for the assessment process should assist the speech-language pathologist to move away from fragmenting language using discrete point testing and toward assessing communication in a realistic manner.

Larson and McKinley (1987) propose a follow-up component to their prototype service delivery model (see Appendix J). In the follow-up component, data regarding the efficacy of services should be collected periodically during the time that speech-language services are being provided and after the services have been terminated.

The discipline of communication sciences and disorders has long recognized the need for follow-up studies, but few have been published. A review of the literature revealed that of those published, only a few studies have been conducted on older students (Aram et al., 1984; DeAjuriaguerra et al., 1976; Garvey and Gordon, 1973; Griffiths, 1969; King et al., 1982; Strominger and Bashir, 1977; Weiss et al., 1979). Weiner (1985) states that retrospective studies, particularly, contain problems in experimental design. Some of the problems he cites in design have been the size of the sample, the kinds of subjects in the sample, the type and consistency of the information available from the initial evaluation, and the follow-up

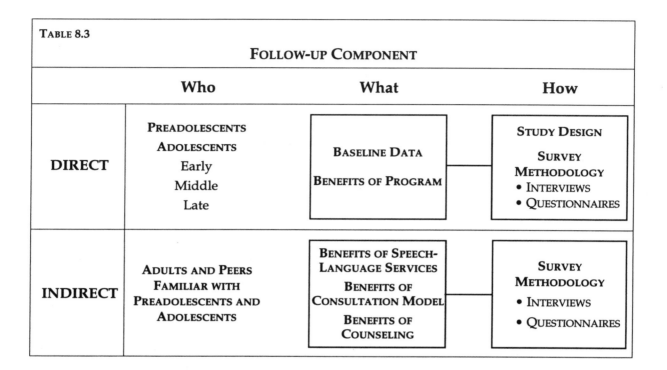

TABLE 8.3			
	FOLLOW-UP COMPONENT		
	Who	**What**	**How**
DIRECT	PREADOLESCENTS ADOLESCENTS Early Middle Late	BASELINE DATA BENEFITS OF PROGRAM	STUDY DESIGN SURVEY METHODOLOGY • INTERVIEWS • QUESTIONNAIRES
INDIRECT	ADULTS AND PEERS FAMILIAR WITH PREADOLESCENTS AND ADOLESCENTS	BENEFITS OF SPEECH-LANGUAGE SERVICES BENEFITS OF CONSULTATION MODEL BENEFITS OF COUNSELING	SURVEY METHODOLOGY • INTERVIEWS • QUESTIONNAIRES

evaluation. Even when the investigators had control over some aspects of the study design, certain factors remained problematic, such as the availability and willingness of the potential subjects to participate and the time and money available for the study. Table 8.3 illustrates comprehensive direct and indirect follow-up procedures.

The speech-language pathologist, during direct follow-up, should work with the recipient of the language assessment and intervention services (i.e., the older student with the language disorder). Initially, it is important to collect baseline data on the student's communication performance across and within a wide variety of communication situations, as well as the case history data that will hopefully provide a historical perspective on the student's communication behavior.

During intervention, the student's communication performance should be evaluated periodically. Once the student has been dismissed from the caseload, periodic checks of the student's progress should be maintained. This is also a time to collect information on the student's perceptions of the benefits of having received intervention. Actual and perceived benefits of language intervention as related to academic, personal-social, and vocational success should be documented on a periodic basis.

Direct follow-up activities should include the selection of study design (i.e., single-subject or group design). Single-subject design as a method to study the clinical process has been well established and presented in the literature (Connell and Thompson, 1986; Kearns, 1986; McReynolds and Kearns, 1983; McReynolds and Thompson, 1986; Vetter, 1985). Vetter (1985) and Larson and McKinley (1987) present information on how to design single-subject and group studies that would assist in demonstrating the efficacy of services provided to students with language disorders. Long-term benefits of services may be investigated using survey methodology such as interviews and questionnaires (Larson and McKinley, 1987). See Appendix K for a sample questionnaire.

During indirect follow-up procedures, the speech-language pathologist should talk with educators, family members, and employers about the older student's communication performance. Likewise, educators should be interviewed to determine the benefits or lack of benefits of a classroom consultation model, if used, as well as any direct services provided to the preadolescent or adolescent. Family members should also be interviewed to determine not only their perceptions of the benefit or lack of benefit of services to their child, but how valuable counseling was for them. Using interviews, questionnaires, and experimental studies, the speech-language pathologist should investigate the benefits, both real and perceived, of the communication services provided to the student with the language disorder.

Once follow-up data have been collected, they must be analyzed carefully. These data should be used to make modifications in the delivery of speech-language services to preadolescents and adolescents with language disorders. Likewise, these data should be shared with colleagues so that they, too, can make appropriate alterations in their programs.

Vetter (1991) proposed two reasons for the lack of investigation of the efficacy of intervention procedures. One, because the research takes so long, most people writing dissertations and those working toward tenure do not have the time for such investigation. Two, the clinicians closest to the students feel that they are not qualified to do clinical research. Vetter presents a strong argument for clinicians conducting research to determine the efficacy of their language intervention activities. She cites several research strategies (i.e., large sample size, precise definitions of what a language disorder is, single-subject designs, practical versus statistical significance, and the use of criterion-referenced tests to replace norm-referenced standardized tests that fragment language).

Regardless of the investigator (Damico, 1988; Larson and McKinley, 1987; Vetter, 1985, 1991; Weiner, 1985), it is clear that speech-language pathologists can no longer fail to investigate and report the efficacy of their services regarding older students with language disorders. To do so is unconscionable.

A CALL TO ACTION

Students Who Can't Communicate: Speech-Language Services at the Secondary Level (McKinley and Larson, 1989) was written as a call to action for secondary school principals. It was reinforced a year later among our own colleagues so that we could become a united voice for older students with language disorders (Larson and McKinley, 1990). We reiterate that call to you now.

Older students with language disorders have a right to services. Speech-language pathologists committed to preadolescents and adolescents should be offering these counter-arguments to administrators and decision makers who challenge older students' need for services (Larson et al., 1993):

1. Many students with language disorders need continued assistance from speech-language pathologists to learn the high-level concepts and vocabulary demanded at each grade.

2. "Turning over" language instruction to other professionals usually ensures that students will be taught communication for academics, but not for social and vocational areas.

3. Students generally make the transition from the concrete into the formal period of cognitive development at the adolescent level (Piaget and Inhelder, 1969).

4. Strong speech-language programs in combination with other special programs (e.g., learning disabilities, vocational education) have proven effective in reducing dropout rates.

5. Speech-language pathologists need to document precisely the changes in growth in language development so proof can be offered that significant progress is being made in oral and written communication skills.

6. Taxpayers will ultimately pay for these students—if not in high school, then during their later years—in the form of adult literacy programs, welfare, basic job training, and many other attempts to reverse the pattern of failure. Businesses are already spending billions of dollars in remedial education each year (Naisbett, 1988; Rukeyser, 1988).

Our society can no longer afford to waste the human potential of youth with language disorders who, given adequate intervention and transition services, can become taxpayers rather than tax takers. Beyond dollars, society can also reap the benefit of creating adult citizens who have problem-solving strategies, communication skills, and increased self-esteem when adequate speech-language services are delivered during their school careers, including during the critical preadolescent and adolescent periods. Once the vision for and the commitment to speech-language services for older students are set, the time and resources needed for implementation become attainable.

The "vision" includes seeing how speech-language pathologists are an integral part of students' school programs, sometimes all the way through to high school graduation. The "commitment" includes standing up for what is fair and just for students with language disorders, even in the face of odds.

"Commitment" may include not dismissing students from intervention when that is clearly the popular choice. It may mean providing advocacy for students at risk of being dropouts or throwaways in our schools. Our level of commitment to at-risk youth needs to intensify. Judge Janice Brice Wellington (1994), speaking at The International Adolescent Conference, stated, "If we continue to operate at the same level of commitment that we currently are, we'll lose more kids than we save." She also explained, "We are engaged in a war [for at-risk youth] where there are few back-up troops. . . . It's a war we won't win unless we do something different [than what we're currently doing]."

By law, all students are entitled to a free, appropriate educational program that meets their individual needs. When the focus is on the needs of students under the existing laws, and when the commitment is there, time and money take care of themselves. High school administrators are not going to invite speech-language pathologists to create jobs for themselves in their buildings. But they will defend those positions once our profession has created them in response to students' needs.

You are needed to apply the vision and the commitment in your community. Keep students' needs first, address those needs, and diminish the waste of human potential of individuals with language disorders. Many preadolescents and adolescents with language disorders are depending on you.

SUMMARY

The roles that speech-language pathologists fill will expand far beyond "direct-service provider" as professionals adjust to a myriad of paradigm shifts and trends. Roles will encompass consultant, teacher, co-teacher, community educator, diversity expert, literacy advocate, researcher, and transition monitor. These expanded roles will help professionals better serve older students with language disorders.

The students themselves face three major transition points as they grow from preadolescence to adolescence to early adulthood. The first is the jump from elementary school to middle or junior high school. The second transition point is marked by entrance into high school. The last transition is high school to a post-school experience, either employment or postsecondary education. Language demands change as settings change, and speech-language pathologists have a responsibility to older students with disorders during these transitions.

Throughout the duration of speech-language services for older students, clinicians should address the effectiveness of those services. This chapter presented various strategies for documenting the efficacy of services.

Finally, we have reiterated a call to action on behalf of older students with language disorders. Since our initial text on adolescents (Boyce and Larson, 1983), we have attempted to persuade our fellow colleagues that serving older students calls for specialized knowledge and techniques to serve the population effectively. We have provided counterarguments for those administrators and school boards who believe speech-language services beyond age 10 are too costly in money and time. And, we have strived to be passionate in this plea so fellow clinicians develop the vision and commitment to create and maintain programs for older students. Failure to heed this plea will result in ongoing waste of our youths' potentials.

DISCUSSION QUESTIONS

1. Describe how you could use computer technology to assist you in following students as they make the transition from:

- the elementary to the middle-school or junior-high level;

- the middle-school or junior-high level to the high-school level; and

- the high-school level to post-school experiences.

2. Assume you have completed some follow-up procedures and have demonstrated the effectiveness of speech-language services for preadolescents and/or adolescents. Discuss what data you would report and to whom (i.e., how you would disseminate the information).

SUGGESTED READINGS

Alexander, W., and McEwin, C. (1989). *Schools in the middle: Status and progress.* Columbus, OH: National Middle School Association.

Heath Resource Center. (1994a). *Make the most of your opportunities: A guide to postsecondary education for adults with disabilities.* Washington, DC: Author.

Vetter, D. K. (1991). Needed: Intervention research. In J. Miller (Ed.), *Research on child language disorders: A decade of progress.* Austin, TX: Pro-Ed.

APPENDICES

DIALECTAL AND BILINGUAL CONSIDERATIONS

PHONEMIC CONTRASTS BETWEEN BLACK ENGLISH AND STANDARD AMERICAN ENGLISH			
SAE PHONEMES	**POSITION IN WORD**		
	INITIAL	**MEDIAL**	**FINAL***
/p/		Unaspirated /p/	Unaspirated /p/
/n/			Reliance on preceding nasalized vowel
/w/	Omitted in specific words (*I 'as, too!*)		
/b/		Unreleased /b/	Unreleased /b/
/g/		Unreleased /g/	Unreleased /g/
/k/		Unaspirated /k/	Unaspirated /k/
/d/	Omitted in specific words (*I 'on't know*)	Unreleased /d/	Unreleased /d/
/ŋ/		/n/	/n/
/t/		Unaspirated /t/	Unaspirated /t/
/l/		Omitted before labial consonants (*help-hep*)	"uh" following a vowel (Bill-Biuh)
/r/		Omitted or /ə/	Omitted or prolonged vowel or glide
/θ/	Unaspirated /t/ or /f/	Unaspirated /t/ or /f/ between vowels	Unaspirated /t/ or /f/ (*bath-baf*)
/v/	Sometimes /b/	/b/ before /m/ and /n/	Sometimes /b/
/ð/	/d/	/d/ or /v/ between vowels	/d/, /v/, /f/
/z/		Omitted or replaced by /d/ before nasal sound (*wasn't-wud'n*)	

BLENDS		FINAL CONSONANT CLUSTERS (second consonant omitted when these clusters occur at the end of a word)		
/str/ becomes /skr/	/ʃr/ becomes /str/	/sk/	/nd/	/sp/
/θr/ becomes /θ/	/pr/ becomes /p/	/ft/	/ld/	/ʤd/
/br/ becomes /b/	/kr/ becomes /k/	/st/	/sd/	/nt/
/gr/ becomes /g/				

*Note weakening of final consonants.

From *Language Disorders: A Functional Approach to Assessment and Intervention* (p. 330), by R. Owens, Jr., 1991, New York: Macmillan. © 1991 by Macmillan Publishing. Reprinted with permission.

GRAMMATICAL CONTRASTS BETWEEN BLACK ENGLISH AND STANDARD AMERICAN ENGLISH		
	BLACK ENGLISH GRAMMATICAL STRUCTURE	**SAE GRAMMATICAL STRUCTURE**
Possessive -'s	Nonobligatory where word position expresses possession. Get *mother* coat. It be mother*'s*.	Obligatory regardless of position. Get mother*'s* coat. It*'s* mother*'s*.
Plural -s	Nonobligatory with numerical quantifier. He got ten *dollar*. Look at the cat*s*.	Obligatory regardless of numerical quantifier. He has ten dollar*s*. Look at the cat*s*.
Regular Past -ed	Nonobligatory; reduced as consonant cluster. Yesterday, I *walk* to school.	Obligatory. Yesterday, I walk*ed* to school.
Irregular Past	Case by case, some verbs inflected, others not. I *see* him last week.	All irregular verbs inflected. I *saw* him last week.
Regular Present Tense Third Person Singular -s	Nonobligatory. She *eat* too much.	Obligatory. She eat*s* too much.
Irregular Present Tense Third Person Singular -s	Nonobligatory. He *do* my job.	Obligatory. He *does* my job.
Indefinite an	Use of indefinite *a*. He ride in *a* airplane.	Use of *an* before nouns beginning with a vowel. He rode in *an* airplane.
Pronouns	Pronominal apposition; pronoun immediately follows noun. Momma *she* mad. She . . .	Pronoun used elsewhere in sentence or in other sentence, not in apposition. Momma is mad. *She* . . .
Future Tense	More frequent use of *be going to* (gonna). I *be going to* dance tonight. I *gonna* dance tonight. Omit *will* preceding *be*. I *be* home later.	More frequent use of *will*. I *will* dance tonight. I *am going to* dance tonight. Obligatory use of *will*. I *will* (I'll) *be* home later.

(continued)

Grammatical Contrasts—*Continued*		
	BLACK ENGLISH GRAMMATICAL STRUCTURE	**SAE GRAMMATICAL STRUCTURE**

Negation	Triple negative.
	    Nobody don't never like me.
	Use of *ain't*.
	    I *ain't* going.
		Absence of triple negative.
		    No one ever likes me.
		Ain't is unacceptable form.
		    I'*m not* going.

Modals	Double modals for such forms as *could* and *should*.
	    I *might could* go.
		Single modal use.
		    I *might be able* to go.

Questions	Same form for direct and and indirect.
	    What *it is*?
	    Do you know what *it is*?
		Different forms for direct and indirect.
		    What *is it*?
		    Do you know what *it is*?

Relative Pronouns	Nonobligatory in most cases.
	    He the one stole it.
	    It the one you like.
		Nonobligatory with *that* only.
		    He's the one *who* stole it.
		    It's the one (that) you like.

Conditional *if*	Use of *do* for conditional *if*.
	    I ask *did* she go.
		Use of *if*.
		    I asked *if* she went.

Perfect Construction	*Been* used for action in the distant past.
	    He *been* gone.
		Been not used.
		    He left a long time ago.

Copula	Nonobligatory when contractible.
	    He sick.
		Obligatory in contractible and uncontractible forms.
		    He's sick.

Habitual or General State	Marked with uninflected *be*.
	    She *be* workin'.
		Nonuse of *be*; verb inflected.
		    She's *working* now.

From *Language Disorders: A Functional Approach to Assessment and Intervention* (p. 331), by R. Owens, Jr., 1991, New York: Macmillan. © 1991 by Macmillan Publishing. Reprinted with permission.

PHONEMIC CONTRASTS BETWEEN HISPANIC ENGLISH AND STANDARD AMERICAN ENGLISH			
SAE Phonemes	**Position in Word**		
	Initial	**Medial**	**Final***
/p/	Unaspirated /p/		Omitted or weakened
/m/			Omitted
/w/	/hu/		Omitted
/b/			Omitted, distorted, or /p/
/g/			Omitted, distorted, or /k/
/k/	Unaspirated or /g/		Omitted, distorted, or /g/
/f/			Omitted
/d/		Dentalized	Omitted, distorted, or /t/
/ŋ/	/n/	/d/	/n/ (*sing-sin*)
/j/	/ʤ/		
/t/			Omitted
/ʃ/	/tʃ/	/s/, /tʃ/	/tʃ/ (*wish-which*)
/tʃ/	/ʃ/ (*chair-share*)	/ʃ/	/ʃ/ (*watch-wash*)
/r/	Distorted	Distorted	Distorted
/ʤ/	/d/	/j/	/ʃ/
/θ/	/t/, /s/ (*thin-tin, sin*)	Omitted	/ʃ/, /t/, /s/
/v/	/b/ (*vat-bat*)	/b/	Distorted
/z/	/s/ (*zip-sip*)	/s/ (*razor-racer*)	/s/
/ð/	/d/ (*then-den*)	/d/, /θ/, /v/ (*lather-ladder*)	/d/

Blends	**Vowels**
/skw/ becomes /eskw/* /sl/ becomes /esl/*	/ɪ/ becomes /i/ (*bit-beet*)

*Separates cluster into two syllables.

From *Language Disorders: A Functional Approach to Assessment and Intervention* (p. 334), by R. Owens, Jr., 1991, New York: Macmillan. © 1991 by Macmillan Publishing. Reprinted with permission.

	HISPANIC ENGLISH GRAMMATICAL STRUCTURE	SAE GRAMMATICAL STRUCTURE
	GRAMMATICAL CONTRASTS BETWEEN HISPANIC ENGLISH AND STANDARD AMERICAN ENGLISH	
Possessive -'s	Use postnoun modifier. This is the homework *of my brother*. Article used with body parts. I cut *the* finger.	Postnoun modifier used only rarely. This is my *brother's* homework. Possessive pronoun used with body parts. I cut *my* finger.
Plural -s	Nonobligatory. The *girl* are playing. The *sheep* are playing.	Obligatory, excluding exceptions. The *girls* are playing. The *sheep* are playing.
Regular Past -ed	Nonobligatory, especially when understood. I *talk* to her yesterday.	Obligatory. I *talked* to her yesterday.
Regular Third Person Singular Present Tense -s	Nonobligatory. She *eat* too much.	Obligatory. She *eats* too much.
Articles	Often omitted. I am going to store. I am going to school.	Usually obligatory. I am going to *the* store. I am going to school.
Subject Pronouns	Omitted when subject has been identified in the previous sentence. Father is happy. Bought a new car.	Obligatory. Father is happy. *He* bought a new car.
Future Tense	Use *go + to*. I *go to* dance.	Use *be + going to*. I *am going* to the dance.
Negation	Use *no* before the verb. She *no* eat candy.	Use *not* (preceded by auxiliary verb where appropriate). She does *not* eat candy.

(continued)

Grammatical Contrasts—*Continued*

	HISPANIC ENGLISH GRAMMATICAL STRUCTURE	SAE GRAMMATICAL STRUCTURE
Question	Intonation; no noun-verb inversion. *Maria is* going?	Noun-verb inversion usually. *Is Maria* going?
Copula	Occasional use of *have*. I *have* ten years.	Use of *be*. I *am* ten years old.
Negative Imperatives	No used for *don't*. *No* throw stones.	*Don't* used. *Don't* throw stones.
***Do* Insertion**	Nonobligatory in questions. You like ice cream?	Obligatory when no auxiliary verb. *Do* you like ice cream?
Comparatives	More frequent use of longer form (more). He is *more* tall.	More frequent use of shorter -er. He is tall*er*.

From *Language Disorders: A Functional Approach to Assessment and Intervention* (p. 335), by R. Owens, Jr., 1991, New York: Macmillan. © 1991 by Macmillan Publishing. Reprinted with permission.

PHONEMIC CONTRASTS BETWEEN ASIAN ENGLISH AND STANDARD AMERICAN ENGLISH			
	POSITION IN WORD		
SAE PHONEMES	INITIAL	MEDIAL	FINAL
/p/	/b/****	/b/****	Omission
/s/	Distortion*	Distortion*	Omission
/z/	/s/**	/s/**	Omission
/t/	Distortion*	Distortion*	Omission
/tʃ/	/ʃ/****	/ʃ/****	Omission
/ʃ/	/s/**	/s/**	Omission
/r/, /l/	Confusion***	Confusion***	Omission
/θ/	/s/	/s/	Omission
/dʒ/	/d/ Or /z/****	/d/ or /z/****	Omission
/v/	/f/***	/f/***	Omission
	/w/**	/w/**	Omission
/ð/	/z/*	/z/*	Omission
	/d/****	/d/****	Omission

BLENDS	VOWELS
Addition of /ə/ between consonants*** Omission of final consonant clusters****	Shortening or lengthening of vowels (seat-sit, it-eat*) Difficulty with /ɪ/, /ɔ/, and /æ/, and substitution of /e/ for /æ/** Difficulty with /ɪ/, /æ/, /ʊ/, and /ə/****

* Mandarin dialect of Chinese only
** Cantonese dialect of Chinese only
*** Mandarin, Cantonese, and Japanese
****Vietnamese only

From *Language Disorders: A Functional Approach to Assessment and Intervention* (p. 337), by R. Owens, Jr., 1991, New York: Macmillan. © 1991 by Macmillan Publishing. Reprinted with permission.

GRAMMATICAL CONTRASTS BETWEEN ASIAN ENGLISH AND STANDARD AMERICAN ENGLISH		
	ASIAN ENGLISH GRAMMATICAL STRUCTURE	**SAE GRAMMATICAL STRUCTURE**
Plural -s	Not used with numerical adjective. 　three *cat* Used with irregular plural. 　three *sheeps*	Used regardless of numerical adjective. 　three *cats* Not used with irregular plural. 　three *sheep*
Auxiliaries *to be* and *to do*	Omission. 　I going home. 　She not want eat. Uninflected. 　I *is* going. 　She *do* not want *eat*.	Obligatory and inflected in the present progressive form. 　I *am going* home. 　She *does* not want *to eat*.
Verb *have*	Omission. 　You been here. Uninflected. 　He *have* one.	Obligatory and inflected. 　You *have* been here. 　He *has* one.
Past Tense -ed	Omission. 　He talk yesterday. Overgeneralization. 　I *eated* yesterday. Double-marking. 　She *didn't ate*.	Obligatory, nonovergeneralization, and single-marking. 　He talk*ed* yesterday. 　I *ate* yesterday. 　She *didn't* eat.
Interrogative	Nonreversal. 　*You are* late? Omitted auxiliary. 　You like ice cream?	Reversal and obligatory auxiliary. 　*Are you* late? 　*Do* you like ice cream?
Perfect Marker	Omission. 　I have write letter.	Obligatory. 　I have writt*en* a letter.
Verb-Noun Agreement	Nonagreement. 　*He go* to school. 　*You goes* to school.	Agreement. 　*He goes* to school. 　*You go* to school.
Article	Omission. 　Please give gift. Overgeneralization. 　She go *the* school.	Obligatory with certain nouns. 　Please give *the* gift. Nonovergeneralization. 　She went to school.

(continued)

	ASIAN ENGLISH GRAMMATICAL STRUCTURE	SAE GRAMMATICAL STRUCTURE

Preposition	Misuse.
	  I am *in* home.
	Omission.
	  He go bus.
		Obligatory specific use.
		  I am *at* home.
		  He goes *by* bus.

Pronoun	Subjective/objective confusion.
	  Him go quickly.
	Possessive confusion.
	  It *him* book.
		Subjective/objective distinction.
		  He gave it to *her*.
		Possessive distinction.
		  It's *his* book.

Demonstrative	Confusion.
	  I like *those* horse.
		Singular/plural distinction.
		  I like *that* horse.

Conjunction	Omission.
	  You I go together.
		Obligatory use between last two items in a series.
		  You *and* I are going together.
		  Mary, John, *and* Carol went.

Negation	Double-marking.
	  I *didn't* see *nobody*.
	Simplified form.
	  He *no* come.
		Single obligatory marking.
		  I *didn't* see anybody.
		  He *didn't* come.

Word Order	Adjective following noun (Vietnamese).
	  clothes new
	Possessive following noun (Vietnamese).
	  dress her
	Omission of object with transitive verb.
	  I want.
		Most noun modifiers precede noun.
		  new clothes
		Possessive precedes noun.
		  her dress
		Use of direct object with most transitive verbs.
		  I want it.

Grammatical Contrasts—*Continued*

From *Language Disorders: A Functional Approach to Assessment and Intervention* (p. 338), by R. Owens, Jr., 1991, New York: Macmillan. © 1991 by Macmillan Publishing. Reprinted with permission.

TEACHER LANGUAGE:
SELF-EVALUATION TECHNIQUE

STUDENT RESPONSE FORM

Name: _____ Date: _____

Teacher: _____ Class: _____

> **THIS IS NOT A TEST! ANSWERS WILL NOT AFFECT YOUR GRADE!**
>
> **PLEASE ANSWER HONESTLY.**

Directions: Use this scale to rate the lecture or instructions your teacher just gave.

> 5—Very easy
>
> 4—Somewhat easy
>
> 3—Neither easy nor hard
>
> 2—Somewhat hard
>
> 1—Very hard

Rate these characteristics of your teacher's language during the lecture or instructions just finished.

_____ Length of instructions or lecture

_____ Complexity of instructions or lecture

_____ Level of vocabulary

_____ Organization of ideas

_____ Ease of listening

_____ Rate of speech

_____ Tone of voice

What would help you to understand class material better?

Do you have other comments about the teacher's language? Write your comments on the back side of this form. Thank you.

© 1995 Thinking Publications. Duplication permitted for educational use only.

ATTITUDINAL SCALE

Date: _____

To: Professional Colleagues

From: _____
Speech-Language Pathologist's Name

Re: Attached Survey

Attached to this memo is a survey called the "Adolescents with Communication Disorders Attitudinal (ACDA) Scale." I would appreciate it if you would complete this survey by _____ and return it to my mailbox.
Date
The survey should take you 5 to 10 minutes to complete.

The purpose of the survey is to provide information that can help me to improve the speech-language program for middle-school and secondary-level students. Data will be treated confidentially. If you wish to receive a copy of the summarized data, please let me know and I'll share the results with you.

Please read the directions carefully before completing the ACDA Scale. If you have any questions or concerns, contact me at

_____.
Address/Phone Number

© 1995 Thinking Publications. Duplication permitted for educational use only.

ACDA SCALE

Directions: Read each statement below. You will be using a number between 1 and 5 to indicate how much you agree or disagree with a set of 20 statements.

All answers will be treated confidentially. No individual data will be reported, only group data from a number of teachers and administrators.

Note: THERE ARE NO CORRECT OR INCORRECT ANSWERS.

Scale: Respond to each of the statements below by choosing the answer that comes closest to how you usually feel or act.

5—I agree strongly.

4—I agree.

3—I neither agree nor disagree.

2—I disagree.

1—I disagree strongly.

_____ 1. Adolescents with communication disorders should be allowed to substitute speech-language intervention for a content area course (e.g., English).

_____ 2. It makes sense to give grades and credit to adolescents receiving speech-language services.

_____ 3. Adolescents with communication disorders should be allowed to take tests orally if written language is severely impaired.

_____ 4. Adolescents with communication disorders should be allowed to tape record class-room lectures and directions given by teachers.

_____ 5. Teachers should provide both oral and written instructions for students.

_____ 6. Teachers should supply written listening guides for students to follow during lectures.

_____ 7. Speech-language programs are a necessary service for adolescents with communication disorders.

© 1995 Thinking Publications. Duplication permitted for educational use only.

_____ 8. Adolescents with communication disorders should be spending full classroom time modules in the speech-language program, not short 15- to 20-minute blocks of time.

_____ 9. Speech-language services are as important for adolescents with mild disorders as for those with severe disorders.

_____ 10. The speech-language program is an important resource for adolescents with communication disorders.

_____ 11. Adolescents with communication disorders should be kept in the educational mainstream as much as possible.

_____ 12. Adolescents who feel they have a problem with communication should be able to refer themselves to the speech-language program for testing.

_____ 13. Adolescents with communication disorders are just as intelligent as adolescents without communication disorders.

_____ 14. Adolescents with communication disorders should be expected to meet the same graduation standards as adolescents without communication disorders.

_____ 15. It is possible for an adolescent with a communication disorder to lead a normal life.

_____ 16. Adolescents with communication disorders should be treated the same as anyone.

_____ 17. Adolescents with communication disorders usually make a contribution to society.

_____ 18. The curriculum should be modified to meet the individual needs of adolescents with communication disorders.

_____ 19. Adolescents with severe disorders deserve more curriculum modifications than adolescents with mild disorders.

_____ 20. Adolescents with communication disorders should be expected to modify their behaviors to meet the demands of the curriculum.

Thank you for your time. Please return this scale to _____.

Person or Location

© 1995 Thinking Publications. Duplication permitted for educational use only.

INCLUSION LIST

The speech-language program is maintaining a list of teachers who are receptive to including students with language disorders in their classrooms and to making modifications in curriculum, when necessary, to meet the students' needs. If this is an interest of yours, and you are willing to have your name added to this list, please share your name below. Detach this information from the rest of the attitudinal scale and return it to _____.

Person or Location

Name: _____

Content area: _____

Grade level(s): _____

© 1995 Thinking Publications. Duplication permitted for educational use only.

CURRICULUM ANALYSIS FORM

Date(s) of Analysis: _____   Examiner Completing Analysis: _____

Student: _____   Class: _____

Grade Level: _____   Instructor: _____

TEXTBOOK ANALYSIS (Use the primary text from the class.)

Identifying Information

1. Title: _____

2. Author(s): _____

3. Copyright: _____

4. Year Adopted by School: _____

5. Readability Level: _____

    a. Is this readability level appropriate for the student?

    _____ No   _____ Yes

    b. Is this readability level similar to that of the student's other textbooks?

    _____ No   _____ Yes

Student Familiarity with the Textbook

1. Is this textbook significantly different from others that the student is reading?

    _____ No   _____ Yes

    If "Yes," how is it different? _____

    _____

© 1995 Thinking Publications. Duplication permitted for educational use only.

2. Check which of the following features are included in the textbook. For any that are present, check whether the student can locate these features upon request and state when they are used.

CHECK IF PRESENT	FEATURES	CAN THE STUDENT LOCATE THE FEATURE?		WHEN IS THE FEATURE USED?
		YES	NO	
	Table of Contents			
	Index			
	Glossary			
	Appendix			
	Bibliography			
	Unit or Chapter Objectives			
	Review Questions and/ or Practice Exercises			
	Italicization of Words (varying print styles)			
	Graphic Aids (charts, tables, graphs, maps)			

CLASSROOM ANALYSIS

Organization of the Class

1. Which topical arrangement typifies this class? (Check one.)

_____ Sequential (independence among topics)   _____ Spiral (dependence among topics)

2. If "sequential" arrangement is primary, have all units been problematic for the student, or only some? (Check one.)

_____ All _____ Some

3. Does the class have significantly different requirements in comparison with the student's other classes?

_____ No _____ Yes

If "Yes," explain: _____

© 1995 Thinking Publications. Duplication permitted for educational use only.

Student's Comprehension of Lecture/Instructions

Enlist the assistance of a "good student" in the classroom. Indicate to that student that you would like him/her to take notes during the first 10 minutes of a lecture or set of instructions given in the class within the next week. These notes should be photocopied by the examiner, then compared with the notes taken by the student undergoing assessment. Use the "good student's" notes to answer questions 1 and 2 below; for question 3, use the notes from the individual being assessed.

1. What was the main idea presented (or sequence of instructions)? _____

   _____

2. What were the relevant supporting ideas? _____

   _____

   _____

3. Answer the following questions:

   a. Did the student's main idea(s) match the one(s) the "good student" identified?

   _____ No _____ Yes

   b. Did the student's relevant supporting details match the ones the "good student" identified?

   _____ No _____ Yes

   c. Did the student indicate verbally or nonverbally any words that were not understood?

   _____ No _____ Yes

   If "Yes," list them: _____

   _____

   d. Does the student report having difficulty comprehending the lectures/instructions only in this class or also in others? (Check one.)

   _____ Only this class _____ This class and others

Student's Comprehension of Tests/Evaluations

Obtain a recent test or other evaluation tool administered to the student. With the student present, ask questions 1 through 4.

1. What questions were most difficult to answer? _____

   Why were they more difficult? _____

   _____

© 1995 Thinking Publications. Duplication permitted for educational use only.

2. What vocabulary items were unfamiliar? _____

_____

3. How well did you prepare for this test? (Circle one.)

    Not at all   Some   Enough   More than usual   A great amount

4. Are the tests in this class significantly different from those in other classes that you are taking?

    _____ No   _____ Yes

    If "Yes," how are they different?

5. Using Bloom's (1956) Taxonomy, what level(s) of thinking was required most often during this test?

    _____ Knowledge   _____ Analysis

    _____ Comprehension   _____ Synthesis

    _____ Application   _____ Evaluation

STUDENT ATTITUDE TOWARD THE CLASS

Ask the student the following questions. The examiner should record responses.

1. Do you think the ideas presented in this class are important to learn?

    _____ No   _____ Yes   _____ Sometimes

2. Do you think this class is interesting?

    _____ No   _____ Yes   _____ Sometimes

3. Do you think this class is taught simply enough so that you can learn the information?

    _____ No   _____ Yes   _____ Sometimes

4. Do you think the information you learn in this class is useful?

    _____ No   _____ Yes   _____ Sometimes

5. Do you think the information in this class is presented clearly by the teacher?

    _____ No   _____ Yes   _____ Sometimes

6. Do you think the information in this class is presented clearly by the textbook?

    _____ No   _____ Yes   _____ Sometimes

7. Do you feel motivated to do well in this class?

    _____ No   _____ Yes   _____ Sometimes

© 1995 Thinking Publications. Duplication permitted for educational use only.

ANALYSIS

Results should be analyzed to determine the following:

1. Does the textbook for the class appear to be interfering significantly with the student's comprehension?

2. Does the student appear to be having difficulty understanding the teacher's lectures/instructions in the classroom compared with other students at the same level?

3. Do the tests in the class seem to be interfering with class performance because the student does not understand the language in them?

4. Does the student show any positive attitude toward the class to attempt to perform as well as possible?

Results should also be compared with the student's performance on informal assessment tasks that require the student to use informational listening for short, simulated lectures by the speech-language pathologist. If the teacher has made use of the "Teacher Language: Self-evaluation Technique" (See Appendix B) in the classroom, results should be compared with those findings (i.e., Is the student undergoing assessment the only student experiencing difficulty understanding the teacher?).

INTERPRETATION

If the "Analysis" questions 1, 2, or 3 above are answered affirmatively, and the data match those obtained during direct assessment of the adolescent, then the problem rests primarily within the student. However, if data mismatch (e.g., the student demonstrated good informational listening skills when the speech-language pathologist delivered the lecture, but poor informational listening skills in the classroom), the problem may lie within the educational system. Students should demonstrate a positive attitude before examiners conclude that the problem rests primarily within the educational system (see "Analysis" question 4).

© 1995 Thinking Publications. Duplication permitted for educational use only.

CASE HISTORY FORM

Interviewer: _____ Date: _____

Personal Information of Interviewee

Name: _____

Birthdate: _____ Age: _____ Sex: _____M _____F

Address: _____

Home Phone: _____ Work Phone of Parent/Guardian: _____

Education: Highest grade completed _____

Environmental History

1. List and describe below all members of your immediate family. Indicate in the far right column any speech, hearing, or language problems present among other members of the household.

Name	Relationship	Communication Problem

2. List two friends with whom you enjoy talking.

_____

_____

© 1995 Thinking Publications. Duplication permitted for educational use only.

Educational and Vocational History

1. List the school subjects that are your best.

   _____

2. List the school subjects you enjoy the most.

   _____

3. List the school subjects that are your most difficult.

   _____

4. Why do you feel you are having difficulty with these subjects?

   _____

5. Are you involved in activities outside of school? _____ No _____ Yes

   If "Yes," describe: _____

6. Do you have any future vocational goals? _____ No _____ Yes

   If "Yes," describe: _____

7. Do you hold a full- or part-time job? _____ No _____ Yes

   If "Yes," describe: _____

Health History

1. List below: (a) major illnesses, diseases, or accidents;

                    (b) age at the time of each; and

                    (c) resulting health complications or handicaps.

Illnesses/diseases/accidents	Age	Resulting handicaps

2. Were you hospitalized for any of the above conditions? _____ No _____ Yes

   If "Yes," where? _____

   For how long? _____

© 1995 Thinking Publications. Duplication permitted for educational use only.

3. Have you received, or are you now receiving rehabilitation treatment such as radiation therapy, physical therapy, or occupational therapy? Describe the reason for, type, duration, and result of treatments:

_____

_____

4. Are you currently under a doctor's care? _____ No _____ Yes

   If "Yes," for what? _____

5. Are you currently taking any medication? _____ No _____ Yes

   If "Yes," what kind? _____

   For what? _____

   How much? _____

   How often? _____

6. Do you have any known allergies? _____ No _____ Yes

   If "Yes," describe: _____

7. Do you have any known drug sensitivities? _____ No _____ Yes

   If "Yes," describe: _____

8. Have you had seizures? _____ No _____ Yes

   If "Yes," how often? _____

   When was the most recent seizure? _____

9. Do you have any known hearing problems? _____ No _____ Yes

   If "Yes," describe: _____

10. Have you had a past history of ear infections? _____ No _____ Yes

    If "Yes," describe: _____

11. Do you have any known visual problems? _____ No _____ Yes

    If "Yes," describe: _____

    Glasses worn? _____ No _____ Yes

© 1995 Thinking Publications. Duplication permitted for educational use only.

Speech, Language, and Hearing History

1. Describe the present problem: _____

   _____

2. How long has there been a problem? _____

   _____

3. What do you think caused the problem? _____

   _____

4. What types of speech and language services have you received? _____

   _____

   How long did you receive them? _____

   How do you feel about the services you received? _____

5. Were you ever dismissed from speech and language services? _____ No _____ Yes

   If "Yes," why? _____

6. How do you feel about your present speech and language problem? _____

   _____

7. Are you understood when you speak? _____ No _____ Yes

   If "No," describe: _____

8. Do you understand when others talk to you? _____ No _____ Yes

   If "No," describe: _____

9. Do you avoid speaking situations? _____ No _____ Yes

   If "Yes," describe: _____

10. Are there times or situations when your problem is better or worse? _____ No _____ Yes

    If "Yes," describe: _____

© 1995 Thinking Publications. Duplication permitted for educational use only.

Please provide in the space below any additional information that may be useful in evaluating your communication skills and in planning an intervention program.

© 1995 Thinking Publications. Duplication permitted for educational use only.

SUPPLEMENTAL FORMS

CASE HISTORY SUPPLEMENT

Student: _____ Age: _____

Examiner: _____ Date: _____

Feelings and Attitudes

Thinking

1. What is thinking? _____

   _____

2. On a scale from 1 to 5, how important is thinking in your life?

1	2	3	4	5
Not at all Important		Sometimes Important		Extremely Important

3. Whom do you know that you consider to be a good thinker? _____

   What makes you feel _(name)_ is a good thinker? _____

   _____

4. Have you ever felt you would like to think better? _____ No _____ Yes

   If "Yes," in what situations? _____

   _____

5. What interferes with your ability to think clearly? _____

   _____

Listening

1. What is listening? _____

   _____

© 1995 Thinking Publications. Duplication permitted for educational use only.

2. On a scale from 1 to 5, how important is listening in your life?

1	2	3	4	5
Not at all Important		Sometimes Important		Extremely Important

3. Whom do you know that you consider to be a good listener? _____

   What makes you feel _(name)_ is a good listener? _____

   _____

4. Have you ever felt you would like to listen better?   _____ No   _____ Yes

   If "Yes," in what situations?   _____

   _____

5. What interferes with your ability to listen? _____

   _____

Speaking

1. What is speaking? _____

   _____

2. How important on a scale from 1 to 5 is speaking in your life?

1	2	3	4	5
Not at all Important		Sometimes Important		Extremely Important

3. Whom do you know that you consider to be a good speaker? _____

   What makes you feel _(name)_ is a good speaker? _____

   _____

4. Have you ever felt you would like to speak better?   _____ No   _____ Yes

   If "Yes," in what situations?   _____

   _____

© 1995 Thinking Publications. Duplication permitted for educational use only.

5. What interferes with your ability to speak? _____

_____

Current Need for Thinking, Listening, and Speaking

Academic Environment

How often are you required to think, listen, and speak in classroom situations? Use this scale:

1 = Frequently	2 = Occasionally	3 = Seldom	4 = Never

Classes/Subjects	**Think**	**Listen**	**Speak**

Comments: _____

_____

Social Environment

How often are you required to think, listen, and speak in daily living situations (e.g., with friends, with family members)? Use this scale:

1 = Frequently	2 = Occasionally	3 = Seldom	4 = Never

Situations	**Think**	**Listen**	**Speak**

Comments: _____

_____

© 1995 Thinking Publications. Duplication permitted for educational use only.

Vocational Environment

How often are you required to think, listen, and speak in a job situation (e.g., with co-workers, with customers)? Use this scale:

1 = Frequently   2 = Occasionally   3 = Seldom   4 = Never

Situations	Think	Listen	Speak

Comments: _____

_____

Intervention: Past and Future

1. What intervention have you received in the past

   For thinking? _____

   _____

   For listening? _____

   _____

   For speaking? _____

   _____

2. Do you feel you need to improve

   Your thinking? _____ No _____ Yes

   Comments: _____

   _____

   Your listening? _____ No _____ Yes

   Comments: _____

   _____

   Your speaking? _____ No _____ Yes

   Comments: _____

   _____

© 1995 Thinking Publications. Duplication permitted for educational use only.

LISTENING QUESTIONNAIRE

The following adaptation of the Personal Analysis Questionnaire proposed by Wolff et al. (1983) can assist adolescents in recognizing their individual beliefs, attitudes, and misconceptions about listening. This questionnaire can be administered orally, requiring the student to listen rather than read.

Mark each statement as true or false.

_____ 1. Teachers or friends who don't listen to me are too stupid to appreciate my ideas.

_____ 2. Teaching students to listen is as foolish as trying to teach them to breathe.

_____ 3. I already have developed good listening skills because I have to listen all the time in school.

_____ 4. It is more important to be good speakers than good listeners because we learn by talking.

_____ 5. It is more important to be good readers than good listeners because we can go back to check material we read.

_____ 6. I think I have been adequately taught to listen at school and home.

_____ 7. Students should not have to work at listening to class lectures.

_____ 8. I can't stand to listen to people who talk about ideas that sound crazy.

_____ 9. It doesn't matter if I stop listening because I don't miss much.

_____ 10. I'm a good listener when I want to be.

Each true answer reveals a misconception about listening. Have students count their number of true responses and compare it to the scale below.

    0, 1 = Free of false information about listening
  2, 3, 4 = Positive attitude toward learning about listening
  5, 6, 7 = Aware of listening as a topic; misconceptions are warping your thinking.
 8, 9, 10 = BRICK WALL. Misconceptions have kept listening information from being useful to you.

Compare and discuss results within the group.

From *Daily Communication: Strategies for the Language Disordered Adolescent* (p. 55–56), by L. Schwartz and N. McKinley, 1984, Eau Claire, WI: Thinking Publications. © 1984 by Thinking Publications. Adapted with permission. Duplication permitted for educational use only.

LEARNING STYLE QUESTIONNAIRE

Directions: This learning style questionnaire attempts to determine how a preadolescent or adolescent learns best a difficult or new subject. This is NOT a learning style preference inventory that assesses how a student likes to learn.

Inform the student that this is NOT a test but rather a survey to find out how he or she best learns a new or difficult subject. Emphasize that there are no right or wrong answers. Read the directions and survey questions to the student. Also, give the questionnaire to the student so that he or she can read along and mark the form.

It is preferable to complete the questionnaire on a one-to-one basis, but small groups of three to seven students may be administered the questionnaire. Rephrase questions and answer students' questions as you proceed through the survey to clarify for better understanding.

Emphasize to students that they are to check and/or rank items as stated. When rankings are requested, be certain that items are ranked and not simply checked. Have the students fill in the identification information (e.g., name, date of birth) before beginning to answer the questions. Stress that students should answer the questions as honestly as possible and that they should give their immediate reaction to each question.

LEARNING STYLE QUESTIONNAIRE

IDENTIFICATION INFORMATION

Name: _____ Current Date: _____

Sex: M _____ F _____ Grade: _____ Birthdate: _____ School District: _____

Parent or Guardian: _____

Address: _____ City: _____

Home Phone: _____ Work Phone: _____

Adult assisting you to complete this questionnaire: _____

Directions: This is NOT a test. There are no right or wrong answers. The following items are simply a way to find out how you learn best. If an item is unclear, feel free to ask questions of the person administering this questionnaire.

The purpose of this questionnaire is to determine how you learn *best*, not how you *like* to learn a subject. For example, you might like to have the TV on while you are studying, but you study best when it is quiet. Also, you might like to study at night, but you are more productive if you study in the morning. "Learn best" means how you remember information the longest, attend to a task the best, or recall details and main ideas most easily. Knowing how you learn best will help us to help you to be more successful in school.

Before you begin to answer the questions, please write your name, current date, address, and other identification information requested in the space provided above.

Answer the following statements honestly about when, how, where, why, and with whom you learn best.

My most difficult subject is: _____

I learn my most difficult subject best:

When?

1. Time (Check only one.)
   _____ Morning
   _____ Afternoon
   _____ Night
   _____ Other (Explain): _____

   _____

© 1995 Thinking Publications. Duplication permitted for educational use only.

2. Timing (Check only one.)

_____ Before meals
_____ After meals

I learn my most difficult subject best:

How?

1. Sound (Check only one.)

_____ Quiet
_____ Radio
_____ Conversation
_____ TV
_____ Music
_____ Noisy
_____ Other (explain): _____

_____

2. Light (Check only one.)
_____ Dim
_____ Moderate
_____ Bright
_____ Other (explain): _____

_____

3. Temperature (Check only one.)
_____ Cold
_____ Cool
_____ Warm
_____ Very Warm
_____ Other (explain): _____

_____

4. Intake (Check only one.)
_____ Eat foods
_____ Drink liquids
_____ Chew on something
_____ Not eat, drink, or chew on anything while learning
_____ Other (explain): _____

_____

© 1995 Thinking Publications. Duplication permitted for educational use only.

I learn my most difficult subject best:

Where?

    1. Place (Indicate your first and second choices.)

        _____ Home _____
                                  Which room/place within your home? (E.g., bedroom, kitchen, living room, etc.)

        _____ School _____
                                  Which room within the school? (E.g., library, study hall, classroom, etc.)

    2. Conditions (Within each place, rank the locations. 1 = The location where you learn best.)

        a. Home

           _____ Desk/Table

           _____ Bed

           _____ Floor

           _____ Straight chair

           _____ Soft chair

           _____ Couch

           _____ Other (explain): _____

                              _____

        b. School

           _____ Desk/Table

           _____ Floor

           _____ Straight chair

           _____ Soft chair

           _____ Other (explain): _____

                              _____

I learn my most difficult subject best:

Why? (Rank these items as to why you learn best. 1 = Your strongest reason for learning.)

       _____ I want to.

       _____ My teacher expects me to/demands it.

       _____ My parent(s) expects me to/demands it.

       _____ I'll get a reward such as:

           _____ money

           _____ better grades

           _____ privileges

       _____ Other (explain): _____

                          _____

© 1995 Thinking Publications. Duplication permitted for educational use only.

I learn my most difficult subject best:

With Whom? (Rank the top four. 1 = The best way to study the subject.)

_____ Alone
_____ A partner
_____ Small group (3–7)
_____ Large group (8 and above)
_____ Teacher(s)
_____ Parent(s)
_____ Sibling(s)
_____ Other (explain): _____
          _____

Given the following situations, rank or check how you learn best.

Inside the Classroom

1. Participating in the class (Rank the ways you learn best in the classroom. 1 = The way you learn difficult material the best.)

   _____ Listening
   _____ Reading
   _____ Writing
   _____ Speaking
   _____ Doing
   _____ Combination of the above
        Please specify: _____
               _____

2. Participating in assignments within the classroom (Rank the top four assignments that help you learn the information best. 1 = The best way to learn via an assignment.)

   _____ Worksheet questions
   _____ Experiments
   _____ Demonstrations
   _____ Group projects
   _____ Individual projects
   _____ Written reports
   _____ Oral reports
   _____ Other (explain): _____
             _____

© 1995 Thinking Publications. Duplication permitted for educational use only.

3. Remembering main points from what the teacher says (Rank the top four. 1 = The best way to remember main points from what the teacher says.)

_____ Repeat the material to yourself

_____ Think of a picture in your mind

_____ Make up words to remember main points in order

_____ Break ideas into smaller chunks

_____ Outline what the teacher says in writing

_____ Follow an outline that the teacher has provided

_____ Use rhyming words to recall main points

_____ Put main points into categories

_____ Audiotape what the teacher is saying and replay it later

_____ Other (explain): _____

_____

4. Taking notes (Check only one.)

While listening to a lecture, I take notes when learning my most difficult subject as follows:

_____ Notes are key words

_____ Notes are attempts at complete sentences

_____ Notes are "doodles"

_____ Other (explain): _____

_____

5. Asking questions of the teacher (Check only one.)

I learn my most difficult subject best if I ask questions:

_____ During class

_____ After class

_____ Before class

_____ Other (explain): _____

_____

© 1995 Thinking Publications. Duplication permitted for educational use only.

6. Remembering main points from a textbook (Rank the top four ways that you learn best from a textbook. 1 = The best way to remember main points from a textbook.)

_____ Look at headings and subheadings within the chapters

_____ Outline important ideas from the textbook

_____ Underline/highlight main points

_____ Write down questions to anticipate what a teacher will ask on a test

_____ Answer questions at the end of each chapter (if available)

_____ Follow along in the textbook while listening to an audiotape of the textbook

_____ Other (explain): _____

_____

Outside the Classroom

1. Participating in outside classroom assignments (Rank the top four assignments that help you to learn a difficult subject best. 1 = The best way to learn via an assignment.)

_____ Preparing a written report

_____ Preparing for an oral report

_____ Answering questions from the textbook or worksheet

_____ Reading assigned information

_____ Other (explain): _____

_____

2. Studying for a test (Rank the top four. 1 = The way you study best for a test.)

I learn best studying for a test in my most difficult subject when I:

_____ Read or reread the textbook the day before

_____ Read or reread the textbook 2–3 days before

_____ Listen or re-listen to audiotapes of what the teacher said

_____ Review the outline of my notes

_____ Review the outline provided by the teacher

_____ Predict questions to be on the test and answer them

_____ Rework problems assigned by the teacher

_____ Other (explain): _____

_____

3. I learn my most difficult subject best when I study for _____ minutes each hour before taking a break.

© 1995 Thinking Publications. Duplication permitted for educational use only.

ADOLESCENT CONVERSATIONAL ANALYSIS

Name: _____ Date: _____

Age: _____ Conversational Partner: _____

Setting of Conversation: _____

Materials Present to Elicit Sample: _____

(Obtain a minimum of 10 minutes of conversational speech with each partner in each setting. Transcribe exactly the conversational units of each participant. Analyze for the behaviors listed below. Circle "A" for appropriate and "I" for inappropriate behaviors. Determine appropriateness and inappropriateness of a behavior by judging whether or not it is penalizing to the adolescent; a behavior perceived by the clinician as penalizing is marked as inappropriate [Prutting and Kirchner, 1983]. Circle "NO" if a behavior is "not observed" during the sample. Probe any behaviors marked "NO" during directed tasks. Compile information on the Adolescent Conversational Analysis Profile on page 291.)

ROLE OF THE LISTENER IN THE CONVERSATION

A   I   NO   1. Appears to understand the vocabulary and syntactical structures of the
conversational partner
Comments:

A   I   NO   2. Appears to follow main idea of conversational topics
Comments:

A   I   NO   3. Appears to listen in a nonjudgmental manner
Comments:

© 1995 Thinking Publications. Duplication permitted for educational use only.

A   I   NO   4. Indicates understanding or lack of understanding of conversational partner by use of verbal and/or nonverbal feedback
Comments:

ROLE OF THE SPEAKER IN THE CONVERSATION

Language Features

A   I   NO   1. Production from a variety of syntactic forms
Comments:

A   I   NO   2. Production of a variety of questions (question forms)
Comments:

A   I   NO   3. Production of figurative language
Comments:

A   I   NO   4. Production of nonspecific language
Comments:

5. Production of precise vocabulary

A   I   NO   a. Word-retrieval skills
Comments:

A   I   NO   b. Verbal mazes
Comments:

© 1995 Thinking Publications. Duplication permitted for educational use only.

A   I   NO   c. False starts
                Comments:

Paralanguage Features

A   I   NO   1. Suprasegmental features (use of vocal inflection, juncture, and rate)
                Comments:

A   I   NO   2. Fluency
                Comments:

A   I   NO   3. Intelligibility
                Comments:

Communication Functions

A   I   NO   1. To give information
                Comments:

A   I   NO   2. To get information
                Comments:

A   I   NO   3. To describe an ongoing event
                Comments:

© 1995 Thinking Publications. Duplication permitted for educational use only.

A I NO   4. To persuade one's listener to do, believe, or feel something
Comments:

A I NO   5. To express one's own intentions, beliefs, and feelings
Comments:

A I NO   6. To indicate a readiness for further communication
Comments:

A I NO   7. To solve problems
Comments:

A I NO   8. To entertain
Comments:

Conversational Rules

     1. Verbal rules governing topics and turns

A I NO   a. Initiation of conversation
Comments:

A I NO   b. Topic choice
Comments:

© 1995 Thinking Publications. Duplication permitted for educational use only.

A I NO   c. Maintenance of conversational topics

                 Comments:

A I NO   d. Switch of topics using direct or indirect cues

                 Comments:

A I NO   e. Turn-taking

                 Comments:

A I NO   f. Repair/revision when necessary

                 Comments:

A I NO   g. Interruptions

                 Comments:

2. Verbal rules of politeness

A I NO   a. Appears not to talk too much or too little in the situation (quantity)

                 Comments:

A I NO   b. Appears to be honest and sincere

                 Comments:

© 1995 Thinking Publications. Duplication permitted for educational use only.

A   I   NO   c. Appears to make relevant contributions
Comments:

A   I   NO   d. Appears to express ideas clearly and concisely
Comments:

A   I   NO   e. Appears to be tactful
Comments:

3. Nonverbal rules

A   I   NO   a. Gestures
Comments:

A   I   NO   b. Facial expressions
Comments:

A   I   NO   c. Eye contact/gazing
Comments:

A   I   NO   d. Physical distance from partner (proxemics)
Comments:

© 1995 Thinking Publications. Duplication permitted for educational use only.

ADOLESCENT CONVERSATIONAL ANALYSIS PROFILE	APPROPRIATE	INAPPROPRIATE	NOT OBSERVED	*Communication Functions—Continued*	APPROPRIATE	INAPPROPRIATE	NOT OBSERVED
ROLE OF LISTENER				To express one's beliefs			
Vocabulary/Syntax				To indicate readiness			
Main Ideas*				To problem solve			
Nonjudgmental Manner				To entertain			
Feedback				**Conversational Rules**			
ROLE OF SPEAKER				Verbal (Topics/Turns)			
Language Features				Initiation			
Syntax				Topic choice			
Questions				Topic maintenance			
Figurative language				Topic switch			
Nonspecific language				Turn-taking*			
Precise vocabulary				Repair/revision			
Word-retrieval skills*				Interruptions			
Verbal mazes				Verbal (Politeness)			
False starts				Quantity			
Paralanguage Features				Sincerity			
Suprasegmental features				Relevance			
Fluency*				Clarity			
Intelligibility*				Tactfulness			
Communication Functions				Nonverbal			
To give information				Gestures			
To get information				Facial expressions			
To describe an event				Eye contact			
To persuade a listener				Proxemics			

_____*38*_____ TOTAL NUMBER OF ITEMS

_____ TOTAL NUMBER OF ITEMS MARKED "NOT OBSERVED"

_____ TOTAL NUMBER OF ITEMS RATED

_____ Number rated as inappropriate ÷ _____ Number of items rated x 100 = _____%

*If consistent problems are evident in this area, conduct additional assessment.

© 1995 Thinking Publication. Duplication permitted for educational use only.

NARRATIVE LEVELS ANALYSIS

Name: _____

Age: _____   Date: _____

Directions: Place check marks to reflect the highest level of narrative development for formulated and reformulated tasks.

COGNITIVE PERIOD	APPROXIMATE AGE OF EMERGENCE	NARRATIVE STAGE	TASKS	
			FORMULATED	REFORMULATED
Preoperational	2 years	Heaps		
	2 to 3 years	Sequences		
	3 to 4 years	Primitive Narratives		
	4 to 4½ years	Unfocused Chains		
	5 years	Focused Chains		
	5 to 7 years	True Narratives		
Concrete	7 to 11 years	Narrative Summaries		
	11 to 12 years	Complex Narratives		
Formal	13 to 15 years	Analysis		
	16 to Adulthood	Generalization		

Description of Formulated Task: _____

Description of Reformulated Task: _____

Comments: _____

_____

_____

© 1995 Thinking Publications. Duplication permitted for educational use only.

PROTOTYPE DELIVERY MODEL

The prototype delivery model that is proposed has evolved out of models previously described (Boyce and Larson, 1983; Larson and McKinley, 1985a; McKinley and Larson, 1985). The model consists of six major components: information dissemination, identification, assessment, program planning, intervention, and follow-up. [See pages 298–299.] All six components must be intact to ensure that appropriate services are provided to adolescents with communication disorders. Mutual interdependency exists among components. A missing component, or lack of coordination, will result in disparate services.

Each of the six components of the delivery model includes direct and indirect services. Direct services refer to activities in which speech-language pathologists have actual contact time with adolescents who are, or may be, viable candidates for speech-language services. For example, selectively screening adolescents with suspected communication disorders, assessing the adolescents, and providing intervention sessions are direct services in the sense that the interactions are between the speech-language pathologist and the adolescent. Indirect services refer to activities in which speech-language pathologists do not have actual contact time with adolescents. Rather, they assist, train, and consult with other persons important to the adolescent (e.g., a teacher, a parent, a friend) for the benefit of the adolescent with a communication disorder. For example, training professionals to utilize a referral form to identify adolescents

with suspected communication disorders and organizing parent support meetings are indirect services.

Whenever indirect services are discussed hereafter, reference will be to the adolescent's environmental and educational systems. The environmental system refers to family members and peers who interact with the adolescent with a communication disorder. The educational system encompasses the adolescent's structured learning situations and the speech-language pathologist's interactions with professionals and paraprofessionals in those settings. Learning situations may be traditional (e.g., a senior high school) or nontraditional (e.g., homebound instruction for hospitalized youth; instruction at a juvenile delinquency center for incarcerated adolescents). The professionals who may be involved within the educational system are classroom teachers, administrators, special educators, social workers, psychologists, guidance and vocational counselors, nurses, and probation officers. The paraprofessionals who may be involved are teacher aides, communication aides, and peer tutors. Obviously, the educational system is a part of the environmental system. However, since the educational system plays a major role during adolescence, that system is presented as a separate area within indirect services.

A comprehensive delivery model includes both direct and indirect services. While an individual adolescent might receive only direct or only indirect services, it is more common that a combination of direct and indirect services is needed.

INFORMATION DISSEMINATION

The first component, information dissemination, refers to educating people about adolescents' communication disorders and varied characteristics. Information dissemination is synonymous with what business calls "marketing the product." Surveys have found limited awareness of speech-language pathology services both in rural (Killarney and Lass, 1981) and large metropolitan areas (Pearlstein, Russell, and Fink, 1977). Van Hattum (1983) wisely asserted:

> No matter how good, how precise, how dependable our product is, it won't sell without marketing. . . . Overall, the person on the street has no more idea what we do than he or she did in 1940. . . . We have maintained our own feelings of professionalism and ethical cleanliness by minimizing our expressions of our importance and of minimizing our public relations effort. . . . People must know we are there, must know what and who we are, must be aware of our competence, must know we do better than anyone else can. (pp. 48–49)

This seems especially true as it relates to speech-language services for adolescents: The average person does not know what can be done. Sometimes, even those within the discipline of communication sciences and disorders do not know what can be done or how best to proceed. Normally, jobs are already in existence, but jobs with the adolescent population frequently need to be created. Professionals need to express with clarity and conviction why a school board should add a new speech-language pathologist to work at the secondary level during hard economic times. (After all, they reason, if the communication disorder was not cured during elementary years, why spend more time and money now?) Perpetuating a lack of visibility makes professionals vulnerable to being considered an expendable service. Thus, it puts at risk any guarantee of appropriate services to adolescents with communication disorders.

Visibility of speech-language pathology must be heightened for adolescents (direct services) as well as for persons important to the adolescent (indirect services). As adolescents and the people around them become aware of what constitutes a communication disorder and how they might benefit from a speech-language program, the identification component is activated. Until people know what constitutes a communication disorder during adolescence, what impact such a problem can have on the individual, and what intervention services can be provided, referral for a suspected disorder will not occur.

IDENTIFICATION

The second component in the delivery model is identification, the process of defining which adolescents have a suspected communication disorder that warrants further evaluation by a speech-language pathologist. Many agencies rely on screening for identification. The term *screening* refers to "the use of a systematic procedure to identify provisionally those [individuals] from a population who manifest, or are likely to manifest, an attribute which is judged to require special attention" (Hill, 1970, p. 1). Complete screening programs involve at least three elements: (1) a goal (i.e., for what are we screening?);

(2) a screening procedure; (3) a criterion against which the effectiveness of the procedure can be measured (Hill, 1970). Unfortunately, a more common practice has been to begin with an instrument, assume the goal is clearly established, and hope that some criterion may be found that will evaluate effectiveness. Models of screening (Hill, 1970) include:

1. The Illness Model

2. The Developmental Model

3. The Crisis Model

4. The Match-Mismatch Model

The Illness Model looks for problematic behaviors regarded as symptoms of underlying pathology. The Developmental Model focuses on delays in the onset of behaviors expected to emerge at a given age. This screening instrument yields information that can be compared with developmental norms. The Crisis Model detects individuals who are having difficulty coping with a crisis (e.g., loss of a parent through death or separation, retention in a class). The Match-Mismatch Model detects students who fail to match the expectations of others who constitute a given social environment (e.g., a high school). This model anchors screening to the social system in which the problematic behavior occurs. We recommend this model as the most appropriate to use with adolescents.

ASSESSMENT

Assessment, the third component in the delivery model, is the thorough documentation of speech-language-hearing performance. A primary question to answer during assessment is where is the problem (i.e., within the

adolescent, within the educational system, and/or within the environmental system). A thorough assessment considers not only the adolescent's performance, but also the contributing factors from other situations (e.g., school, home).

The adolescent's school experience must be considered, to determine if the problem may be within the educator and/or the curriculum. The educator may lack the ability to teach. The curriculum may not be sequentially organized or at an appropriate developmental level. The educator's inability to teach and inappropriate curriculum should not be misdiagnosed as a language disorder within the adolescent. For example, if many students are struggling to comprehend the content presented by a specific teacher, it would be erroneous to diagnose those students as having language disorders. At the same time, the student with a language disorder within such a classroom is likely to experience extreme frustration. A thorough assessment isolates how much of the academic difficulty can be attributed to the student and how much to flaws within the educational system.

Professionals must consider the environmental system during assessment, to rule out the possibility that a language difference exists. Students with adequate language for their primary linguistic community risk being labeled as disordered if environmental conditions are ignored.

The adolescent's evaluation (direct services) may include obtaining appropriate case history data and administering instruments and informal testing procedures, such as analysis of a representative spontaneous language sample (Boyce and Larson, 1983; Loban, 1976). Indirect assessment services may include analysis of curricula materials for language, surveying teacher attitudes toward communication disorders, and observing how peers with normal language interact.

Assessment should confirm or reject initial impressions of a communication disorder observed during identification and determine if it constitutes a handicapping condition that warrants special services. Assessment should also document the awareness that adolescents have about their communication disorder, and their motivation to modify their communication behaviors. Adolescents with documented communication disorders who acknowledge their problem, and are willing to work to improve their communication, may be better candidates for program planning than adolescents without these traits.

PROGRAM PLANNING

The fourth component, program planning, is the connecting link between assessment and intervention. Before effective intervention can occur, an appropriate individual plan must be drafted. This planning might involve the adolescent directly. For example, adolescents may offer suggestions for their own goals and objectives (e.g., Individualized Educational Program in the schools). Indirect services related to program planning might include planning with teachers on how to modify curricula or how to modify the learning environment for the benefit of the adolescent.

Program planning occurs both before an adolescent's entrance into intervention as well as during the adolescent's involvement. Ongoing program planning might involve contracting with the adolescent to learn specific behaviors, or earning points toward a quarterly grade for speech and language.

INTERVENTION

Intervention, the fifth component in the delivery model, refers to any method of ameliorating or reducing the communication disorder within the adolescent. One of the primary goals of intervention during the period of adolescence is acquisition of functional communication for academic, personal-social, and vocational settings. As such, intervention will involve a coordination of efforts among a variety of professionals who may be working with the adolescent in different environments. The *Stage I*—early adolescent will tend to have intervention goals and activities directed toward functional communication for academic and personal-social settings. The *Stage II*—middle adolescent will often have functional communication goals for all three settings: academic, personal-social, and vocational. By *Stage III*—late adolescence, goals of intervention usually focus upon personal-social and vocational settings.

Intervention for a given adolescent may include direct or indirect services, or a combination. Direct services may be delivered through an itinerant program, a resource room, or a self-contained classroom (Committee on Language, Speech, and Hearing Services in Schools, 1983). Indirect services frequently employ a consultation model. Such a model has become a viable and important alternative to direct services. Frassinelli, Superior, and Meyers (1983) define consultation as "a three person chain of service in which a consultant interacts with a caregiver (consultee) to benefit an individual (client) for whom the caregiver is responsible" (p. 25). Consultation enables a larger population to be served, and it retains a natural environmental setting for communication. Consultation may be combined with some direct services, periodic or ongoing (Frassinelli, Superior, and Meyers, 1983).

While consultation is typically thought of in conjunction with teachers, the families of adolescents cannot be forgotten. The families are an essential link to the generalization of newly acquired functional communication. At the same time, families may need information about the adolescent's communication deficits, and assistance in coping with their feelings.

Intervention will vary in intensity and content, depending upon the individual needs of the adolescent. Ongoing assessment and program planning during intervention, whether it be direct or indirect, are necessary to remain most responsive to the changing needs and abilities of youth with communication disorders.

FOLLOW-UP

The last component in the prototype delivery model is follow-up. Follow-up refers to any activity designed to measure the real and perceived benefits of speech-language programs. We believe that the discipline of communication sciences and disorders has not validated its intervention approaches. For a given communication disorder, little evidence exists that approach X is more successful than approach Y.

Current research shows a "continuum of failure" as children grow older, i.e., young children with language deficits often have residual problems during adolescence. If they do receive intervention during the secondary level, will these youth continue to experience significant communication problems during their post high school years? Only valid follow-up studies will begin to answer this question.

Adolescents who receive speech-language services might be involved in follow-up activities (direct services), or other adults might be used as informants (indirect services). If follow-up activities are used, they should occur both during speech-language services and after services are terminated.

From *Communication Assessment and Intervention Strategies for Adolescents* (pp. 56–61) by V. L. Larson and N. L. McKinley, 1987, Eau Claire, WI: Thinking Publications. © 1987 by Thinking Publications. Reprinted with permission.

PROTOTYPE DELIVERY MODEL						
WHO?	INFORMATION DISSEMINATION		IDENTIFICATION		ASSESSMENT	
	WHAT?	HOW?	WHAT?	HOW?	WHAT?	HOW?
DIRECT — Adolescents Early Middle Late	Expections and problems; Normal developmental data; Benefits of adequate communication; Self-referral process; Prevention	Publications; Career days, job fairs; Classroom lectures; Intake screening	Match-mismatch with expectations for communication	Self-referral; Selective screening	History; Learning style; Cognition; Comprehension and production of linguistic features; Discourse; Nonverbal communication; Survival language skills	Informal assessment (administration, analysis, interpretation) A. Case history form B. Learning style questionnaire C. Discourse samples 1. Conversations 2. Narrations D. Directed tasks; Formal assessment instruments (administration, analysis, interpretation)
INDIRECT — Educational System Members	Expectations and problems; Normal developmental data; Benefits of adequate communication; Referral process; How related professionals can help the adolescent; Prevention	Inservice; Media; Telecom-muni-cations	Match-mismatch with expectations for communication	Observational checklist referral forms	Structure of system; Teacher's language; Teachers' and administrators' attitudes; Curriculum variables	Structure of educational system checklist; Self-evaluation technique; Attitudinal scale; Curriculum analysis form
INDIRECT — Environmental System Members	Expectations and problems; Normal developmental data; Benefits of adequate communication; Referral process; How family and friends can help the adolescent; Prevention	Media; Telecom-muni-cations; Informational and support meetings	Match-mismatch with expectations for communication	Observational checklist referral forms	Family members' perceptions of the adolescent; Environmental system members' feelings and attitudes; Communication styles	Interviews; Obervation

(continued)

PROTOTYPE DELIVERY MODEL—*Continued*									
		PROGRAM PLANNING			**INTERVENTION**			**FOLLOW-UP**	
	WHO?	**WHAT?**	**HOW?**		**WHAT?**	**HOW?**		**WHAT?**	**HOW?**
DIRECT	Adolescents Early Middle Late	Adolescent's involvement; Adolescent's attitude; Group versus individual sessions; Program selection	Writing goals and objectives; Motivational procedures; Group characteristics; Selecting programs		Thinking; Listening; Speaking; Nonverbal communication; Survival language	General procedures A. Mediation B. Bridging C. Discussion; Selected specific methods A. Referential communication activities B. Simulation and role-playing activities C. Narrative skill building activities; Commercial resources		Baseline data; Benefits of program	Study design; Survey methodology A. Interviews B. Questionnaires
INDIRECT	Educational System Members	Educational policies and procedures; Consultation; Peer involvement and attitude modification	Administrator's involvement; Collaborative approach; Peer tutoring		Modifications of the system	Consultation A. Curriculum committee participation B. Content area tutoring C. Adaptation of classroom discourse D. Adaptation of materials		Benefits of services for adolescents; Benefits of consultation model; Benefits of counseling	Survey methodology A. Interviews B. Questinnaires
	Environmental System Members	Alteration or maintenance of parents' attitudes and behaviors; Awareness of referral agencies; Sibling acceptance and involvement	Informational and support meetings; Newsletters, phone campaigns, home visits; Sibling tutoring		Modifications of the system	Counseling		Benefits of services for adolescents; Benefits of consultation model; Benefits of counseling	Survey methodology A. Interviews B. Questionnaires

FOLLOW-UP QUESTIONNAIRE

COVER LETTER

Dear _____:

    We are collecting information from people who were in the speech-language program in high school. We have very little information about people like you. We would like you to help with a project that will study the benefits of the speech-language program while you were in high school. It will take you about _____ minutes to complete the questionnaire I have sent.

    This questionnaire has been approved by the Review Board for the Protection of Human Subjects. If you have any complaints about your participation in this study, please contact _____ at _____.

    Your participation in the project is completely voluntary. You may refuse to participate. It will not be held against you. If you decide not to participate, throw the questionnaire away.

    It is all right to ask for help to read the questionnaire. You may also ask someone to explain unfamiliar words. However, you should decide the answers to the questions by yourself. Send your questionnaire back to me in the self-addressed envelope.

    The questionnaire is anonymous. Please do not write your name or address anywhere on the questionnaire or the return envelope. Your information will be combined with that of others. Your cooperation is very important for the success of this study. I hope you will participate in the study. If you have any questions about this study, contact me at _____. Thank you for your cooperation.

Sincerely,

_____
Speech-Language Pathologist

© 1995 Thinking Publications. Duplication permitted for educational use only.

SPEECH-LANGUAGE FOLLOW-UP QUESTIONNAIRE

PERSONAL DATA

Date of Follow-up: _____

Middle/Junior High School Attended: _____

High School Attended: _____

Number of Years in Secondary-Level Speech-Language Programs:

_____ years, from calendar year _____ to _____

Are you the sole head of the household for tax purposes?

_____ No   _____ Yes

Are you living independently from your parents?   _____ No   _____ Yes

Number of Dependents: _____

Age at Time of this Follow-up:

_____ less than 20 years of age

_____ 20 to 25 years of age

_____ 25 to 30 years of age

_____ more than 30 years of age

EDUCATIONAL/EMPLOYMENT DATA

Educational Status: (Check one.)

_____ Credits toward high school diploma, but diploma is not yet earned

_____ High school diploma

_____ 1 to 2 years of vocational/technical education after high school

_____ 1 to 3 years of college education

_____ Earned B.S. or B.A. degree from college

_____ Other (Specify: _____)

© 1995 Thinking Publications. Duplication permitted for educational use only.

Work Experience: (Check one.)

_____ Fewer than 3 years of part-time employment

_____ More than 3 years of part-time employment

_____ Fewer than 3 years of full-time employment

_____ More than 3 years of full-time employment

_____ Other (Specify: _____)

Employment Skill Level: (Check one.)

_____ Primarily unskilled (little or no training required for the job)

_____ Semi-skilled (trained on the job)

_____ Vocationally/technically skilled (trained in school 1 to 3 years after high school)

_____ Professional (trained at the bachelor's degree level or more)

_____ Other (Specify: _____)

Number of Paid Jobs (held at the same time, or at different times): (Check one.)

_____ 3 or fewer jobs

_____ 4 to 6 jobs

_____ 7 to 10 jobs

_____ More than 10 jobs

Average Income Earned:

1. Per Hour: (Check one.)

_____ Minimum wage

_____ Between minimum wage and $1 beyond minimum wage

_____ $1 to $2 beyond minimum wage

_____ $2 to $3 beyond minimum wage

_____ $3 to $4 beyond minimum wage

_____ More than $4 beyond minimum wage

© 1995 Thinking Publications. Duplication permitted for educational use only.

2. Per Year (Individual): (Check one.)

_____ Less than $5,000

_____ $5,000 to $10,000

_____ $10,001 to $15,000

_____ $15,001 to $20,000

_____ $20,001 to $25,000

_____ Over $25,001

3. Per Year (Joint Income): (Check one, if applicable.)

_____ Less than $5,000

_____ $5,000 to $10,000

_____ $10,001 to $15,000

_____ $15,001 to $20,000

_____ $20,001 to $25,000

_____ Over $25,001

BENEFITS RECEIVED FROM THE SPEECH-LANGUAGE PROGRAM

Use this scale for the questions below.

1	2	3	4	5
Not at all	A little bit	Some	Quite a bit	A great amount

1. On a scale from 1 to 5, how much do you think your participation in the speech-language program helped you in school? _____

2. On a scale from 1 to 5, how much do you think your participation in the speech-language program helped you to relate better to people? _____

3. On a scale from 1 to 5, how much do you think your participation in the speech-language program helped you to perform better at work? _____

ADDITIONAL COMMENTS (Please note on the back of this sheet.)

© 1995 Thinking Publications. Duplication permitted for educational use only.

REFERENCES

Abel, E. (1990). *Fetal alcohol syndrome.* Oradell, NJ: Medical Economics Books.

Abkarian, G., Jones, A., and West, G. (1992). Young children's idiom comprehension: Trying to get the picture. *Journal of Speech and Hearing Research, 35,* 580–587.

Ackerman, B. (1982). On comprehending idioms: Do children get the picture? *Journal of Experimental Child Psychology, 33,* 439–454.

Adams, G., Montemayor, R., and Gullotta, T. (1989). *Biology of adolescent behavior and development.* London: Sage Publications.

Adams, W. (1980). Adolescence. In S. Gabel and M. Erickson (Eds.), *Child development and developmental disabilities* (pp. 59–84). Boston, MA: Little, Brown, and Company.

Agency for Instructional Technology. (1984). *Solutions unlimited* [Computer software]. Bloomington, IN: Author.

Alexander, F. (1993). National standards: A new conventional wisdom. *Educational Leadership, 50*(5), 9–10.

Alexander, W., and McEwin, C. (1989). *Schools in the middle: Status and progress.* Columbus, OH: National Middle School Association.

Alley, G., and Deshler, D. (1979). *Teaching the learning disabled adolescent: Strategies and methods.* Denver, CO: Love Publishing.

Allington, R., and Fleming, J. (1978). The misreading of high-frequency words. *Journal of Special Education, 12,* 417–421.

American Educational Research Association, American Psychological Association, and National Council on Measurement in Education. (1985). *Standards for educational and psychological testing.* Washington, DC: American Psychological Association.

American Speech-Language-Hearing Association. (1985). Clinical management of communicatively handicapped minority language populations. *Asha, 27*(6), 29–32.

American Speech-Language-Hearing Association. (1988). Inside the national office: Office of minority concerns. *Asha, 30*(8), 23–25.

American Speech-Language-Hearing Association. (1992a). Communication and the ADA. *Asha, 34*(6/7), 62–67.

American Speech-Language-Hearing Association. (1992b). The dream . . . an accessible America. *Asha, 34*(6/7), 35–61.

American Speech-Language-Hearing Association Ad Hoc Committee on Instrument Evaluation. (1986, August). *Report of the committee submitted to the Executive Board.* Rockville, MD: Author.

Applebee, A. (1978). *The child's concept of story.* Chicago, IL: University of Chicago Press.

Applebee, A. (1981). *Writing in the secondary school*. Urbana, IL: National Council of Teachers of English.

Applebee, A., Auten, A., and Lehr, F. (1981). *Writing in the secondary school: English and the content areas*. Urbana, IL: National Council of Teachers of English.

Aram, D., and Hall, N. (1989). Longitudinal follow-up of children with preschool communication disorders: Treatment implications. *School Psychology Review, 18*, 487–501.

Aram, D., Ekelman, B., and Nation, J. (1984). Preschoolers with language disorders: 10 years later. *Journal of Speech and Hearing Research, 27*, 232–244.

Arlin, P. (1975). Cognitive development in adulthood: "A fifth stage?" *Developmental Psychology, 11*, 602–606.

Arwood E. (1983). *Pragmaticism: Theory and application*. Rockville, MD: Aspen.

Asch, S., and Nerlove, H. (1960). The development of double function terms in children: An exploratory investigation. In B. Kaplan and S. Wapner (Eds.), *Perspectives in psychological theory: Essays in honor of Heinz Werner* (pp. 47–60). New York: International Universities Press.

Ashear, V., and Snortum. J. (1971). Eye contact in children as a function of age, sex, social and intellectual variables. *Developmental Psychology, 4*, 479.

Associated Press. (1992, September 21). Communication skills said lacking: Businesses say workers need help. *Oshkosh Northwestern*, p. 12.

Atkins, C., and Cartwright, L. (1982). Preferred language elicitation procedures used in five age categories. *Asha, 24*, 321–323.

Austin, J. (1962). *How to do things with words*. London: Oxford University Press.

Bakan, D. (1971). Adolescence in America: From ideal to social fact. *Daedalus, 100*, 981.

Bandura, A., and Walters, R. (1963). *Social learning and personality development*. New York: Holt, Rinehart and Winston.

Barber, L., and McClellan, M. (1987). Looking at America's dropouts: Who are they? *Phi Delta Kappan, 69*(4), 264–267.

Barker, L. (1971). *Listening behavior*. Englewood Cliffs, NJ: Prentice-Hall.

Bart, W. (1971). The factor structure of formal operations. *British Journal of Educational Psychology, 41*, 40–77.

Benedict, R. (1954). Continuities and discontinuities in cultural conditioning. In W. Martin and C. Stendler (Eds.), *Readings in child development* (pp. 142–148). New York: Harcourt, Brace.

Bergman, M. (1987). Social grace or disgrace: Adolescent social skills and learning disability subtypes. *Reading, Writing, and Learning Disabilities, 3*, 161–166.

Bernstein, D. (1989). Assessing children with limited English proficiency: Current perspectives. *Topics in Language Disorders, 9*(3), 15–20.

Berzonsky, M. (1978). Formal reasoning in adolescence: An alternate view. *Adolescence, 13*, 279–290.

Birdwhistell, R. (1970). *Kinesics and context.* Philadelphia, PA: University of Pennsylvania Press.

Blackwell, P., Engen, E., Fischgrund, J., and Zarcadoolas, C. (1978). *Sentences and other systems: A language and learning curriculum for hearing-impaired children.* Washington, DC: Alexander Graham Bell Association.

Blalock, J. (1981) Persistent problems and concerns of young adults with learning disabilities. In W. Cruickshank and A. Silver (Eds.), *Bridges to tomorrow: Vol. 2* (pp. 35–56). Syracuse, NY: Syracuse University Press.

Blalock, J. (1982). Persistent auditory language deficits in adults with learning disabilities. *Journal of Learning Disabilities, 15,* 604–609.

Blanck, P., and Rosenthal, R. (1982). Developing strategies for decoding "leaky" messages: On learning how and when to decode discrepant and consistent social communications. In R. Feldman (Ed.), *Development of nonverbal behavior in children* (pp. 203–229). New York: Springer-Verlag.

Bliss, L. (1993). *Pragmatic language intervention: Interactive activities.* Eau Claire, WI: Thinking Publications.

Bloom, B. (Ed.). (1956). *Taxonomy of educational objectives: The classification of education goals. Handbook I—Cognitive domain.* New York: Longman.

Bloom, L., and Lahey, M. (1978). *Language development and language disorders.* New York: John Wiley.

Blosser, J., and DePompei, R. (1989). The head-injured student returns to school: Recognizing and treating deficits. *Topics in Language Disorders, 9*(2), 67–77.

Blue, C. (1975). The marginal communicator. *Language, Speech, and Hearing Services in Schools, 6,* 32–37.

Botvin, G., and Sutton-Smith, B. (1977). The development of structural complexity in children's fantasy narratives. *Developmental Psychology, 13,* 377–388.

Boyce, N., and Larson, V. L. (1983). *Adolescents' communication: Development and disorders.* Eau Claire, WI: Thinking Publications.

Boyett, J., and Conn, H. (1992). *Workplace 2000: The revolution reshaping American business.* New York: Plume Publishing.

Bracewell, R., Scardamalia, M., and Bereiter, C. (1982). Cognitive processes in composing and comprehending discourse. *Educational Psychologist, 17*(3), 146–164.

Broughton, J. (1977). Beyond formal operations: Theoretical thoughts in adolescence. *Teachers College Record, 79,* 87–97.

Brown, A., and Smiley, S. (1977). Rating the importance of structural units of prose passages: A problem of metacognitive development. *Child Development, 48,* 1–8.

Brown, B. Byers, and Beveridge, M. (1979). *Language disorders in children, Monograph, No. 1.* London: College of Speech Therapists.

Brown, B. Byers, and Edwards, M. (1989). *Developmental disorders of language.* San Diego, CA: Singular.

Brown, R. (1973). *A first language: The early stages*. Cambridge, MA: Harvard University Press.

Brown, V., Hammill, D., and Wiederholt, J. (1986). *Test of reading comprehension* (Rev. ed.). Austin, TX: Pro-Ed.

Bryan, T. (1977). Children's comprehension of nonverbal communication. *Journal of Learning Disabilities, 10*, 501–506.

Bryan, T., Donahue, M., and Pearl, R. (1981). Studies of learning disabled children's pragmatic competence. *Topics in Learning and Learning Disabilities, 1*(2), 29–39.

Bryant, B., and Wiederholt, J. (1991). *Gray oral reading tests—Diagnostic*. Austin, TX: Pro-Ed.

Budoff, M. (1987). Measures for assessing learning potential. In C. Lidz (Ed.), *Dynamic assessment: An interactional approach to evaluating learning potential* (pp. 173–195). New York: Guilford Press.

Bunce, B. (1989). Using a barrier game format to improve children's referential communication skills. *Journal of Speech and Hearing Disorders, 54*, 33–43.

Byrne, S., Constant, A., and Moore, G. (1992). Making transitions from school to work. *Educational Leadership, 49*(6), 23–26.

Campione, J., and Brown, A. (1987). Linking dynamic assessment with school achievement. In C. Lidz (Ed.), *Dynamic assessment: An interactional approach to evaluating learning potential* (pp. 82–115). New York: Guilford Press.

Carey, A. (1992a). Get involved: Multiculturally. *Asha, 34*(5), 3–4.

Carey, A. (1992b). Americans with disabilities act and you. *Asha, 34*(6/7), 5–6.

Carlson, A. (1993, January 26). *State of the state address*. St. Paul, MN: Minnesota Public Radio.

Carpenter, L. (1990). *Including multicultural content in the undergraduate communication disorders curriculum: A resource guide and reference document*. Unpublished manuscript, University of Wisconsin at Eau Claire.

Casby, M. (1988). Speech-language pathologists' attitudes and involvement regarding language and reading. *Language, Speech, and Hearing Services in Schools, 19*, 352–358.

Casby, M. (1992). The cognitive hypothesis and its influence on speech-language services in schools. *Language, Speech, and Hearing Services in Schools, 23*, 198–202.

Case, R. (1984). The process of stage transition: A neo-Piagetian view. In R. Sternberg (Ed.), *Mechanisms of cognitive development* (pp. 19–44). New York: Freeman.

Case, R. (1985). *Intellectual development: Birth to adulthood*. Orlando, FL: Academic Press.

Cetron, M., and Gayle, M. (1990, September/October). Educational renaissance: 43 trends for U.S. schools. *The Futurist*, pp. 33–40.

Chall, J. (1983). *Stages of reading development*. New York: McGraw-Hill.

Chamberlain, P., and Medinos-Landurand, P. (1991). Practical considerations for the assessment of LEP students with special needs. In E. Hamayan and J. Damico (Eds.), *Limiting bias in the assessment of bilingual students* (pp. 111–156). Austin, TX: Pro-Ed.

Chapman, R. (1972). Some simple ways of talking about normal language and communication. In J. McLean, D. Yoder, and R. Schiefelbusch (Eds.), *Language intervention with the retarded: Developing strategies* (pp. 17–32). Baltimore, MD: University Park Press.

Chapman, R. (1981). Exploring children's communicative intents. In J. Miller (Ed.), *Assessing language production in children* (pp. 111–136). Baltimore, MD: University Park Press.

Chappell, G. (1980). Oral language performance of upper elementary school students obtained via story reformulation. *Language, Speech, and Hearing Services in Schools, 11*, 236–250.

Chomsky, C. (1969). *The acquisition of syntax in children from 5 to 10.* Cambridge, MA: MIT Press.

Clark, D. (1988). *Dyslexia: Theory and practice of remedial instruction.* Parkton, MD: York Press.

Coats, D. (1991). America's youth: A crisis of character. *Imprimis: Journal of Hillsdale College, 20*(9), 1–6.

Cole, K., Mills, P., and Kelley, D. (1994). Agreement of assessment profiles used in cognitive referencing. *Language, Speech, and Hearing Services in Schools, 25*, 25–31.

Cole, L. (1983). Implications of the position on social dialects. *Asha, 25*(9), 25–27.

Coles, R. (1983, September 4). The age of insolence: Those terrible teens. *Family Weekly,* pp. 4–5.

Committee on Language, Speech, and Hearing Services in Schools. (1983). Recommended service delivery models and caseload sizes for speech-language pathology services in the schools. *Asha, 25*, 65–70.

Committee on the Status of Racial Minorities. (1983). Social dialects: Position paper. *Asha, 25*(9), 23–24.

Conger, J. (1973). *Adolescence and youth psychological development in a changing world.* New York: Harper and Row.

Costa, A. (1993). How world-class standards will change us. *Educational Leadership, 50*(5), 50–51.

Council for Exceptional Children. (1994). *Teaching Exceptional Children, 26*(3) (Suppl.), 1–4.

Crager, R., and Spriggs, A. (1969). Development of concept utilization. *Developmental Psychology, 1*, 415–424.

Crago, M. (1990, April). Professional gatekeeping: The multicultural, multilingual challenge. *Communique,* pp. 10–13.

Crago, M., and Cole, E. (1991). Using ethnography to bring children's communicative and cultural worlds into focus. In T. Gallagher (Ed.), *Pragmatics of language: Clinical practice issues* (pp. 99–131). San Diego, CA: Singular.

Craig, H. (1983). Applications of pragmatic language models for intervention. In T. Gallagher and C. Prutting (Eds.), *Pragmatic assessment and intervention issues in language* (pp. 101–128). San Diego, CA: College-Hill.

Crais, E. (1990). World knowledge to word knowledge. *Topics in Language Disorders, 10*, 45–62.

Creaghead, N. (1992). Classroom interactional analysis/script analysis. In J. Damico (Ed.), *Best practices in school speech-language pathology* (pp. 65–72). San Antonio, TX: Psychological Corporation.

Creaghead, N., and Tattershall, S. (1991). Observation and assessment of classroom pragmatic skills. In C. Simon (Ed), *Communication skills and classroom success: Assessment and therapy methodologies for language and learning disabled students* (pp. 106–122). Eau Claire, WI: Thinking Publications.

Cruttenden, A. (1985). Intonation comprehension in ten-year-olds. *Journal of Child Language, 12*, 643–661.

Crystal, D. (1982). *Profiling linguistic disability.* London: Edward Arnold.

Crystal, D., Fletcher, P., and Garman, M. (1991). *The grammatical analysis of language disability: A procedure for assessment and remediation.* San Diego, CA: Singular.

Culatta, B., Page, J., and Ellis, J. (1983). Story retelling as a communicative performance screening tool. *Language, Speech, and Hearing Services in Schools, 14*, 66–78.

Cummins, J. (1989). A theoretical framework for bilingual special education. *Exceptional Children, 56*(2), 111–119.

Damico, J. (1988). The lack of efficacy in language therapy: A case study. *Language, Speech, and Hearing Services in Schools, 19*(1), 51–66.

Damico, J. (1991). Clinical discourse analysis: A functional approach to language assessment. In C. Simon (Ed.), *Communication skills and classroom success: Assessment and therapy methodologies for language and learning disabled students* (pp. 125–150). Eau Claire, WI: Thinking Publications.

Damico, J. (1992). Using a whole language framework for language intervention. *The Clinical Connection, 6*(1), 10–13.

Damico, J. (1993). Language assessment in adolescents: Addressing critical issues. *Language, Speech, and Hearing Services in Schools, 24*, 29–35.

Damico, J., and Armstrong, M. (1991). Empowerment in the clinical context: The speech-language pathologist as advocate. *The NSSLHA Journal, 18*, 34–43.

Damico, J., and Damico, S. (1993). Language and social skills from a diversity perspective: Considerations for the speech-language pathologist. *Language, Speech, and Hearing Services in Schools, 24*, 236–243.

Davelaar, E. (1977). Formal operational reasoning and its relationship to complex speech patterns and tentative statement use. *Language and Speech, 20*(1), 73–79.

Davis, A. (1944). Socialization and adolescent personality. In N. Henry (Ed.), *Adolescence, yearbook of the national society for the study of education: Volume 43. Part 1* (pp. 198–216). Chicago, IL: University of Chicago, Department of Education.

DeAjuriaguerra, J., Jaeggi, A., Guignard, F., Kocher, F., Maguard, M., Roch, S., and Schmid, E. (1976). The development and prognosis of dysphasia in children. In D. Morehead and A. Morehead (Eds.), *Normal and deficient child language* (pp. 345–386). Baltimore, MD: University Park Press.

de Bettencourt, L. (1987). Strategy training: A need for clarification. *Exceptional Children, 54*(1), 24–30.

DePaulo, B., and Jordan, A. (1982). Age changes in deceiving and detecting deceit. In R. Feldman (Ed.), *Development of nonverbal behavior in children* (pp. 151–180). New York: Springer-Verlag.

Deshler, D., and Schumaker, J. (1983). Social skills of learning disabled adolescents: Characteristics and intervention. *Topics in Learning and Learning Disabilities, 3*(2), 15–23.

Dimitrovsky, L. (1964). The ability to identify the emotional meaning of vocal expressions at successive age levels. In J. Davitz (Ed.), *The communication of emotional meaning* (pp. 69–86). New York: McGraw-Hill.

DiSimoni, F. (1978). *Token test for children.* Chicago, IL: Riverside.

Dittman, A. (1972). Developmental factors in conversational behavior. *Journal of Communication, 22,* 404–423.

Dollaghan, C. (1987). Comprehension monitoring in normal and language-impaired children. *Topics in Language Disorders, 7*(2), 45–60.

Dolphin C. (1991). Variables in the use of personal space. In *Intercultural communication: A reader* (pp. 320–329). Belmont, CA: Wadsworth.

Donahue, M. (1984). Learning disabled children's conversational competence: An attempt to activate the inactive listener. *Applied Psycholinguistics, 5,* 21–35.

Donahue, M. (1985). Communicative style in learning disabled children: Some implications for classroom discourse. In P. Ripich and F. Spinelli (Eds.), *School discourse problems* (pp. 97–124). San Diego, CA: College-Hill.

Donahue, M., and Bryan, T. (1984). Communicative skills and peer relations of learning disabled adolescents. *Topics in Language Disorders, 4,* 10–21.

Donahue, M., Pearl, R., and Bryan, T. (1980). Learning disabled children's conversational competence: Responses to inadequate messages. *Applied Psycholinguistics 1,* 387–403.

Donahue, M., Pearl, R., and Bryan, T. (1982). Learning disabled children's syntactic proficiency on a communicative task. *Journal of Speech and Hearing Disorders, 47,* 397–403.

Dore, J. (1974). A pragmatic description of early language development. *Journal of Psycholinguistics, 3,* 343–350.

Dore, J. (1975). Holophrases, speech acts, and language universals. *Journal of Child Language, 2,* 21–40.

Dorval, B. (1980, April). *The development of conversation.* Paper presented at the Biennial Southeastern Conference on Human Development, Alexandria, VA.

Douglas, J., and Peel, B. (1979). The development of metaphor and proverb translation in children grades one through seven. *Journal of Educational Research, 73,* 116–119.

Duncan, D. M. (1989). *Working with bilingual language disability.* London: Chapman and Hall.

Duncan, S., Jr., and Fiske, D. (1977). *Face to face interaction: Research, methods, and therapy.* New York: John Wiley.

Duranti, A. (1988). Ethnography of speaking: Toward a linguistics of praxis. In F. Newmeyer (Ed.), *Linguistics: The Cambridge survey: Vol. 4. Language: The socio-cultural context* (pp. 210–228). Cambridge, UK: Cambridge University Press.

Edmondson, W. (1981). *Spoken discourse: A model for analysis.* New York: Longman.

Eisenberg, L. (1965). A developmental approach to adolescence. *Children, 12,* 131–135.

Eisner, E. (1965). Critical thinking: Some cognitive components. *Teachers College Record, 66,* 624–634.

Elder, G. (1975). Adolescence in the life cycle: An introduction. In S. Dragastin and G. Elder, Jr. (Eds.), *Adolescence in the life cycle: Psychological change and social context* (pp. 1–22). Washington, DC: Hemisphere Publishing.

Elkind, D. (1974). *Children and adolescents: Interpretive essays on Jean Piaget.* New York: Oxford University Press.

Elkind, D. (1975). Recent research on cognitive development in adolescents. In E. Sigmund, S. Dragastin, and G. Elder, Jr. (Eds.), *Adolescence in the life cycle: Psychological change and social context* (pp. 49–62). New York: John Wiley.

Elkind, D. (1978). Understand the young adolescent. *Adolescence, 13*(49), 127–134.

Elkind, D., Barocas, R., and Johnsen, R. (1969). Concept production in children and adolescents. *Human Development, 12,* 10–21.

Ellis, E. (1989). A metacognitive intervention for increasing class participation. *Learning Disabilities Focus, 5*(1), 36–46.

Ellis, E., and Friend, P. (1991). Adolescents with learning disabilities. In B. Wong (Ed.), *Learning about learning disabilities* (pp. 506–563). San Diego, CA: Academic Press.

Ellsworth, P., and Sindt, V. (1991). *What every teacher should know about how students think: A survival guide for adults.* Eau Claire, WI: Thinking Publications.

Engler, L., Hannah, E., and Longhurst, T. (1973). Linguistic analysis of speech samples: A practical guide for clinicians. *Journal of Speech and Hearing Disorders, 38,* 192–204.

Epstein, H. (1974). Phrenoblysis: Special brain and mind growth periods. I. Human brain and skill development. *Developmental Psychobiology, 7,* 207–216.

Epstein, H. (1978). Growth spurts during brain development: Implications for educational policy and practice. In J. Chall and A. Mirsky (Eds.), *Education and the brain: The seventy-seventh yearbook of education* (pp. 343–370). Chicago, IL: University of Chicago Press.

Epstein, H. (1979). Cognitive growth and development: Brain growth and cognitive functions. *Colorado Journal of Educational Research, 19*(1), 4–5.

Epstein, J., and MacIver, D. (1990). *Education in the middle grades: Overview of national practices and trends.* Columbus, OH: National Middle School Association.

Epstein, H., and Toepfer, C. (1978). A neuroscience basis for reorganizing middle grades education. *Educational Leadership, 35*(8), 656–660.

Erikson, E. (1968). *Identity: Youth and crisis.* New York: W.W. Norton.

Everson, J., and Goodall, D. (1991). School-to-work transition for youth who are both deaf and blind. *Asha, 33*(11) 45–47.

Fawcett, G. (1994). Debatable issues underlying whole language philosophy: A literacy instructor's perspective. *Language, Speech, and Hearing Services in Schools, 25,* 37–39.

Fein, D. (1983). The prevalence of speech and language impairments. *Asha, 25*(2), 37.

Feldman, R., White, J., and Lobato, D. (1982). Social skills and nonverbal behavior. In R. Feldman (Ed.), *Development of nonverbal behavior in children* (pp. 257–274). New York: Springer-Verlag.

Ferguson, L. (1970). *Personality development.* Belmont, CA: Brooks/Cole.

Fersh, D., and Thomas, P. (1993). *Complying with the Americans with disabilities act: A guidebook for people with disabilities.* Westport, CT: Quorum Books.

Feuerstein, R. (1979). *The dynamic assessment of retarded performers: The learning potential assessment device. Theory instruments, and techniques.* Chicago, IL: Scott Foresman.

Feuerstein, R. (1980). *Instrumental enrichment.* Chicago, IL: Scott Foresman.

Feuerstein, R. (1983, November). *Instrumental enrichment training workshop.* Toronto, Ontario.

Fischer, K. (1980). Learning as the development of organized behavior. *Journal of Structural Learning, 3,* 253–267.

Fischer, K., and Corrigan, R. (1981). A skill approach to language development. In R. Stark (Ed.), *Language behavior in infancy and early childhood* (pp. 245–275). New York: Elsevier/North Holland.

Fischer, K., Hand, H., and Russell, S. (1984). The development of abstractions in adolescence and adulthood. In M. Commons, F. Richards, and C. Armon (Eds.), *Beyond formal operations* (pp. 43–73). New York: Praeger Scientific.

Fischer, K., and Pipp, S. (1984). Processes of cognitive development: Optimal level and skill acquisition. In R. Sternberg (Ed.), *Mechanisms of cognitive development* (pp. 45–81). New York: Freeman.

Flavell, J. (1976). Metacognitive aspects of problem solving. In L. Resnick (Ed.), *The nature of intelligence* (pp. 231–236). Hillsdale, NJ: Erlbaum.

Flavell, J. (1977). *Cognitive development.* Englewood Cliffs, NJ: Prentice-Hall.

Fonosch, G., and Schwab, L. (1981). Attitudes of selected university faculty members toward disabled students. *Journal of College Student Personnel, 22,* 229–235.

Frassinelli, L., Superior, K., and Meyers, J. (1983). A consultation model for speech and language intervention. *Asha, 25*(11), 25–30.

Freeman, D. (1983). *Margaret Mead and Samoa: The making and unmaking of an anthropological myth.* Cambridge, MA: Harvard University Press.

French, R. (1978). Nonverbal patterns in youth culture. *Educational Leadership, 35*(7), 541–546.

Freud, A. (1948). *The ego and the mechanism of defense.* New York: International Universities Press.

Freud, S. (1953). *A general introduction to psychoanalysis.* New York: Permabooks.

Furlong, M., and Morrison, G. (1994). Introduction to miniseries: School violence and safety in perspective. *School Psychology Review, 23*(2), 139–150.

Gajewski, N., and Mayo, P. (1989a). *SSS: Social skill strategies (Book A).* Eau Claire, WI: Thinking Publications.

Gajewski, N., and Mayo, P. (1989b). *SSS: Social skill strategies (Book B).* Eau Claire, WI: Thinking Publications.

Galda, S. (1981, April). *The development of the comprehension of metaphor.* Paper presented at the Annual Meeting of the American Educational Research Association, Los Angeles, CA.

Gall, M. (1981). *Handbook for evaluating and selecting curricula materials.* Boston, MA: Allyn and Bacon.

Gallagher, T. (1983). Pre-assessment: A procedure for accommodating language use variability. In T. Gallagher and C. Prutting (Eds.), *Pragmatic assessment and intervention issues in language* (pp. 1–28). San Diego, CA: College-Hill.

Gallagher, T. (1991). Language and social skills: Implications for assessment and intervention with school-age children. In T. Gallagher (Ed.), *Pragmatics of language: Clinical practice issues* (pp. 11–41). San Diego, CA: Singular.

Gardner, J. (1982). *The turbulent teens.* San Diego, CA: Oak Tree Publications.

Garnett, K. (1986). Telling tales: Narratives and learning-disabled children. *Topics in Language Disorders, 6,* 44–56.

Garvey, J., and Gordon, N. (1973). A follow-up study of children with disorders of speech and development. *British Journal of Disorders of Communication, 8,* 17–28.

Gates, G. (1923). An experimental study of the growth of social perception. Journal of *Educational Psychology, 14,* 449–461.

Geers, A., and Moog, J. (1978). Syntactic maturity of spontaneous speech and elicited imitations of hearing-impaired children. *Journal of Speech and Hearing Disabilities, 43,* 380–391.

George, P., Stevenson, C., Thomason, J., and Beane, J. (1992). *The middle school—and beyond*. Alexandria, VA: Association for Supervision and Curriculum Development.

German, D. (1992). Word-finding intervention for children and adolescents. *Topics in Language Disorders, 13*(1), 33–50.

German, D. (1993). *Word finding intervention program*. Tucson, AZ: Communication Skill Builders.

Gesell, A., Ilg, F., and Ames, L. (1956). *Youth: The years from ten to sixteen*. New York: Harper.

Getzel, E. Evans. (1990). Entering postsecondary programs: Early individualized planning. *Teaching Exceptional Children, 23*, 51–53.

Gillam, R., and Johnston, J. (1992). Spoken and written language relationships in language/learning-impaired and normally achieving school-age children. *Journal of Speech and Hearing Research, 35*, 1303–1315.

Gillespie, D. (1990). Involving business and education. *National Dropout Prevention Newsletter, 3*(1), 1–3.

Gillespie, S., and Cooper, E. (1973). Prevalence of speech problems in junior and senior high schools. *Journal of Speech and Hearing Research, 16*(4), 739–743.

Gilligan, C. (1982). New map of development: New vision of maturity. *American Journal of Orthopsychology, 52*(2), 199–212.

Goldstein, H., Arkell, C., Ashcroft, S., Hurley, O., and Lilly, M. (1975). In N. Hobbs (Ed.), *Issues in the classification of children* (Vol. 2, pp. 4–61). San Francisco, CA: Jossey-Bass.

Golumbia, L., and Hillman, S. (1990, August). *A comparison of learning disabled and nondisabled adolescent motivational processes*. Paper presented at the Annual Meeting of the American Psychological Association, Boston, MA.

Gray, L., and House, R. (1989). No guarantee of immunity: Aids and adolescents. In D. Capuzzi and D. Gross (Eds.), *Youth-at-risk: A resource for counselors, teachers, and parents* (pp. 231–270). Alexandria, VA: American Association for Counseling and Development.

Greenberg, K. (1990). Combining research and theoretical application: The cognet project. *International Journal of Cognitive Education and Mediated Learning, 1*(3), 237–244.

Greenfield, P., and Smith, J. (1976). *The structure of communication in early language development*. New York: Academic Press.

Greer, J., and Wethered, C. (1984). Learned helplessness: A piece of the burnout puzzle. *Exceptional Children, 50*(6), 524–531.

Gregg, N. (1983). College learning disabled writer: Error patterns and instructional alternatives. *Journal of Learning Disabilities, 16*, 334–338.

Grice, H. (1975). Logic and conversation. In P. Cole and J. Morgan (Eds.), *Syntax and semantics: Vol. 3. Speech acts* (pp. 41–58). New York: Academic Press.

Griffiths, C. (1969). A follow-up study of children with disorders in speech. *British Journal of Disorders of Communication, 4*, 46–56.

Gross, D., and Capuzzi, D. (1989). Defining youth at risk. In D. Capuzzi and D. Gross (Eds.), *Youth at risk: A resource for counselors, teachers, and parents* (pp. 3–18). Alexandria, VA: American Association for Counseling and Development.

Gross, T. (1985). *Cognitive development.* Monterey, CA: Brooks/Cole.

Gruen, A., and Gruen, L. (1994). *Daily problem solving activities: Transitioning to independence.* Eau Claire, WI: Thinking Publications.

Gruenewald, L., and Pollak, S. (1984). *Language interaction in teaching and learning.* Baltimore, MD: University Park Press.

Grunwell, P. (1986). Aspects of phonological development in later childhood. In K. Durkin (Ed.), *Language development in the school years* (pp. 34–56). Cambridge, MA: Brookline.

Hahn, A. (1987). Reaching out to America's dropouts: What to do? *Phi Delta Kappan, 69*(4), 256–263.

Hains, A., and Miller, D. (1980). Moral and cognitive development in delinquent and nondelinquent children and adolescents. *Journal of General Psychology, 137,* 21–35.

Hakes, D. (1980). *The development of metalinguistic abilities in children.* New York: Springer-Verlag.

Hall, G. (1904). *Adolescence: Its psychology and its relations to physiology, anthropology, sociology, sex, crime, religion, and education.* New York: Appleton.

Hallahan, D. (Ed.). (1980). Teaching exceptional children to use cognitive strategies. *Exceptional Education Quarterly, 1*(1), ix–xv.

Halliday, M. (1975). *Learning how to mean: Explorations in the development of language.* New York: Elsevior-North Holland.

Hamburg, D. (1992). *Today's children: Creating a future for a generation in crisis.* New York: Times Books.

Hamby, J. (1989, May). National dropout rates: Sources, problems, and efforts toward solutions. *A Series of Solutions and Strategies, 1,* pp. 1–8.

Hammill, D., and Larsen, S. (1988). *Test of written language* (2nd ed.). Austin, TX: Pro-Ed.

Harter, S., and Connell, J. (1984). A comparison of alternative models between academic achievement and children's perceptions of competence, control, and motivated orientation. In J. Nicholls (Ed.), *The development of achievement-related cognitions and behaviors* (pp. 214–250). Greenwich, CT: J.A.I. Press.

Hathaway, W., Sheldon, C., and McNamara, P. (1989). The solution lies in programs that work. In D. Capuzzi and D. Gross (Eds.), *Youth at risk: A resource for counselors, teachers, and parents* (pp. 367–394). Alexandria, VA: American Association for Counseling and Development.

Havertape, J., and Kass, C. (1978). Examination of problem solving in learning disabled adolescents through verbalized self-instructions. *Learning Disability Quarterly, 1*(4), 94–100.

Havighurst, R. (1953). *Human development and education*. New York: Longmans, Green.

Hayes, J. (1981). *The complete problem solver*. Philadelphia, PA: Franklin Institute Press.

Hayes, J., and Flower, L. (1987). On the structure of the writing process. *Topics in Language Disorders, 7*(4), 19–30.

Hayes, J., Flower, L., Schriver, K., Stratman, J., and Carey, L. (1985). *Cognitive processes in revision* (Tech. Rep. No. 12). Pittsburgh, PA: Carnegie Mellon University, Communication Design Center.

Heath Resource Center. (1985). *Measuring student progress in the classroom*. Washington, DC: Author.

Heath Resource Center. (1992). *Transition resource guide*. Washington, DC: Author.

Heath Resource Center. (1993). *Heath resource directory*. Washington, DC: Author.

Heath Resource Center. (1994a). *Make the most of your opportunities: A guide to postsecondary education for adults with disabilities*. Washington, DC: Author.

Heath Resource Center. (1994b). *Getting ready for college: Advising high school students with learning disabilities*. Washington, DC: Author.

Hechinger, F. (1992). *Fateful choices: Healthy youth for the 21st century*. New York: Hill and Wang.

Hedberg, N., and Westby, C. (1993). *Analyzing storytelling skills: Theory to practice*. Tucson, AZ: Communication Skill Builders.

High school dropout rates, 1990. (1993, August 25). *The Chronicle of Higher Education Almanac, XL*(1), p. 7.

Hill, J. (1970, April). *Models for screening*. Paper presented at the Annual Meeting of the American Educational Research Association, Minneapolis, MN.

Hoggan, K., and Strong, C. (1994). The magic of "once upon a time": Narrative teaching strategies. *Language, Speech, and Hearing Services in Schools, 25*(2), 76–89.

Hoskins, B. (1993, May). *In the midst of a paradigm shift: Implications for language and education*. Paper presented at the Van Riper Lecture Series, Kalamazoo, MI.

Hull, G. (1987). Current views of error and editing. *Topics in Language Disorders, 7*, 55–64.

Hymes, D. (1971). Competence and performance in linguistic theory. In R. Huxley and E. Ingram (Eds.), *Language acquisition: Models and methods* (pp. 3–28). New York: Academic Press.

Hymes, D. (1972). Introduction. In C. Cazden, V. John, and D. Hymes (Eds.), *Functions of language in the classroom* (pp. xi–lvii). New York: Teachers College Press.

Hymes, D. (1974). The ethnography of speaking. In B. Blount (Ed.), *Language, culture, and society: A book of readings* (pp. 189–223). Cambridge, MA: Winthrop.

Ingram, D. (1981). *Assessing communication behavior: Procedures for the phonological analysis of children's language* (Vol. 2). Baltimore, MD: University Park Press.

Inhelder, B., and Piaget, J. (1958). *The growth of logical thinking from childhood to adolescence—an essay on the construction of formal operational structures.* New York: Basic Books.

Isaacson, S. (1991). Assessing written language skills. In C. Simon (Ed.), *Communication skills and classroom success: Assessment and therapy methodologies for language and learning disabled students* (pp. 224–237). Eau Claire, WI: Thinking Publications.

Jackson, S. (1965). The growth of logical thinking in normal and subnormal children. *British Journal of Educational Psychology, 35,* 255–258.

James, S. (1990). *Normal language acquisition.* Austin, TX: Pro-Ed.

Jastak, S., and Wilkinson, G. (1984). *Wide range achievement test* (Rev. ed.). Wilmington, DE: Jastak Associates.

Johnson, D. (1985). Using reading and writing to improve oral language skills. *Topics in Language Disorders, 5,* 55–69.

Johnson, R., Greenspan, S., and Brown, G. (1980, September). *Children's ability to recognize and improve upon socially inept communications.* Paper presented at the 88th Annual Convention of the American Psychologists Association, Montreal, Canada.

Johnston, J. (1982). Narratives: A new look at communication problems in older language-disordered children. *Language, Speech, and Hearing Services in Schools, 13,* 144–155.

Johnston, J. (1985). *Doing things with words.* Madison, WI: Educational Teleconferencing Network.

Johnston, W., and Packer, A. (1987). *Workforce 2000: Work and workers for the 21st century.* Indianapolis, IN: Hudson Institute.

Jones, J., and Stone C. (1989). Metaphor comprehension by language learning disabled and normally achieving adolescent boys. *Learning Disability Quarterly, 12,* 251–260.

Jones, P. (1972). Formal operational reasoning and the use of tentative statements. *Cognitive Psychology, 3,* 467–471.

Kagan, J., Rosman, B., Day, D., Albert, J., and Phillips, W. (1964). Information processing in the child: Significance of analytic and reflective attitudes. *Psychology Monographs, 78*(1), 1–37.

Kamhi, A. (1987). Metalinguistic abilities in language-impaired children. *Topics in Language Disorders, 7,* 1–12.

Kamhi, A. (1991). Specific language impairment as a clinical category: An introduction. *Language, Speech, and Hearing Services in Schools, 22,* 65.

Kamhi, A., and Catts, H. (1986). Toward an understanding of developmental language and reading disorders. *Journal of Speech and Hearing Disorders, 51,* 337–347.

Kamhi, A., and Catts, H. (Eds.) (1989). *Reading disabilities: A developmental language perspective.* Austin, TX: Pro-Ed.

Kamhi, A., and Lee, R. (1988). Cognition. In M. Nippold (Ed.), *Later language development: Ages nine through nineteen* (pp. 127–158). Boston, MA: Little, Brown and Company.

Kaufer, D., Hayes, J., and Flower, L. (1986). Composing written sentences. *Research in the Teaching of English, 20*(2), 121–140.

Kerr, M., and Nelson, C. (1989). *Strategies for managing behavior problems in the classroom.* Columbus, OH: Merrill.

Kett, J. (1977). *Rites of passage: Adolescence in America, 1790 to the present.* New York: Basic Books.

Killarney, G., and Lass, N. (1981). A survey of rural public awareness of speech-language pathology and audiology. *Asha, 23,* 415–419.

Killian, C. (1979). Cognitive development of college freshmen. *Journal of Research in Science Teaching, 16,* 347–350.

King, R., Jones, C., and Lasky, E. (1982). In retrospect: A fifteen-year follow-up report of speech-language disordered children. *Language, Speech, and Hearing Services in Schools, 13,* 24–32.

Kirp, D. (1974). Student classification, public policy, and the courts: The rights of children. *Harvard Educational Review, 44*(1), 7–52.

Kishta, M. (1979). Proportional and combinatorial reasoning in two cultures. *Journal of Research in Science Teaching, 16,* 439–443.

Knapp, M. (1978). *Nonverbal communication in human interaction.* New York: Holt, Rinehart and Winston.

Knight-Arest, I. (1984). Communicative effectiveness of learning disabled and normally achieving 10- to 13-year-old boys. *Learning Disability Quarterly, 7,* 237–245.

Knowles, M. (1973). *The adult learner: A neglected species.* Houston, TX: Gulf Publishing.

Kohlberg, L. (1975). The cognitive-developmental approach to moral education. *Phi Delta Kappan, 56*(10), 670–677.

Konopka, G. (1971). Adolescence in the 1970s. *Child Welfare, 50*(10), 553–559.

Konopka, G. (1973). Requirements for healthy development of adolescent youth. *Adolescence, 8*(3), 291–316.

Kosel, M., and Fish, M. (1984). *The factory* [Computer software]. Pleasantville, NY: Sunburst Communications.

Kramer, P., Koff, E., and Luria, Z. (1972). The development of an exceptional language structure in older children and young adults. *Child Development, 43,* 121–130.

Kretschmer, E. (1951). *Korperbau and character.* Berlin, Germany: Springer-Verlag.

Kriegler, S., and van Niekerk, H. (1993). IE–A contribution to cultivating a culture of learning? *International Journal of Cognitive Education and Mediated Learning, 3*(1), 21–26.

Kroh, O. (1944). *Entwicklungspsychologic des Grundschulkindes.* Langensalza, Germany: Herman Beyer.

Kuhn, T.S. (1970). *The structure of scientific revolutions.* Chicago, IL: University of Chicago Press.

Labinowicz, E. (1980). *The Piaget primer.* Menlo Park, CA: Addison-Wesley.

Lahey, M. (1988). *Language disorders and language development.* New York: Macmillan.

Lahey, M. (1990). Who shall be called language disordered? Some reflections and one perspective. *Journal of Speech and Hearing Disorders, 55,* 612–620.

Lapadat, J. (1991). Pragmatic language skills of students with language and/or learning disabilities: A quantitative synthesis. *Journal of Learning Disabilities, 24*(3), 147–158.

Larson, M., and Dittman, F. (1975). *Compensatory education and early adolescence: Reviewing our national strategy.* Menlo Park, CA: Stanford Research.

Larson, V. L., and McKinley, N. (1985a, November). *Innovative service delivery models for adolescents with language disorders.* Paper presented at the Annual Convention of the American Speech-Language-Hearing Association, Washington, DC.

Larson, V. L., and McKinley, N. (1985b). General intervention principles with language impaired adolescents. *Topics in Language Disorders, 5,* 70–77.

Larson, V. L., and McKinley, N. (1987). *Communication assessment and intervention strategies for adolescents.* Eau Claire, WI: Thinking Publications.

Larson, V. L., and McKinley, N. (1990, November). *Adolescents with language disorders: An "action plan" for service delivery.* Poster session at the Annual Convention of the American Speech-Language-Hearing Association, Seattle, WA.

Larson, V. L., McKinley, N., and Boley, D. (1993). Service delivery models for adolescents with language disorders. *Language, Speech, and Hearing Services in Schools, 24,* 36–42.

Lawson, A., and Wollman, W. (1976). Encouraging the transition from concrete to formal cognitive functioning—An experiment. *Journal of Research in Science Teaching, 13,* 413–430.

Leadbeater, B., and Dionne, J. (1981). The adolescent's use of formal operational thinking in solving problems related to identify resolution. *Adolescence, 16*(61), 111–121.

Lee, L. (1974). *Developmental sentence analysis.* Evanston, IL: Northwestern University Press.

Leiter, R. (1979). *Leiter international performance scale* (Rev. ed.). Wood Dale, IL: Stoelting Company.

Leonard, L. (1991). Specific language impairment as a clinical category. *Language, Speech, and Hearing Services in Schools, 22,* 66–68.

Levin, J. (1976). What have we learned about maximizing what children learn? In J. Levin and V. Allen (Eds.), *Cognitive learning in children: Theories and strategies* (pp. 105–134). New York: Academic Press.

Levine, J., and Sutton-Smith, B. (1973). Effects of age, sex, and task on visual behavior during dyadic interaction. *Developmental Psychology, 9,* 400–405.

Lewin, K. (1939). Field theory and experiment in social psychology concepts and methods. *American Journal of Sociology, 44,* 868–897.

Lewis, B., and Freebairn, L. (1992). Residual effects of preschool phonology disorders in grade school, adolescence, and adulthood. *Journal of Speech and Hearing Research, 35*, 819–831.

Lidz, C. (1991). *Practitioner's guide to dynamic assessment.* New York: Guilford Press.

Lipsitz, J. (1979). Adolescent development: Myths and realities. *Children Today, 8*(5), 2–7.

Lipsitz, J. (1980). *Growing up forgotten: A review of research and programs concerning early adolescence.* New Brunswick, NJ: Transaction.

Loban, W. (1976). *Language development: Kindergarten through grade twelve.* Urbana, IL: National Council of Teachers of English.

Lochhead, J., and Clement, J. (Eds.). (1979). *Cognitive process instruction: Research on teaching thinking skills.* Philadelphia, PA: Franklin Institute Press.

Logemann, J. (1994). Treatment efficacy and outcome: Everyone's job. *Asha, 36*(6/7), 3.

Long, S., and Fey, M. (1989). *Computerized language profiling* (Version 6.1.) [Computer software]. Ithaca, NY: Ithaca College.

Long, S., and Fey, M. (1993). *Computerized profiling* [Computer software]. San Antonio, TX: Psychological Corporation.

Long, S., and Masterson, J. (1993). Use in language analysis. *Asha, 35*(8), 40–41.

Lund, N., and Duchan, J. (1983). *Assessing children's language in naturalistic contexts.* Englewood Cliffs, NJ: Prentice-Hall.

Lutzer, V. (1988). Comprehension of proverbs by average children and children with learning disorders. *Journal of Learning Disabilities, 21*, 104–108.

MacLachlan, B., and Chapman, R. (1988). Communication breakdowns in normal and language learning-disabled children's conversation and narration. *Journal of Speech and Hearing Disorders, 53*, 2–7.

Madaus, G., and Tan, A. (1993). The growth of assessment. In G. Cawelti (Ed.), *Challenges and achievements of American education* (pp. 53–79). Alexandria, VA: Association for Supervision and Curriculum Development.

Maeroff, G. (1988). Withered hopes, stillborn dreams: The dismal panorama of urban schools. *Phi Delta Kappan, 69*(9), 632–638.

Mandler, J., and Johnson, N. (1977). Remembrance of things parsed: Story structure and recall. *Cognitive Psychology, 9*, 111–151.

Mann, V., Cowin, E., and Schoenheimer, J. (1989). Phonological processing, language comprehension and reading ability. *Journal of Learning Disabilities, 22*, 76–89.

Marcia, J. E. (1980). Identity in adolescence. In J. Adelson (Ed.), *Handbook of adolescent psychology* (pp. 159–187). New York: John Wiley.

Markgraf, B. (1966). An observational study determining the amount of time that students in the 10th and 12th grades are expected to listen in the classroom. In S. Duker (Ed.), *Listening readings* (pp. 90–101). New York: Scarecrow Press.

Martorano, S. (1977). A developmental analysis of performance on Piaget's formal operations tasks. *Developmental Psychology, 13*(6), 666–672.

Mason, W. (1976). Specific (developmental) dyslexia. *Developmental Medicine and Child Neurology, 9*, 183–190.

Maxwell, W. (Ed.). (1983). *Thinking: The expanding frontier.* Philadelphia, PA: Franklin Institute Press.

McCarthy, D. (1930). *The language development of the preschool child* (Institute of Child Welfare Monograph Series No. 4). Minneapolis, MN: University of Minnesota Press.

McFadden, T. (1991). Narrative and expository language: A criterion-based assessment procedure for school-age children. *Journal of Speech-Language Pathology and Audiology, 15*(4), 57–63.

McKinley, N., and Larson, V. L. (1983, November). *Adolescents' conversations with a friend and an unfamiliar adult.* Paper presented at the Annual Convention of the American Speech-Language-Hearing Association, Cincinnati, OH.

McKinley, N., and Larson, V. L. (1985). Neglected language disordered adolescents: A delivery model. *Language, Speech, and Hearing Services in Schools, 16*, 2–15.

McKinley, N., and Larson, V. L. (1989). Students who can't communicate: Speech-language services at the secondary level. *National Association of Secondary School Principals Curriculum Report, 19*(2), 1–8.

McKinley, N., and Larson, V. L. (1990). Language and learning disorders in adolescents. *Seminars in Speech and Language, 11*, 182–191.

McKinley, N., and Larson, V. L. (1991, November). *Seventh, eighth, and ninth graders' conversations in two experimental conditions.* Poster session presented at the Annual Convention of the American Speech-Language-Hearing Association, Atlanta, GA.

McLean, J., and Snyder-McLean, L. (1978) *A transactional approach to early language training.* Columbus, OH: Merrill.

MDC. (1988). *America's shame, America's hope: Twelve million youth at risk.* Chapel Hill, NC: Author.

Mead, M. (1950). *Coming of age in Samoa.* New York: New American Library.

Mehrabian, A. (1968). Communication without words. *Psychology Today, 2*, 51–52.

Mendelberg, H. (1984). Split and continuity in language use of Mexican-American adolescents of migrant origin. *Adolescence, 19*(73), 171–182.

Menyuk, P. (1991). Metalinguistic abilities and language disorder. In J. Miller (Ed.), *Research on child language disorders: A decade of progress* (pp. 387–397). Austin, TX: Pro-Ed.

Mercer, J. (1975). Psychological assessment and the rights of children. In N. Hobbs (Ed.), *Issues in the classification of children.* (Vol. 1, pp. 130–159). San Francisco, CA: Jossey-Bass.

Merritt D., and Liles, B. (1987). Story grammar ability in children with and without language disorder: Story generation, story retelling, and story comprehension. *Journal of Speech and Hearing Research, 30,* 539–552.

Miller, J. (1981). *Assessing language production in children: Experimental procedures.* Baltimore, MD: University Park Press.

Miller, J., and Chapman, R. (1983). *Systematic analysis of language transcripts (SALT)* [Computer software]. Madison, WI: University of Wisconsin, Waisman Center.

Miller, J. and Chapman, R. (1991). *SALT: A computer program for the systematic analysis of language transcripts.* Madison, WI: University of Wisconsin, Waisman Center.

Miller, N., and Dollard, J. (1941). *Social learning and imitation.* New Haven, CT: Yale University Press.

Miller, P. (1989). Theories of adolescent development. In J. Worell and F. Danner (Eds.), *The adolescent as decision-maker: Applications to development and education* (pp. 13–49). San Diego, CA: Academic Press.

Mitchell, J. (1979). *Adolescent psychology.* Toronto, Canada: Holt, Rinehart and Winston.

Montague, M., and Lund, K. (1991). *Job-related social skills: A curriculum for adolescents with special needs.* Ann Arbor, MI: Exceptional Innovations.

Montemeyor, R., and Eisen, M. (1977). The development of self-conceptions from childhood to adolescence. *Developmental Psychology, 13,* 314–319.

Montgomery, J., and Herer, G. (1994). Future watch: Our schools in the 21st century. *Language, Speech, and Hearing Services in Schools, 25,* 130–135.

Mordecai, D., Palin, M., and Palmer, C. (1985). *Lingquest 1: Computer assisted language sample analysis* [Computer software]. Columbus, OH: Merrill.

Morris, M., Leuenberger, J., and Aksamit, D. (1985, November). *Language learning disabled students in the college setting.* Paper presented at the Annual Convention of the Speech-Language-Hearing Association, Washington, DC.

Muma, J. (1978). *Language handbook: Concepts, assessment, intervention.* Englewood Cliffs, NJ: Prentice-Hall.

Muuss, R. (1975). *Theories of adolescence.* New York: Random House.

Naisbitt, J. (1988). Back to basics: U.S. businesses tackle remedial education. *John Naisbitt's Trend Letters, 7*(15), 8.

National Commission on Youth. (1980). *The transition of youth to adulthood: A bridge too long.* Boulder, CO: Westview Press.

National Institutes of Health. (1984). *Head injury: Hope through research.* (NIH Publication No. 84-2478, pp. 1–37). Bethesda, MD: Author.

Neimark, E. (1979). Current status of formal operations research. *Human Development, 22,* 60–67.

Neimark, E. (1980). Intellectual development in the exceptional adolescent as viewed within a Piagetian framework. *Exceptional Education Quarterly, 1*(2), 47–56.

Nelson, N. (1984). Beyond information processing: The language of teachers and textbooks. In G. Wallach and K. Butler (Eds.), *Language learning disabilities in school-age children* (pp. 154–178). Baltimore, MD: Williams and Wilkins.

Nelson, N. (1988). The nature of literacy. In M. Nippold (Ed.), *Later language development: Ages nine to nineteen* (pp. 11–28). Boston, MA: Little, Brown and Company.

Nelson, N. (1989). Curriculum-based language assessment and intervention. *Language, Speech, and Hearing Services in Schools, 20,* 170–184.

Nelson, N. (1992). Targets of curriculum-based language assessment. In J. Damico (Ed.), *Best practices in school speech-language pathology* (pp. 73–86). San Antonio, TX: Psychological Corporation.

Nelson, N. (1993). *Childhood language disorders in context: Infancy through adolescence.* New York: Macmillan.

Nelson, N. (1994). School-age language: Bumpy road or super-expressway to the next millennium? *American Journal of Speech-Language Pathology, 3*(3), 29–31.

Nelson, N., and Friedman, K. (1988). *Development of the concept of story in narratives written by older children.* Unpublished paper, Western Michigan University, Kalamazoo.

Newcomer, P. (1990). *Diagnostic achievement battery* (2nd ed.). Austin, TX: Pro-Ed.

Newcomer, P., and Bryant, B. (1993). *Diagnostic achievement test for adolescents* (2nd ed.). Chicago, IL: Riverside.

Nichols, R., and Lewis, T. (1954). *Listening and speaking: A guide to effective oral communication.* Dubuque, IA: Wm. C. Brown.

Nichols, R., and Stevens, L. (1957). Listening to people. *Harvard Business Review, 35*(5), 85–92.

Nicholson, C., and Hibpshman, T. (1990). *Slosson intelligence test* (Rev. ed.). East Aurora, NY: Slosson Educational Publications.

Nippold, M. (1985). Comprehension of figurative language in youth. *Topics in Language Disorders, 5*(3), 1–20.

Nippold, M. (1988a). Introduction. In M. Nippold (Ed.), *Later language development: Ages nine to nineteen* (pp. 1–10). Boston, MA: Little, Brown and Company.

Nippold, M. (1988b). The literate lexicon. In M. Nippold (Ed.), *Later language development: Ages nine to nineteen* (pp. 29–48). Boston, MA: Little, Brown and Company.

Nippold, M. (1988c). Figurative language. In M. Nippold (Ed.), *Later language development: Ages nine through nineteen* (pp. 179–210). Boston, MA: Little, Brown and Company.

Nippold, M. (Ed.) (1988d). *Later language development: Ages nine through nineteen.* Boston, MA: Little, Brown and Company.

Nippold, M. (1988e). Linguistic ambiguity. In M. Nippold (Ed.), *Later language development: Ages nine to nineteen* (pp. 211–224). Boston, MA: Little, Brown and Company.

Nippold, M. (1991). Evaluating and enhancing idiom comprehension in language disordered students. *Language, Speech, and Hearing Services in Schools, 22,* 100–106.

Nippold, M. (1993). Developmental markers in adolescent language: Syntax, semantics, and pragmatics. *Language, Speech, and Hearing Services in Schools, 24,* 21–28.

Nippold, M., and Fey, M. (1983). Metaphoric understanding in preadolescents having a history of language acquisition difficulties. *Language, Speech, and Hearing Services in Schools, 14,* 171–180.

Nippold, M., and Martin, S. (1989). Idiom interpretation in isolation versus context: Developmental study with adolescents. *Journal of Speech and Hearing Research, 32,* 59–66.

Nippold, M., Martin, S., and Erskine, B. (1988). Proverb comprehension in context: A developmental study with children and adolescents. *Journal of Speech and Hearing Research, 31,* 19–28.

Nippold, M., Schwarz, I., and Undlin, R. (1992). Use and understanding of adverbial conjuncts: A developmental study of adolescents and young adults. *Journal of Speech and Hearing Research, 35,* 108–118.

Nisbet, J., Zanella, K., and Miller, J. (1984). An analysis of conversations among handicapped students and a non-handicapped peer. *Exceptional Children, 51*(2), 156–162.

Noel, M. (1980). Referential communication abilities of learning disabled children. *Learning Disability Quarterly, 3,* 70–75.

Offer, D., Ostrov., E., and Howard, K. (1977). *The Offer self-image questionnaire for adolescents: A manual.* Chicago, IL: Michael Reese Hospital.

Offer, D., Ostrov, E., and Howard, K. (1981). The mental health professional's concept of the normal adolescent. *American Medical Association Archives of General Psychiatry, 38*(2), 149–153.

Offer, D., Ostrov, E., Howard, K., and Atkinsen, R. (1988). *The teenage world: Adolescents' self-image in ten countries.* New York: Plenum.

Olver, R., and Hornsby, J. (1966). On equivalence. In J. Bruner, R. Olver, and P. Greenfield (Eds.), *Studies in cognitive growth* (pp. 68–85). New York: John Wiley.

O'Malley, R., and Bachman, J. (1983). Self-esteem: Change and stability between 13 and 23. *Developmental Psychology, 19,* 257–268.

O'Neil, J. (1992). Preparing for the changing workplace. *Educational Leadership, 49*(6), 6–9.

O'Neil, J. (1993). Can national standards make a difference? *Educational Leadership, 50*(5), 4–8.

Overton, W., and Meehan, A. (1982). Individual differences in formal operational thought: Sex role and learned helplessness. *Child Development, 53,* 1536–1543.

Owens, R., Jr. (1991). *Language disorders: A functional approach to assessment and intervention.* New York: Macmillan.

Pacheco, R. (1983). Bilingual mentally retarded children: Language confusion or real deficits? In D.R. Omark and J.G. Erickson (Eds.), *The bilingual exceptional child* (pp. 233–254). San Diego, CA: College-Hill.

Page, J., and Stewart, S. (1985). Story grammar skills in school-age children. *Topics in Language Disorders, 5,* 16–30.

Papalia, D., and Olds, S. (1975). *A child's world—Infancy through adolescence.* New York: McGraw-Hill.

Parrill-Burnstein, M. (1981). *Problem solving and learning disabilities: An information processing approach.* New York: Grune and Stratton.

Pascual-Leone, J. (1980). Constructive problems for constructive theories: The current relevance of Piaget's work and a critique of information processing simulation psychology. In H. Speda and P. Kluwe (Eds.), *Psychological models of thinking* (pp. 176–203). New York: Academic Press.

Paulson, F., Paulson, P., and Meyer, C. (1991). What makes a portfolio a portfolio? *Educational Leadership, 48*(5), 60–63.

Pearlstein, E., Russell, L., and Fink, R. (1977, November). *Speech/language pathology and audiology: The public's view.* Paper presented at the Annual Convention of the American Speech-Language-Hearing Association, Chicago, IL.

Peck, M. (1982). Youth suicide. *Death Education, 6,* 29–47.

Perera, K. (1986). Language acquisition and writing. In P. Fletcher and M. Garman (Eds.), *Language acquisition: Studies in first language acquisition* (2nd ed.) (pp. 494–519). New York: Cambridge University Press.

Perl, S. (1979). The composing processes of unskilled college writers. *Research in the Teaching of English, 13*(4), 317–336.

Peters-Johnson, C. (1994). Action: School services. *Language, Speech, and Hearing Services in Schools, 25,* 121–127.

Piaget, J. (1959). *The language and thought of the child* (Reprint of 1926 edition). London: Routledge and Kegan Paul.

Piaget, J. (1970). Piaget's theory. In P. Mussen (Ed.), *Carmichael's manual of child psychology* (Vol. 1, pp. 703–732). New York: John Wiley.

Piaget, J., and Inhelder, B. (1969). *The psychology of the child.* New York: Basic Books.

Prutting, C., and Kirchner, D. (1983). Applied pragmatics. In T. Gallagher and C. Prutting (Eds.), *Pragmatic assessment and intervention issues in language* (pp. 29–64). San Diego, CA: College-Hill.

Pye, C. (1987). *Pye analysis of language* [Computer software]. Lawrence, KS: University of Kansas.

Rank, O. (1945). *Will therapy and truth and reality.* New York: Knopf.

Rankin, R. (1926). *The measurement of the ability to understand spoken language.* Unpublished doctoral dissertation, University of Michigan, Ann Arbor.

Ratner, V., and Harris, L. (1994). *Understanding language disorders: The impact on learning.* Eau Claire, WI: Thinking Publications.

Reed, N. (1977). *An analysis of comprehension levels of an ask/tell syntactic structure in a group of adolescents, aged ten to eighteen years.* Unpublished master's thesis, University of Ohio, Cincinnati.

Reed, V. (1994). *An introduction to children with language disorders* (2nd ed.). New York: Macmillan.

Rees, N. (1974). The speech pathologist and the reading process. *Asha, 16,* 255–258.

Rees, N., and Wollner, S. (1982, February). *A taxonomy of pragmatic abilities.* (Teleconference program). Madison, WI: Educational Teleconferencing Network.

Remplein, H. (1956). *Die seelische enturcklung in der kindheit und reifezeit.* Munchen, Germany: Ernst Reinhard.

Retherford, K. (1993). *Guide to analysis of language transcripts* (2nd ed.). Eau Claire, WI: Thinking Publications.

Rice, M. (1983). Contemporary accounts of the cognition/language relationship: Implications for speech-language clinicians. *Journal of Speech and Hearing Disorders, 48,* 347–359.

Riedlinger-Ryan, K., and Shewan, C. (1984). Comparison of auditory language comprehension skills in learning-disabled and academically achieving adolescents. *Language, Speech, and Hearing Services in Schools, 15,* 127–136.

Ritter, E. (1979). Social perspective taking ability, cognitive complexity and listener adapted communication in early and late adolescence. *Communication Monographs, 46,* 40–51.

Rivers, L., Henderson, D., Jones, R., Ladner, J., and Williams, R. (1975). Mosaic of labels for Black children. In N. Hobbs (Ed.), *Issues in the classification of children* (Vol. 2, pp. 213–245). San Francisco, CA: Jossey-Bass.

Robinson, E. (1981). The child's understanding of inadequate messages and communication failure: A problem of ignorance or egocentrism? In W. Dickson (Ed.), *Children's oral communication skills* (pp. 167–187). New York: Academic Press.

Rosenberg, M. (1979). *Conceiving the self.* New York: Basic Books.

Rosenberg, M. (1986). Self-concept from middle childhood through adolescence. In J. Suls and A.G. Greenwald (Eds.), *Psychological perspectives on the self* (Vol. 3, pp. 107–135). Hillsdale, NJ: Erlbaum.

Rosenthal, D. (1979). Language skills and formal operations. *Merrill-Palmer Quarterly, 25*(2), 133–143.

Roth, F., and Spekman, N. (1986). Narrative disclosure: Spontaneously generated stories of learning disabled and normally achieving students. *Journal of Speech and Hearing Disorders, 51,* 8–23.

Rubin, D. (1987). Divergence and convergence between oral and written communication. *Topics in Language Disorders, 7,* 1–18.

Rukeyser, L. (1988, August 30). U.S. firms make it their business to help ease the dropout dilemma. *Minneapolis Star Tribune,* p. 2D.

Rumelhart, D. (1975). Notes on a schema for stories. In D. Bobrow and A. Collins (Eds.), *Representation and understanding: Studies in cognitive science* (pp. 211–236). New York: Academic Press.

Rutherford, R. (1976). Talk about pop. In S. Rogers (Ed.), *They don't speak our language: Essays on the language world of children and adolescents* (pp. 106–127). London: Edward Arnold.

Rutherford, R., Freeth, M., and Mercer, E. (1969). *Topics of conversation in 15-year-old children.* London: The Nuffield Foundation.

Samovar, L., and Porter, R. (1991a). *Communication between cultures.* Belmont, CA: Wadsworth.

Samovar, L., and Porter, R. (1991b). *Intercultural communication: A reader.* Belmont, CA: Wadsworth.

Sanders, L. (1971). The comprehension of certain syntactic structures by adults. *Journal of Speech and Hearing Disorders, 14,* 739–745.

Scheiber, B., and Talpers, J. (1987). *Unlocking potential: College and other choices for learning disabled people—A step-by-step guide.* Bethesda, MD: Adler and Adler.

Schlesinger, I. (1977). The role of cognitive development and linguistic input in language acquisition. *Journal of Child Language, 4,* 153–169.

Schory, M. (1990). Whole language and the speech-language pathologist. *Language, Speech, and Hearing Services in Schools, 21,* 206–211.

Schubert, R., and Gates, M. (1990). *Making the grade: A report card on American youth.* Washington, DC: National Collaboration for Youth.

Schuele, C., and van Kleeck, A. (1987). Precursors to literacy: Assessment and intervention. *Topics in Language Disorders, 7,* 32–44.

Schumaker, J., and Hazel, J. (1984). Social skills assessment and training for the learning disabled: Who's on first and what's on second? Part II. *Journal of Learning Disabilities, 17*(8), 492–499.

Schumaker, J., Sheldon-Wildgen, J., and Sherman, J. (1980). *An observational study of the academic and social behavior of learning disabled adolescents in the regular classroom* (Research Report 22). Lawrence, KS: University of Kansas, Institute for Research in Learning Disabilities.

Schwartz, A. (1985). Microcomputer-assisted assessment of linguistic and phonological processes. *Topics in Language Disorders, 6,* 26–40.

Schwartz, L., and McKinley, N. (1984). *Daily communication: Strategies for the language disordered adolescent.* Eau Claire, WI: Thinking Publications.

Scott, C. (1988). Spoken and written syntax. In M. Nippold (Ed.), *Later language development: Ages nine through nineteen* (pp. 49–96). Boston, MA: Little, Brown and Company.

Scott, C.M., and Erwin, D.L. (1992). Descriptive assessment of writing: Process and products. In W. Secord and J. Damico (Eds.), *Best practices in school speech-language pathology* (pp. 87–98). San Antonio, TX: Psychological Corporation.

Search Institute. (1990). The troubled journey: New light on growing up healthy. *Source, 6*(3), 1–4.

Search Institute. (1991). Backbone: Essential for survival on the troubled journey. *Source, 7*(1), 1–4.

Searle, J. (1965). What is a speech act? In M. Black (Ed.), *Philosophy in America* (pp. 221–239). New York: Allen and Union, Cornell University Press.

Seidenberg, P. (1988). Cognitive and academic instructional intervention for learning-disabled adolescents. *Topics in Language Disorders, 8*, 56–71.

Selman, R.L. (1980). *The growth of interpersonal understanding: Developmental and clinical analyses.* New York: Academic Press.

Shantz, C. (1981). The role of role-taking in children's referential communication. In W. Dickson (Ed.), *Children's oral communication skills* (pp. 85–102). New York: Academic Press.

Sheehy, G. (1981). *Pathfinders: Overcoming the crises of adult life and finding your own path to well-being.* New York: Bantam Books.

Sheldon, A. (1977). On strategies for processing relative clauses: A comparison of children and adults. *Journal of Psycholinguistic Research, 6*, 305–318.

Shewan, C. (1989). American Speech-Language-Hearing Association data: Speech-language pathologists in the schools. *Asha, 31*(1), 56.

Siegal, M. (1980). Kohlberg versus Piaget: To what extent has one theory eclipsed the other? *Merrill-Palmer Quarterly, 26*(4), 285–297.

Siegel, L., and Ryan, E. (1988). Development of grammatical-sensitivity, phonological, and short-term memory skills in normally achieving and learning disabled children. *Developmental Psychology, 2*(1), 28–37.

Simmons, R., Blyth, D., Van Cleave, E., and Bush, D. (1979). Entry into early adolescence: The impact of school structure, puberty, and early dating on self-esteem. *American Sociological Review, 44*, 948–967.

Simon, C. (1979). *Communicative competence: A functional-pragmatic approach to language therapy.* Tucson, AZ: Communication Skill Builders.

Simon, C. (1990, Fall/Winter). Fracture in the collaborative process: Anatomy of a resignation. *Hearsay: Journal of the Ohio Speech and Hearing Association,* 112–119.

Simon, C. (Ed.). (1991). *Communication skills and classroom success: Assessment and therapy methodologies for language and learning disabled students.* Eau Claire, WI: Thinking Publications.

Simon, C. (1994). *Evaluating communicative competence: A language sampling procedure* (Rev. 2nd ed.). Tempe, AZ: Communi-Cog Publications.

Simon, C., and Holway, C. (1991). Presentation of communication evaluation information. In C. Simon (Ed.), *Communication skills and classroom success: Assessment and therapy methodologies for language and learning disabled students* (pp. 151–199). Eau Claire, WI: Thinking Publications.

Simon, C., and Myrold-Gunyuz, P. (1990). *Into the classroom: The SLP in the collaborative role.* Tucson, AZ: Communication Skill Builders.

Simpson, R. (1982). *Conferencing parents of exceptional children.* Rockville, MD: Aspen.

Sizer, T. (1991). No pain, no gain. *Educational Leadership, 48*(8), 32–34.

Skinner, B. (1957). *Verbal behavior.* New York: Appleton-Century Crofts.

Smith, S., Mann, V., and Shankweiler, D. (1986). Spoken sentence comprehension by good and poor readers: A study with the token test. *Cortex, 22,* 627–632.

Snyder, L., and Downey, D. (1991). The language-reading relationship in normal and reading-disabled children. *Journal of Speech and Hearing Research, 34,* 129–140.

Snyder, L., and Godley, D. (1992). Assessment of word-finding disorders in children and adolescents. *Topics in Language Disorders, 13,* 15–32.

Sparks, S. (1993). *Children of prenatal substance abuse.* San Diego, CA: Singular.

Spekman, N. (1981). A study of the dyadic verbal communication abilities of learning disabled and normally achieving 4th and 5th grade boys. *Learning Disability Quarterly, 4,* 139–151.

Spranger, E. (1955). *Psychologie des jugendalters* (24th ed.). Heidelberg, Germany: Quelle and Meyer.

Stein, N., and Glenn, C. (1979). An analysis of story comprehension in elementary school children. In R. Freedle (Ed.), *New directions in discourse processing* (Vol. 2, pp. 53–120). Norwood, NJ: Ablex.

Stemmer, P., Brown, B., and Smith, C. (1992). The employability skills portfolio. *Educational Leadership, 49*(6), 32–35.

Sternberg, R. (1985). *Beyond IQ: A triarchic theory of human intelligence.* New York: Cambridge University Press.

Stewart, S. (1991). Development of written language proficiency. Methods for teaching text structure. In C. Simon (Ed.), *Communication skills and classroom success: Assessment and therapy methodologies for language and learning disabled students* (pp. 419–433). Eau Claire, WI: Thinking Publications.

Stone C.A., and Forman E.A. (1988). Differential patterns of approach to a complex problem-solving task among learning disabled adolescents. *Journal of Special Education, 22*(2), 167–185.

Strain, P., Guralnick, M., and Walker, H. (Eds.). (1986). *Children's social behavior: Development, assessment, and modification.* New York: Academic Press.

Strominger, A., and Bashir, A. (1977, November). *A nine-year follow-up of language-delayed children.* Paper presented at the Annual Convention of the American Speech and Hearing Association, Chicago, IL.

Sue, D. (1981). *Counseling the culturally different: Theory and practice.* New York: John Wiley.

Suls, J. (1989). Self-awareness and self-identity in adolescence. In J. Worrell and F. Danner (Eds.), *The adolescent as decision maker: Applications to development and education* (pp. 144–179). San Diego, CA: Academic Press.

Sunburst Communications. (1988). Failure: Why schools must help children at risk. *Solutions: News for Computer Educators, 3*(2), 1–12.

Tanner, J. (1974). Sequence and tempo in the somatic changes in puberty. In M. Grumbach, G. Grave, and F. Mayer (Eds.), *Control of the onset of puberty* (pp. 448–470). New York: John Wiley.

Task Force on Secondary Programs for the Speech-Language Impaired. (April, 1983). *Project adolang: Identification of adolescent language problems and implications for education.* Tallahassee, FL: Florida Department of Education, Bureau of Education for Exceptional Students.

Taylor, D. (1988). Ethnographic educational evaluation for children, families, and schools. *Theory into Practice, 27*(1), 67–76.

Taylor, J. (1969). *The communicative abilities of juvenile delinquents: A descriptive study.* Unpublished doctoral dissertation. Columbia, MO: University of Missouri.

Taylor, O., and Peters, C. (1982). Sociolinguistics and communication disorders. In N. Lass, L. McReynolds, J. Northern, and D. Yoder (Eds.), *Speech, language, and hearing: Vol. II. Pathologies of speech and language* (pp. 802–818). Philadelphia, PA: W.B. Saunders.

Taylor, O. (in press). Clinical practice as a social occasion. In L. Cole and V. Deal (Eds.), *Communication disorders in multicultural populations.* Rockville, MD: American Speech-Language-Hearing Association.

Teale, W., and Sulzby, E. (1986). Introduction: Emergent literacy as a perspective for examining how young children become writers and readers. In W. Teale and E. Sulzby (Eds.), *Emergent literacy: Writing and reading* (pp. vii–xxv). Norwood, NJ: Ablex.

Terman, L., and Merrill, M. (1973). *Stanford-Binet intelligence scale* (Form L-M). Chicago, IL: Riverside.

Thomas, E., and Walmsley, S. (1976, August). *Some evidence of continuing linguistic acquisition in learning disabled adolescents.* Paper presented at the International Federation of Learning Disabilities Third International Scientific Conference, Montreal, Canada.

Thorndike, R., Hagen, E., and Sattler, J. (1986). *Stanford-Binet intelligence scale* (4th ed.). Chicago, IL: Riverside.

Thorndyke, P. (1977). Cognitive structures in comprehension and memory of narrative discourse. *Cognitive Psychology, 9,* 77–110.

Turner, J., and Helms, D. (1979). *Life span development.* Philadelphia, PA: W.B. Saunders.

Tyack, D., and Gottsleben, R. (1974). *Language sampling, analysis and training: A handbook for teachers and clinicians.* Palo Alto, CA: Consulting Psychologists Press.

U.S. Department of Education, Office of Special Education. (1993). *Fifteenth annual report to Congress on the implementation of the individuals with disabilities education act.* Washington, DC: Author.

Valens, E. (1975). *The other side of the mountain.* New York: Warner Books.

Vallett, R. (1981). *Vallett inventory of critical thinking abilities.* Novata, CA: Academic Therapy Publications.

Valletutti, P., and Bender, M. (1982). *Teaching interpersonal and community living skills: A curriculum model for handicapped adolescents and adults.* Baltimore, MD: University Park Press.

Van Hattum, R. (1983). Public information: More is not enough. *Asha, 25*(2), 29–34.

van Kleeck, A. (1987). Foreword. The metas: Implications for the language impaired. *Topics in Language Disorders, 7*(2), vi–vii.

Velluntino, F. (1978). Toward an understanding of dyslexia: Psychological factors in specific reading disability. In A. Benton and D. Pearl (Eds.), *Dyslexia: An appraisal of current knowledge* (pp. 61–111). New York: Oxford University Press.

Vetter, D. K. (1985). Evaluation of clinical intervention: Accountability. *Seminars in Speech and Language, 6*(1), 55–64.

Vetter, D. K. (1991). Needed: Intervention research. In J. Miller (Ed.), *Research on child language disorders: A decade of progress* (pp. 243–252). Austin, TX: Pro-Ed.

Vogel, S. (1974). Syntactic abilities in normal and dyslexic children. *Journal of Learning Disabilities, 7,* 47–53.

Vygotsky, L. (1962). *Thought and language.* Cambridge, MA: MIT Press.

Walker, H., Schwarz, I., Nippold, M., Irvin, L., and Noell, J. (1994). Social skills in school-age children and youth: Issues and best practices in assessment and intervention. *Topics in Language Disorders, 14*(3), 70–82.

Wallach, G. (1990). Magic buries Celtis: Looking for broader interpretations of language learning and literacy. *Topics in Language Disorders, 10*(2), 63–80.

Wallach, G., and Miller, L. (1988). *Language intervention and academic success.* Boston, MA: Little, Brown and Company.

Warden, M., and Hutchinson, T. (1992). *Writing process test.* Chicago, IL: Riverside.

Weaver, C. (1993). Understanding and educating students with attention deficit hyperactivity disorder: Toward a system theory and whole language perspective. *American Journal of Speech-Language Pathology, 2*(2), 79–89.

Weaver, H. (1972). *Human listening: Processes and behavior.* Indianapolis, IN: Bobbs-Merrill.

Weaver, P., and Dickinson, D. (1982). Scratching below the surface structure: Exploring the usefulness of story grammars. *Discourse Processes, 5,* 225–243.

Wechsler, D. (1981). *Wechsler adult intelligence scale* (Rev. ed.). San Antonio, TX: Psychological Corporation.

Wechsler, D. (1991). *Wechsler intelligence scale for children* (3rd ed.). San Antonio, TX: Psychological Corporation.

Weiner, F. (1984). *Computerized language sample analysis* [Computer software]. State College, PA: Parrot Software.

Weiner, F. (1985). The value of follow-up studies. *Topics in Language Disorders, 5*(3), 78–92.

Weiner, F. (1988). *Parrot easy language sample analysis* [Computer software]. State College, PA: Parrot Software.

Weiss, R., Hansen, K., and Heubelein, T. (1979, November). *Pragmatic psycholinguistic therapy for language disorders in early childhood.* Short course presented at the Annual Convention of the American Speech-Language-Hearing Association, Atlanta, GA.

Wellborn, S. (1981, December 14). Special report: Troubled teenagers. *U.S. News and World Report, 91,* 40–43.

Weller, C. (1989). *Investigation of subtypes and severities of learning disabled adults* (Report No. 133FH80023). Washington, DC: National Institute for Disability and Rehabilitation Research.

Weller, C., Crelly, C., Watteyne, L., and Herbert, M. (1992). *Adaptive language disorders of young adults with learning disabilities.* San Diego, CA: Singular.

Weller, C., and Strawser, S. (1987). Adaptive behavior of subtypes of learning disabled individuals. *Journal of Special Education, 21*(1), 102–115.

Wellington, J. (1994, September). *Reflections of a juvenile court judge: Problems and prospects.* Paper presented at The International Adolescent Conference, Miami, FL.

Wells, S., Bechard, S., and Hamby, J. (1989, July). How to identify at-risk students. *A Series of Solutions and Strategies, 2,* 1–6.

Werner, E. (1975). *A study of communication time.* Unpublished master's thesis, University of Maryland, College Park.

Westby, C. (1984). Development of narrative language abilities. In G. Wallach and K. Butler (Eds.), *Language learning disabilities in school-age children* (pp. 103–127). Baltimore, MD: Williams and Wilkins.

Westby, C. (1989). Assessing and remediating text comprehension problems. In A. Kamhi and H. Catts (Eds.), *Reading disabilities: A developmental language perspective* (pp. 199–259). Austin, TX: Pro-Ed.

Westby, C. (1990). The role of the speech-language pathologist in whole language. *Language, Speech, and Hearing Services in Schools, 21,* 228–237.

Westby, C. (1991a). Learning to talk—talking to learn: Oral-literate language differences. In C. Simon (Ed.), *Communication skills and classroom success: Assessment and therapy methodologies for language and learning disabled students* (pp. 334–357). Eau Claire, WI: Thinking Publications.

Westby, C. (1991b). *Steps to developing and achieving language-based curriculum in the classroom.* Rockville, MD: American Speech-Language-Hearing Association.

Westby, C., and Erickson, J. (1992). Prologue. *Topics in Language Disorders, 12*(3), v–viii.

Wiederholt, J., and Bryant, B. (1992). *Gray oral reading tests* (3rd ed.). Austin, TX: Pro-Ed.

Wiggins, G. (1989). Teaching to the (authentic) test. *Educational Leadership, 46*(7), 41–47.

Wiig, E. (1982, May) *Identifying language disorders in adolescents.* LaCrosse, WI: Oral presentation at Gunderson Clinic.

Wiig, E. (1983, October/November). *Assessment and development of social communication skills in adolescents with language-learning disabilities.* Madison, WI: Educational Teleconferencing Network.

Wiig, E., and Becker-Caplan, L. (1984). Linguistic retrieval strategies and word-finding difficulties among children with language disabilities. *Topics in Language Disorders, 4*(3), 1–18.

Wiig, E., and Harris, S. (1974). Perception and interpretation of nonverbally expressed emotions by adolescents with learning disabilities. *Perceptual and Motor Skills, 38,* 239–245.

Wiig, E., Kutner, S., Florence, D., Sherman, B., and Semel, E. (1977). Perception and interpretation of explicit negations by learning-disabled children and adolescents. *Perceptual and Motor Skills, 44,* 1251–1257.

Wiig, E., and Secord, W. (1992). From word knowledge to world knowledge. *The Clinical Connection, 6*(3), 12–14.

Wiig, E., and Semel, E. (1975). Productive language abilities in learning disabled adolescents. *Journal of Learning Disabilities, 8*(9), 45–53.

Wiig, E., and Semel, E. (1976). *Language disabilities in children and adolescents.* Columbus, OH: Charles E. Merrill.

Wiig, E., and Semel, E. (1980). *Language assessment and intervention for the learning disabled.* Columbus, OH: Charles E. Merrill.

Williams, J. (1992). What do you know? What do you need to know? *Asha, 34,* 54–61.

Willig, A., and Greenberg, H. (1986). *Bilingualism and learning disabilities.* New York: American Library.

Wittebols, J. (1986). *Improving universe data on schools and school districts: Collecting national dropout statistics.* Washington, DC: Council of Chief State School Officers.

Wolf, D. (1989). Portfolio assessment: Sampling student work. *Educational Leadership, 46*(7), 35–39.

Wolff, F., Marsnik, N., Tacey, W., and Nichols, R. (1983). *Perceptive listening.* Chicago, IL: Holt, Rinehart and Winston.

Wong, B. (Ed.) (1991). *Learning about learning disabilities.* San Diego, CA: Academic Press.

Wood, F. (1988). Learners at risk. *Teaching Exceptional Children, 20*(4), 4–9.

Woodcock, R., and Johnson, M. (1990). *The Woodcock-Johnson psycho-educational battery* (Rev. ed.). Chicago, IL: Riverside.

Woodcock, R., McGrew, K., and Werder, J. (1993). *Mini-battery of achievement.* Chicago, IL: Riverside.

Worden, P., Malmgren, I., and Gabourie, P. (1982). Memory for stories in learning disabled adults. *Journal of Learning Disabilities, 15*(3), 145–152.

Worden, P., and Nakamura, G. (1982). Story comprehension and recall in learning-disabled versus normal college students. *Journal of Educational Psychology, 74*(5), 633–641.

Worthen, B., and Spandel, V. (1991). Putting the standardized test debate in perspective. *Educational Leadership, 48*(5), 65–69.

Zeller, W. (1952). *Konstitution und entwicklung.* Gottingen, Germany: Psychologische Rundschau.

Zessoules, R., and Gardner, H. (1991). Authentic assessment: Beyond the buzzword and into the classroom. In V. Perrone (Ed.), *Expanding student assessment* (pp. 47–71). Alexandria, VA: Association for Supervision and Curriculum Development.

AUTHOR INDEX

SUBJECT INDEX

Nonverbal communication *(continued)*
    during language sampling, 121
    encoding, decoding of cues, 61
    evolution of adolescent patterns, 61
    eye contact, 61, 75
    facial expressions, 60
    importance and functions, 115
    listener feedback, 61
    observation of, 133
Nonverbal organizational disorder, 68

Objectivity of assessment procedures, 118
Older students. *See also* Adolescence; Youth at risk
    cultural and linguistic diversity among, 57–59
    with disabilities, percentage graduating, 234
    how they learn, 174
    importance of speech-language intervention for, 153
    inadequate detection of language deficits among, 14–15
    involvement in intervention planning, 159
    language disordered, 77–79
    language expectations of, 77–79
    need for speech-language services, 77–78
    nonverbal communication problems, 75
    participation in assessment, 88–89, 121
    prevalence of communication disorders among, 15–17
    and school-life transitions, 221–225
    and school-to-work transitions, 225–232
    six major environments of, 117
    and transition to postsecondary education, 232–239
    written language deficits among, 76–77
Oral communication, intervention approaches, 180–182
Organization, informal assessment task for, 131–132
Output phase of cognition, 107, 168
    functions of, 108

Paradigm, defined, 82
Paradigm shifts
    affecting assessment, 82
    affecting speech-language pathologist role, 219–221
    affecting speech-language services, 156–157

Paralanguage
    as category of nonverbal communication, 59
    expected features, 116
Peer group, assessment as part of student's environmental system, 97
Physical development of adolescents, 35–37
Phonetic transcription, of language samples, 123
Phonology, addressed in oral language intervention, 180
Physical development of adolescents, 11–12
Piagetian approach to cognition, 42–44
Piagetian theory, 27–30, 42–44, 174
Pictures, use of in obtaining language samples, 127
Portfolios, as method of informal assessment, 120–121
Postsecondary education
    guidelines for success in, 237–239
    planning for transition to, 235–237
    resource for students considering, 239
    transition to from high school setting, 232–239
Postsecondary students
    with language disorders, assessing, 93–94
    and Section 504, 94
Pragmatics, 52
    emphasized in oral language intervention, 180–181
Preadolescence. *See also* Adolescence
    age span for, 1
    transitions during, 221–224
Preadolescents. *See* Older students
Problem-solving model chart, for intervention, 166–167
Production deficit disorder, 67–68
Production deficits
    in conversations, 73–74
    evidence of, 71–72
    in narrations, 74–75
Production of linguistic features, 47, 48–51, 132–133
    assessment of, 109–110, 133–135, 137
    evidence of deficits, 71–75
    figurative language, 51
    skills to address in intervention, 170
    speaking, writing compared, 51
    verbal maze behavior, 50–51, 112
    words per oral communication unit, 49–50